This book is a nourishing banquet of play and healing. It offers great resources for those who connect children, families, and communities to the natural world.

—**Richard Louv**, *author of* Last Child in the Woods, Vitamin N, *and* Our Wild Calling

Brilliant! Blending the powers of play and expressive therapies with the robust healing of the natural world is a groundbreaking contribution! Highly recommended!

—**David A. Crenshaw, PhD, ABPP, RPT-S,** *author and board-certified clinical psychologist*

Ready for an adventure? *Nature-Based Play and Expressive Therapies* guides you through the rationale, explores the research base for nature play, and reveals vital cultural considerations to meaningfully integrate the wisdom of the natural world into your practice. Offering abundant and detailed case studies and compelling interventions, the authors walk readers through a verdant landscape of techniques and models of using nature to nurture healing and growth. In addition, authors describe both individual and family interventions, address nature-based play therapy in urban environments and discuss how to bring nature into the therapy room. Readers of this inspiring anthology are invited into the woods to explore relationships, process trauma, and promote emotional well-being with nature as their co-therapist!

—**Anne Stewart, PhD**, *professor of graduate psychology at James Madison University and registered play therapist supervisor*

Nature-Based Play and Expressive Therapies

Nature-Based Play and Expressive Therapies addresses a wide range of healing modalities and case studies that can be used in both indoor and outdoor environments.

Each chapter includes vignettes to support the interventions and approaches presented. Readers will find a diverse array of helpful handouts and topics explored, including tips for creating outdoor healing gardens and labyrinths, guidelines for using nature to address trauma, working with sandplay and storytelling in nature, adapting nature-based interventions via telehealth, and much more.

Chapters focus on work with young children and teens in individual settings as well as work with families and groups, making this book an important read for a wide range of mental health professionals.

Janet A. Courtney, PhD, RPT-S is founder of FirstPlay® Therapy and author of *Healing Child and Family Trauma Through Expressive and Play Therapies, Infant Play Therapy,* and *Touch in Child Counseling and Play Therapy.*

Jamie Lynn Langley, LCSW, RPT-S maintains a private practice and is teaching faculty at Middle Tennessee State University. She is president of the Tennessee Association for Play Therapy and provides play therapy training and supervision.

Lynn Louise Wonders, LPC, RPT-S is a child and family counselor, professional trainer, consultant, and author of *When Parents Are at War: A Child Therapist's Guide to Navigating High Conflict Divorce* and the *Miss Piper's Playroom* series of therapeutic children's books.

Rosalind Heiko, PhD, ISST, RPT-S is a sandplay therapist, founding board member of the World Association of Sand Therapy Professionals and author of *A Therapist's Guide to Mapping the Girl Heroine's Journey in Sandplay.*

Rose LaPiere, LPC, RPT-S, ACS is a trauma therapist and is past president of NJCA-Creativity Division and currently serving on the board for the World Association of Sand Therapy Professionals.

Nature-Based Play and Expressive Therapies

Interventions for Working with Children, Teens, and Families

Edited by Janet A. Courtney, Jamie Lynn Langley, Lynn Louise Wonders, Rosalind Heiko, and Rose LaPiere

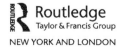
Routledge
Taylor & Francis Group

NEW YORK AND LONDON

First published 2022
by Routledge
605 Third Avenue, New York, NY 10158

and by Routledge
4 Park Square, Milton Park, Abingdon, Oxon, OX14 4RN

Routledge is an imprint of the Taylor & Francis Group, an informa business

Library of Congress Cataloging-in-Publication Data
Names: Courtney, Janet A., editor. | Langley, Jamie Lynn, editor. | Wonders, Lynn Louise, editor. | Heiko, Rosalind, editor. | LaPiere, Rose, editor.
Title: Nature-based play and expressive therapies : interventions for working with children, teens, and families / edited by Janet A. Courtney, Jamie Lynn Langley, Lynn Louise Wonders, Rosalind Heiko, Rose LaPiere.
Description: New York, NY : Routledge, 2022. | Includes bibliographical references and index.
Identifiers: LCCN 2021041669 (print) | LCCN 2021041670 (ebook) | ISBN 9780367712693 (hardback) | ISBN 9780367712679 (paperback) | ISBN 9781003152767 (ebook)
Subjects: LCSH: Arts--Therapeutic use. | Psychotherapy. | Family psychotherapy. | Art therapy for children. | Nature.
Classification: LCC RC489.A72 N385 2022 (print) | LCC RC489.A72 (ebook) | DDC 616.89/1656--dc23/eng/20211014
LC record available at https://lccn.loc.gov/2021041669
LC ebook record available at https://lccn.loc.gov/2021041670

ISBN: 978-0-367-71269-3 (hbk)
ISBN: 978-0-367-71267-9 (pbk)
ISBN: 978-1-003-15276-7 (ebk)

DOI: 10.4324/9781003152767

Typeset in Times New Roman
by MPS Limited, Dehradun

Access the Support Material: www.Routledge.com/9780367712679

To my nature loving grandchildren, Sophia, Abigail, Jacob, and Ezra
who make my heart melt at just the word Mimi.
Janet A. Courtney

To my husband, Charley, and our two sons, Justin and Andrew. I fondly remember that time we found ourselves at the end of a rainbow on my birthday. Yes, our family is my treasure.
Jamie Lynn Langley

I dedicate this book to my three young adult children, Jonathan, Patrick, and Madeline, with whom I enjoyed many years playing in nature.
Lynn Louise Wonders

To my four-year-old grandson Noah, who gently holds roly-polies and fireflies;
plays fiercely in dirt, water, and mud; and reminds me every day about
how extraordinary our connection to nature can be.
Roz Heiko

In loving memory of my father, John J. Esposito, and his love for reading and writing.
Rose LaPiere

Contents

Appendices and Handouts

Vignettes and Case Studies

Chapter 1
Case Vignette of Anna

Chapter 2
Case Vignette of Sharon

Chapter 3
Case Vignette of Markus
Case Vignette of Sarah

Chapter 4
Case Vignette of Jose

Chapter 5
Case Vignette of Aponi

Chapter 6
Case Vignette of Rainey
Case Vignette of Sally

Chapter 7
Case Vignette of Lemont
Case Vignette of Janice
Case Vignette of Matt
Case Study of Shante

Chapter 8
Case Study of Grace

Chapter 9
Case Study of Carla

Chapter 10
Case study of Peter

Chapter 11
Case study of Sarina

Chapter 12
Case study of Elizabeth and Grace

Figures and Tables

Figures

Tables

Foreword

Eliana Maria Vedruna Gil

My father died when he was 56 and I was 23. I have increasingly more vague memories of him and many of those who could fill in the blanks are now also long gone. I have small snapshot memories, with one monumental exception. The snapshots are of a kind, melancholy, tender man, who was thought of by his family as marching to his own drum. One of the ways he did that was to maintain a creative approach to work: He followed dreams, passions, and less tradition. In this way, I feel his blood running through my body.

In this book, and for the purpose of introducing this book, I will turn my attention to the monumental exception: a long, detailed, and rich memory of my father. The reader will likely connect the dots about why I'm sharing this story in this book, long before I make them explicit.

My memories of my father are separate from those of my mother. They divorced when I was young, and after that I spent time with each of them separately. My father always liked to show me new places, those he loved and cherished. This memory is foundational and life-altering. It is my memory alone, as my brothers were not present, and as happens with memory, there are likely aspects that are romanticized, expanded, or sprinkled with love facts I have had vivid dreams about this extended experience, and more recently, wrote a fairy tale in a workshop I took with Dr. Roz Heiko.

My parents are both Ecuatorianos, from Ecuador, South America. Ecuador is a third-world country, rich with incredible tourist attractions, most notably the Galapagos Islands. My father's family habitated the Galapagos Islands for generations. As a matter of fact, when tourists visit the tourism center in the Galapagos, there is a plaque that mentions my great-great-grandfather and the fact that he brought the giant sea turtles to the Islands.

My adventure begins when I was seven years old and my father took me to the Island Isabella. We lived there in a small wooden cottage for a period of time, maybe three or four months. I remember we took a small plane from Guayaquil, and then a boat over to the Island. My father seemed to know everyone and he stopped for long introductions of his daughter: My father was so proud of his four children!!!

We always returned to the same small, wooden cottage. I believe I have a picture with my dad at age three, in front of the cottage. The entrance to the front door was created by people walking, not by a formal walk-way like the ones I had seen in the city. As far as your eyes could see there were tropical plants, tall trees, rainbow flowers, and creatures, big and small: I loved traveling by donkey everywhere we went. I also loved the fish jumping, the chickens laying eggs, the penguins that made me laugh, the beautiful reptiles that looked prickly but loved you if you simply brought them fruit or vegetables. There was always a lovely breeze, a bright sun, and the most gorgeous rain falls I've ever experienced. There were boundless places to explore, rocks to climb, and mosquito bites to nurse. When I went home, my mother and grandmother were aghast at what looked like a multicolored map of bruises and scrapes. To me, each one held a lovely memory of my active participation with life!

On this particular summer visit, my father said he had a surprise for me and took my hand as we went around back. There was a fenced in area, which was different, and my eyes darted around. My dad took me to a little structure and inside, there was a giant Galapagos turtle. My father said it had been living here for quite a time because it had gotten hurt during a fire nearby. He told me that she was getting well enough to go wherever she wanted to go, but that he thought I would enjoy spending time with her.

I quickly became obsessed with the turtle and called her DARIA. It was the first place I went in the morning, where I spent most of my days, and last thing I did at night. I quickly learned that she was very shy and my goal in life became to make her comfortable enough to put her head out. My dad noticed that I was "trying too hard" and he pointed out that maybe I was standing too close, reaching inside her shell too much, talking too loud in her ears, and generally "in her face" too much. He also didn't think it was useful to try to push her to take steps when she didn't want to. I was so frustrated that she would move when I wasn't looking, and seemed to move the most in the night, while I slept.

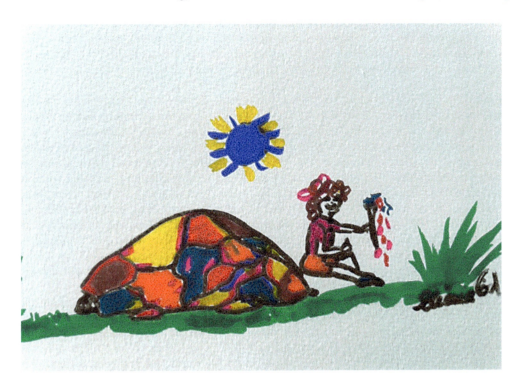

Figure F.1 "Sweet memories of childhood friends."
Courtesy of Eliana Maria Vedruna Gil.

With my dad's prompting, I tried new tactics. I read a book next to her (not in front), and sometimes I whispered the story. When I drew pictures of her, I left them out for her to see, but I didn't put them in front of her face. I prepared and brought her food but put it away from her, rather than trying to make her chew it. I ate my breakfast sitting next to her, but she never loved the smells of pancakes and cereal and fresh papaya or pineapple, the way I did. I brought a little radio out so she could hear music and I set up my paint set so that I could paint whatever I wanted. Like an uncle painter I had, I learned to put shells, and nuts and sticks into the paint. I was very proud of my creations, as was my dad. I used to go on walks with a basket (as I do now) and collect whatever little treasures the land offered. One day I was so excited to have found these perfectly round little balls, and my father laughed hilariously as he told me they were Iguana droppings! I still found a way to use them in my art, maybe just out of spite.

A turtle does not give you much feedback I learned, not like a dog that greets you at the door, or the parrots who flew onto my shoulder. Even the donkey seemed somewhat happy to see me in the morning, but the turtle was a tough customer, and I learned to love her despite her not showing outward signs of loving me. She was one of my favorite animal relationships.

I have another striking memory of using my paints to fill in the squares the turtle had on her shell. She did not seem to care one way or the other, and I had a field day creating a symmetrical, aesthetically pleasing piece of art. When my dad came home, he smiled, thanked me, and said we would now bathe her in case the paint could hurt her in any way. Washing her shell with bubbly soap was truly great fun. This was the first time my dad lifted me up to get on the top of her shell so that I could pour water down both sides of the shell. I loved being up on her shell and fancied myself riding around the fenced-in area as if the turtle was the donkey. It never happened, but my dad made me a little wooden staircase, and he placed it next to the turtle so that I could climb up and down. Sometimes, I fell asleep on a comfy towel that I put on the shell.

Eventually, when I least expected it, she began to eat while I was with her, and I got a close up and personal look at her wrinkled face, her teeth, and her stretchy neck. She never did let me touch or pet her but as time went on, she let me see her walking with her big curvy legs. "She's getting stronger every day," my dad would say, and he began to prepare me for two inevitable happenings: We would be leaving the Island and going back home to Guayaquil, and we would be opening the fence for her so that she could venture out if she wanted. I had seen lots of other turtles in the woods as I walked around, and my dad told me that these turtles were Daria's big family, and they would be happy to have her join the family again.

When I took Dr. Heiko's fairy-tale course, she asked two questions that have stayed with me and caused a deepening of my own reflection: The first one was to think of something that my family always said about me growing up, and the second was to connect the fairy tale to something about my work. I promptly remembered something people said a lot about me growing up: "She's so patient, and she loves being outdoors." The second question made me smile. The thing about the fairy tale I wrote about the turtle, and the memory of my magical time with my father in the Island Isabella, now revealed some of my most important reflections that have guided my clinical work: I have always valued therapeutic patience. I have always felt it critical to "be with" a child client, never rush ahead, do parallel play instead of "getting in his/her face," and allow clients to pace themselves. These things that I prioritize as a therapist seem to be strongly and inherently connected to my experience with Daria, and it makes me happy to know that Daria and my dad taught those early lessons that have served me well.

When Janet and Jamie asked me to write this foreword, I thought the best thing I could do was chronicle the important lessons about my time in the Island Isabella.

This book is a glorious confirmation of the power of nature in healing in providing life lessons, and in helping us interact with deeper aspects of self. More and more research is being developed to affirm what many of us have known our whole lives: Children's exploration of nature is a vast oasis of life affirming experiences. We can likely do nothing more important with our child clients than to help them value the life cycles that appear in nature, the seasons, and allow children to discover the transformation constantly occurring in nature, and how nature touches our souls.

I'm so excited that Janet and her colleagues have prioritized this work and I highly encourage readers to go on their own journeys, integrating past memories with present affirmations and future activities. During this writing, I added one additional thing to my bucket list: Return to the Isla Isabella and see if Daria is still hanging around. These Galápagos turtles are believed to live for hundreds of years. I will look forward to our reconnecting and believe that it is truly possible.

Acknowledgements

Janet A. Courtney, PhD

I want to give a heartfelt thank you to my dear coeditors, Roz Heiko, Jamie Lynn Langley, Rose LaPiere, and Lynn Louise Wonders, who immediately said YES to this project when I discussed approaching Routledge with the idea of an edited nature-based book. It is with deep gratitude that I thank Eliana Maria Vedruna Gil, Larry Rubin, and all the book authors for their outstanding contributions. And a huge thank you to Anna Moore at Routledge who immediately recognized the uniqueness of a therapeutic book related to nature. I feel deep love and gratitude to my husband, Robert Nolan, sons, Jesse and Austin, my daughter-in-law, Stephanie, my sister, Carol, and brother, Allen. And many hugs to my grandchildren, Sophia, Abigail, Jacob, and Ezra, who make my heart leap with joy when we spend time together especially in nature.

Rosalind Heiko, PhD

Here's to the 2019 Nature Play Retreat Faculty and Participants—what a wonderful nurturing heartfelt inspiring time! This experience nurtured and enhanced my love of nature—internal and in the world—bringing forth the gifts of community and inventiveness in abundance. Gratitude for you all. And to my fellow editors: Janet, Lynn, Rose, and Jamie, who have inspired a deep and abiding respect for working to heal trauma and suffering in natural settings—gratitude for your generosity and wisdom.

Jamie Lynn Langley, LCSW

My mom was always my loudest cheerleader and I know how proud she would be. Thank you, Mom. I am also grateful for my husband, Charley, and our two sons, Justin and Andrew. Our family adventures together have often included nature excursions. These are cherished memories that have also helped me introduce nature play for the children and families I work with. Thank you to Janet for bringing this shared passion to fruition and for guidance in this endeavor. Also, much appreciation to our colleagues who have participated in this collaboration to encourage nature play as a healing way.

Rose LaPiere, LPC, RPT-C

I am grateful to many people for their encouragement and wisdom in this project. My parents and siblings who were my first teachers. The love and support from my husband and children and all our special moments in nature. To Janet, Lynn, Roz, and Jamie, who shared a passion for nature and worked hard to help bring this book to life. Lisa Dion, I am thankful for your guidance and collaboration in our chapter. I am humbled by the families who allowed me into their lives and let me walk with them in their journey to heal.

Lynn Louise Wonders, LPC

For our lead editor Dr. Janet A. Courtney; my fellow coeditors Jamie, Rose, and Dr. Roz; and all the therapists who have embraced the magical combination of nature and play for therapeutic change in the work we do for children and families, I am so grateful. I am thankful for my three children and husband who are all avid nature lovers and certainly all know how to play well in nature. I'm thankful to all my own teachers, particularly Wong Loh Sin See and Leong Tan, who have taught me how to harmonize with all of nature.

About the Editors

Janet A. Courtney, PhD, LCSW, is founder of FirstPlay® Therapy, an Infant Play Therapy model. Dr. Courtney is author of *Healing Child Trauma Through Expressive & Play Therapies: Art, Nature, Storytelling Body & Mindfulness*, and editor of, *Infant Play Therapy: Foundations, Models, Programs and Practice* and *Touch in Child Counseling and Play Therapy: An Ethical and Clinical Guide*. She has been an adjunct professor at Barry University School of Social Work, Miami, Florida, since 1997. Learn more: www.firstplaytherapy.com

Rosalind Heiko, PhD, RPT-S (aka "Dr. Roz"), is a child and family licensed psychologist, and Sandplay teacher, training therapists nationally and internationally for over 35 years. She is an executive board member of the World Association of Sand Therapy Professionals. Her most recent book is *A Therapist's Guide to Mapping the Girl Heroine's Journey in Sandplay* (Rowman & Littlefield) and has published chapters in books edited by Eliana Maria Vedruna Gil and Eric Green.

Jamie Lynn Langley, LCSW, RPT-S, is a licensed clinical social worker and registered play therapist-supervisor. She has been in practice for over 30 years, first in community mental health and then private practice since late 2016. Jamie integrates nature-based interventions and creativity in play therapy, supervision, and training provided and has authored several articles and chapters on these considerations. She is the cofounder and president of the Tennessee Association for Play Therapy and on faculty at Middle Tennessee State University. Learn more: www.jamielynnlangley.com

Rose LaPiere, LPC, RPT-S, is a trauma therapist who has helped children and families for over 20 years. She is a writer, presenter, EMDR consultant, registered play therapist-supervisor and mother of two boys. She works with children and adults through the lens of attachment, mindfulness, therapeutic powers of play, interpersonal neurobiology, and family system theory. She is past president of NJCA-Creativity Division, currently serving on the board for the World Sand Therapy Professionals. Learn more: www.RoseLaPiere.com

Lynn Louise Wonders, LPC, RPT-S, CPCS, has provided counseling for children and families for over 20 years. She is a licensed professional counselor, certified counselor supervisor, and registered play therapist-supervisor. She is the author of *When Parents Are at War: A Child Therapist's Guide to Navigating High Conflict Divorce & Custody Cases*, The Miss Piper's Playroom therapeutic book series and a mindfulness book for children called *Breathe*. Learn more: www.WondersCounseling.com

Contributors

Angela M. Cavett, PhD, LP, RPT-S, is a licensed psychologist, registered play therapist-supervisor, and clinical director at Chrysalis Behavioral Health Services and Training Center in Fargo, North Dakota, where she has created Healing Gardens. A novice gardener, *Beginners Mind* has allowed her to learn from others across disciplines in order to develop a natural healing environment.

Bree Conklin LCSW, DSW, utilizes neurosequential model of therapeutics, EMDR, compassionate bereavement care, TF-CBT, child–parent psychotherapy, circle of security, and play therapy. In addition to her clinical practice, Bree serves as contributing faculty at the University of Tennessee, University of West Florida, and Walden University.

Lisa Dion, LPC, RPT-S, is an international teacher, creator of Synergetic Play Therapy, founder and president of the Synergetic Play Therapy Institute, and host of the Lessons from the Playroom podcast. She is the author of *Aggression in Play Therapy: A Neurobiological Approach for Integrating Intensity* and is the 2015 recipient of the APT Professional Education and Training Award of Excellence.

Megan Ellard, is a Qualified Early Childhood Teacher and Play Therapist. She is currently pursuing her MCPT at Deakin University, Australia and serves her community as a Nature Play facilitator and advocate as well as an Early Childhood Consultant.

Jackie Flynn Ed.S, LMHC-S, RPT, is the founder of *EMDR and Play Therapy Integrated Support*, as well as the host of Play Therapy Community® Podcast. She is registered play therapist, certified EMDR therapist, EMDRIA-approved consultant, and a couples counselor. She provides counseling to individuals, families, couples, and groups in her private practice in Central Florida.

Eliana Maria Vedruna Gil, PhD, ATR, RPT-S, LMFT, is a founding partner of Gil Institute for Trauma Recovery & Education, LLC, a group private practice in Fairfax, Viriginia. She currently works as senior clinical and research consultant. Former president of the Association for Play Therapy, she is an approved MFT supervisor as well as a registered play therapist-supervisor and registered art therapist.

Paris Goodyear-Brown, LCSW, RPT-S, is founder and director of Nurture House and an adjunct instructor at Vanderbilt University. She is the author of several books, including *Tackling Touchy Subjects, Handbook of Child Sexual Abuse: Identification, Assessment, and Treatment, Play Therapy with Traumatized Children: A Prescriptive Approach,* and *The Worry Wars: An Anxiety Workbook for Kids and their Helpful Adults.*

Harleen Hutchinson, Psy.D., IMH-®, is a psychologist, an endorsed infant mental health clinician, executive director of the Journey institute, Inc., and an adjunct professor at Barry University School of Social Work. She provides reflective supervision, lectures, and consults locally and nationally on issues relating to trauma, maternal mental health, attachment, and pediatric bereavement.

Susan Jung, EdS, earned her counseling from the University of Florida. She opened Winning Strides to serve clients with equine-assisted therapy and learning. Susan is a licensed professional counselor and certified professional counselor supervisor in Georgia. As adjunct instructor at Wesleyan College in Macon, she teaches Equine-assisted therapy courses.

Ashley S. Lingerfelt, LPC, specializes in infant, early childhood, and perinatal mental health. She is the clinical director and founder of Playtime Therapy of Georgia, LLC, and serves on the board of directors for the Georgia Birth Network and the Georgia Chapter of Postpartum Support International.

Joyce C. Mills, PhD, LMFT, RPT-S, is the founder of StoryPlay® model, a resiliency-focused Ericksonian model of play therapy, and teaches worldwide. She is the recipient of the 1997 Annual Play Therapy International Award. She has authored *Therapeutic Metaphors for Children and the Child Within* (2nd ed.); *Reconnecting to the Magic of Life*; and *Butterfly Wisdom: Four Passages to Transformation.*

Judi A. Parson, PhD, is a pediatric qualified registered nurse and play therapist. She is the founding director of Australasia Pacific Play Therapy Association and serves as the discipline lead, course director and senior lecturer in play therapy for Deakin University, Australia.

Meyleen Velasquez, LCSW, LICSW, PMH-C, RPT-S, is a psychotherapist specializing in perinatal and infant mental health and play therapy. Her practice supports young children, individuals identifying as women, and clinicians practicing from an anti-oppressive framework. In the past, she served as president of the FAPT and chair for the Florida chapter of Postpartum Support International.

Cyndera Quackenbush, MA, graduated from Pacifica Graduate Institute with a degree in clinical psychology. Having been given a unique stone inheritance from her father, Cyndera is the creator of the *Story Through Stone Reflection Cards.* Cyndera facilitates workshops in California and internationally on the topics of therapeutic use of card imagery and archetypes.

Lawrence Rubin, Ph.D., ABPP, LMHC, RPT-S, a Florida-based clinician who directs the counseling programs at St. Thomas University, is past APT chair, editor for Psychotherapy.net, on the editorial board of the International Journal of Play, and has published several popular books, including *Handbook of Medical Play Therapy and Child Life.*

Sang Min Shin, PhD, NCC, LPC, RPT, is an assistant professor in Mental Health Counseling Program of Educational Psychology Special Service Department in the College of Education at the University of Texas at El Paso. Dr. Shin earned her PhD in counseling and counselor education from the University of Florida. Her research interests include play therapy, nature-based play therapy, and multiculturalism.

Jacqueline M. Swank, PhD, LMHC, LCSW, RPT-S, is an associate professor of counselor education at the University of Florida. She uses nature and play-based interventions in working with children and adolescents and their families in various treatment settings. Her research interests include the efficacy of nature and play-based interventions with children and adolescents and their families.

Jennifer Taylor, LCSW, RPT-S, is a certified EMDR therapist. She received her master's degree in Social Work from Florida State University. She is an adjunct instructor for the University of Memphis. She is in private practice in Honolulu, Hawaii, and specializes in treating trauma in children, families and caregivers.

Danielle Woods, MC, NCC, LPC, LISAC, is a StoryPlay® facilitator and director of Faith Works, LLC in Scottsdale, Arizona. She is a Certified Mental Health and Integrated Medicine Provider and a "Working with Parents in Recovery" coach. She coauthored the chapter "Touch in StoryPlay®," in *Touch in Child Counseling and Play Therapy, an Ethical and Clinical Guide.*

Introduction

Lawrence C. Rubin

My family and I recently moved. The very last "thing" I bid farewell to was the mango tree that had preceded our arrival some 20 years before, and that would hopefully greet new families for years to come. As I hugged it, I thanked it for its many sweet bounties, fondly recalled the blossoming mess that heralded its fruiting, the awe and satisfaction it offered as those fruits grew to maturity, shedding the smaller and weaker ones as it did, and how its final farewell after harvest was yet another mess, but one scented with fond memories of the picking, the gifting, the pruning and the eager anticipation of next year's renewal.

It was my personal timepiece—not one driven by atomic exactitude, but by the random whims of a larger and unseen force with which it communicated and from which it drew its own personal rhythm and nourishment—one well beyond my ken. What I found fascinating, as did Eliana Maria Vedruna Gil in describing her relationship with Daria, the Galapagos tortoise, was that I was simply the observer, the guardian and its admiring companion, eagerly awaiting its simple gifts and always receptive to whatever wisdom, insights, and wonders it could impart to me. And there were many of those, well beyond its tangible and tasty fruits.

It taught me, or perhaps reminded me of, the fine lines that separate living from dying, predictability form uncertainty, and the ever-present impact of the unseen on the seen. It reminded me of the inescapable fact that life does indeed always push through and that our natural world is a wonderland, and that while nature can wreak havoc, bring destruction, and inspire horror; that it also carries with it the seeds of its own renewal and rebirth.

Clearly, I've always taken every opportunity to enjoy the sensory and physical aspects of the natural world in all spheres of my life; personal, professional, emotional, and intellectual. I have long been enthralled with Howard Gardner's notion of multiple intelligences (2006), and in particular his concept of "naturalistic intelligence"—the ability to connect with, attend to and engage with the natural world, and in so doing categorize, experience, and abstract meaning from our interactions with it. In its spirit, I have always found ways to incorporate children's appreciation for nature into my assessment and play therapy. But it wasn't until happening across Richard Louv's work and his fascinating premise of nature-deficit disorder (2006) that I fully and deeply appreciated just how critical our and our children's relationship with nature truly was. Louv's book resonated with me as I have always found comfort, grounding and meaning in the natural world, in spite of having grown up in Brooklyn's perfect cement symmetry.

As a therapist, I have always attempted to bring the outdoors inside with my clients as I lined the shelves of my sandtray miniature collection with every imaginable natural object I could find—rocks, wood, leaves, bark, and shells; and when possible taking "nature walks" with them to look at the sky, the trees, the birds and the plants in order to link those sensory experiences with the challenges they might be struggling with at the time. Freed from the confines of the air-conditioned fluorescent office, clients and I often found ourselves in powerful therapeutic conversations walking through a field, examining a plant, marveling at a tree or watching (and of course, projectively giving shape to) the clouds.

As a college teacher, I often struggled to enliven classroom discussions, so often found escape to the natural beauty of our campus liberating of both body and mind. Gathering cell phones at the door and offering the simple directive, "go explore," my students brought back fascinating insights and newfound appreciation for everything from the geometric and tactile wonder of a pinecone, the sound and feel of pine needles beneath their feet, the wordlessness of a gentle breeze and the discovery of an unfamiliar scent. Insights into the natural world and connections between those insights and their own inner awakening made for wonderful classroom discussions. Lessons were abounding.

As a parent, I never wanted to impose my appreciation for nature on our children but did manage to sneak in a few lessons and conversations about life, death and renewal, as well as beauty and awe during frequent walks through the woods off the Blue Ridge Parkway in North Carolina. My son, who has struggled with inattention, impulsivity and distractibility has recently relocated to the slower pace and boundless vistas of Kentucky; while our daughter, a digital native to be sure, recently lagged behind on a walkabout to take a picture of a budding tree. My lessons had taken root in both of our children, perhaps not surprising given that they have always been encouraged to get their feet wet, skin their knees, and get their hands dirty. See where I'm going here?

When Janet privileged me with the task of writing this introduction, my mind raced with all of these thoughts and memories, but I specifically recalled a workshop that she and her husband, Bob, offered about using rocks, gems, and minerals in play therapy. They were onto something I remember thinking. For them, as I imagine it is for you, the playroom is, or at least can be, a microcosm of the natural world, and the natural world a macrocosm for the rich bounty of experiences you have and will continue to have as you open your playroom doors to nature, whether you are a native or an immigrant.

It is probably no coincidence that you have decided to engage with the many fine scholarly thoughts, clinical insights, case examples, experiential exercises, and "questions for thought" that accompany each chapter in this book. You have probably already found a way to connect the natural world, either on a small or large scale, in either a "real" or simulated fashion with your clinical work with children, teens, and families. And if you haven't, perhaps you will after reading this wonderful book, and even more so, necessary volume.

In the spirit of this book, I like to think of what Janet has done is to create a journey for you by mapping out several realms (what she calls "sections") of interest and then providing you with able guides—the authors. And whether you are a clinician, educator, researcher, or simply a curious citizen of the natural world, I trust there will be something waiting for you in the pages to come.

The first of these realms, "Essential Nature Foundations," introduces us to the core concepts around integrating nature into play and expressive therapies. In Chapter 1, entitled "An Introduction to the Emerging Practice of Nature-Based Play and Expressive Therapies," Janet A. Courtney and Jamie Lynn Langley identify what they call the 12 Cs of nature-based play therapy that link to Charles Schaefer's therapeutic powers of play. In Chapter 2, entitled "Not Just a Walk in the Park: Complex Layers of Integrating Nature into Play Therapy Practice," Judi A. Parson and Megan Ellard review the literature integrating nature and nature-based therapies within tested theoretical perspectives and then take us through the assessment and treatment of foster child Sharon as she finds her own secret garden. In Chapter 3, entitled "Creation of Safe Space for Transformation and Healing: The Chrysalis Model of Intentional Design for Healing Gardens," Angela M. Cavett introduces us to the healing power of Healing Gardens based upon her own personal experiences in nature, Buddhist teachings, and the lived and metaphoric power of the chrysalis.

The second of these realms, "Cultural Considerations," introduces us to the notion of nature-based play therapy that is grounded in an appreciation for culture and humility when addressing it therapeutically. In Chapter 4, entitled "Let's Go Outside: Nature-Based Play Therapy Through the Lens of Cultural Humility," Meyleen Velasquez introduces us to eight-year-old Jose, a Honduran immigrant with whom she channels newfound insights about racism, colorism, and xenophobia for his care and betterment. In Chapter 5, entitled "Sacred Ground: The Cultural Implication of Nature-Based Therapy with Young Children and the Intersection of Culture," Harleen Hutchinson blends different treatment modalities to help a mother understand how maternal stress and affect regulation have influenced her baby's social emotional functioning.

The third of these realms, "Healing Nature-Based Trauma Therapies," helps us to understand the powerful role that nature and nature-based treatment can play in the healing of trauma in children. In Chapter 6, entitled "The Nature of TraumaPlay®: Incorporating Nature into the Seven Key Components," Paris Goodyear-Brown describes her "flexibly sequenced play therapy model" for treating trauma through vivid descriptions and images of nature/outdoor-based therapeutic activities with children. In Chapter 7, entitled "Using Nature to Create Safety for Medical Trauma Integration," Rose LaPiere and Lisa Dion share the moving story of eight-year-old Lemont's use of a "nature hut" to deal with the pain and trauma that accompanied the assessment and treatment of his Celiac disease. In Chapter 8, entitled "The Integration of Nature-Based Play and EMDR Therapies in the Aftermath of Trauma," Jackie Flynn combines practical play-based and expressive interventions with EMDR to create a path of healing for 13-year-old Grace who is struggling to grow in the shadow of childhood trauma.

The fourth of these realms, "Nature Play Therapy Models and Other Individual Therapeutic Applications," expands our awareness of nature-based play therapy by focusing on several popular theoretical modalities. In Chapter 9, entitled "Cultivating Mindfulness Through Use of Nature in Play Therapy," Lynn Louise Wonders offers us the compelling composite case of seven-year-old Carla and her parents who, together, are struggling with family dissolution and who benefit from an integration of nature-based mindfulness and creative play-based interventions.

In Chapter 10, entitled "Nature-Based Child-Centered Play Therapy: Taking the Playroom Outside," Jacqueline M. Swank and Sang Min Shi introduce us to Nature-Based Child-Centered Play Therapy (NBCCPT), its empirical and ethical foundations, and application to the case of six-year-old Peter whose adjustment difficulties nicely yielded to the opportunity to play in and with nature. In Chapter 11, entitled "Equine-Assisted Psychotherapy and Learning for Children: Why Horses?", Susan Jung shares her expertise and clinical wisdom earned in the course of utilizing horses in therapy and how Equine-assisted therapy helped young Serena who was abandoned at five, twice fostered, and now seeking the security of a forever home.

The fifth of these realm, "Nature-Based Family Interventions," helps us to appreciate the many ways that nature and nature-based interventions can be used in the service of treating family systems. In Chapter 12, entitled "Tiny Hearts and Hands: Nature Sensory Play Promotes Infant Mental Health," Janet A. Courtney and Ashely S. Lingerfelt utilize a variety of nature-based, sensorimotor exercises to help young mother Elizabeth enhance her infant child's emotional and social development. In Chapter 13, entitled "Nature Play Therapy as a Healing Way for Children, Teens, and Families: Incorporating Nature with Play and Expressive Therapies," Jamie Lynn Langley provides us with a roadmap for the use of both structured and unstructured NaturePlay experiences for children and teens and their families to connect, thrive, and heal. In Chapter 14, entitled "Using Nature-Based Interventions in Family Play Therapy," Jennifer Taylor and Bree Conklin teach us how to introduce nature-based play and expressive arts interventions within sessions that can be developed into action plans for use by parents and their children's in-between therapeutic visits.

The sixth and final realm, "Nature-Based Storytelling Interventions," regrounds us, so to speak, by showing how storytelling can unlock the implicit therapeutic healing energy of nature. In Chapter 15, entitled "Into the Great Forest: Fairy-Tale Themes of the Wild Take Shape in Sandplay," Rosalind Heiko demonstrates through lively clinical vignettes to engage with children in the natural world within the sheltered container of our offices; employing fairy-tale themes in storytelling and Sandplay about the Great Forest and some of its inhabitants. In Chapter 16, entitled "The Wisdom of Nature: StoryPlay®, Connecting Nature's Gifts of Thriving and Resiliency to Play," Danielle Woods and Joyce C. Mills show us through word, image, and clinical vignettes how the natural world can be adapted to provide pathways to healing through a combination of metaphor, story, and Milton Ericson's concept of utilization. In Chapter 17, entitled "Story Stone Play: Embodied Imagination in Virtual Therapy and Beyond," Cyndera Quackenbush and Janet A. Courtney introduce us to a creative and playful 10-step intervention called Story Stone Play, which encourages children to find their own imagery in each stone picture and to tell stories that tap into their feelings, memories, and embodied imagination. The book closes with a final section on nature gratitude and appreciation.

So, with all that said, come on in, I assure you that the water is more than fine, and so are the many lessons, stories, and clinical adventures of growth, healing, and resilience upon which you are about to embark.

References

Gardner, H. E. (2006). *Multiple intelligences: New horizons in theory and practice*. Basic Books.
Louv, R. (2006). *Last child in the woods: Saving our children from nature-deficit disorder*. Algonquin Books.

PART I
Essential Nature Foundations

1 An Introduction to the Emerging Practice of Nature-Based Play and Expressive Therapies

Janet A. Courtney and Jamie Lynn Langley

Anna, a 14-year-old teen on the autism spectrum, entered the play therapy room very anxious and dysregulated. The therapist made several attempts to help focus and calm her by offering different sensory-based activities, which only worked to increase her agitation. The therapist, armed with the understanding that nature can play a role in assisting to regulate emotional states, suggested to Anna that they could go outside for a nature walk. Anna agreed and a brief walk led to a huge strong oak tree. The therapist encouraged Anna to place her hands on the trunk of the tree while listening to the surrounding sounds and breathing in the scents of nature. Spontaneously, Anna decided to remove her shoes so she could feel the ground beneath her feet. The therapist invited Anna to imagine that she was also a beautiful strong tree with deep roots going into the ground. She was encouraged to feel the support of the earth beneath her feet. Like a quick shift in the wind, Anna's emotional state instantly calmed. Sitting now under the shelter of the tree branches with her back leaning against the trunk of the tree, Anna was able to share her inner thoughts and feelings. During the next session, Anna drew an image of the tree that became a central healing metaphor in her on-going therapy.

Introduction

The case in vignette of Anna illustrates how utilizing the elements of nature's resources to calm and heal resonated with a teenage client. Beginning with a simple nature walk and a grounding connection with a tree, this led to subsequent nature-based play and expressive art experiences (see Appendix A). This client experience speaks to our innate desire to commune with nature at a deeper level. Biologist E. O. Wilson (1993) formulated a widely accepted construct related to our human connection to nature, which he labeled the "biophilia hypothesis" that postulated a pervasive attraction or curiosity—an "emotional affiliation" (P. 31)—that draws people to nature. Kellert (1993) defined it as a "human dependence on nature that extends far beyond the simple issues of material and physical sustenance to encompass the human craving for aesthetic, intellectual, cognitive, and even spiritual meaning and satisfaction" (p. 20).

Nature has been long known and described as a healing balm throughout the ages. Human beings have evolved very closely with nature since time immemorial and many cultural traditions around the world are deeply rooted in nature. Mills and Crowley (2014) noted that in all indigenous healing philosophies and stories there is a deep-seated belief in the healing power of nature:

> The natural world is our relative, our teacher, and our healer, and that everything is sacred. In these wisdom teachings, the earth, sky, moon, sun, and stars are not viewed through a scientific lens... Instead, they are experienced as our Mother Earth, Father Sky, Grandmother Moon, Grandfather Sun, and the Star Nation—as relatives guiding, protecting, and teaching us many lessons along life's physical and spiritual paths.
>
> (Mills & Crowley, 2014, p. 3)

Given the opportunity to be exposed to nature at a young age, children have an instinctive yearning to intimately connect with the environment around them. They are multisensory engrossed, and for everything that calls their attention they want to touch, smell, listen, and yes even for the wee ones, taste (yikes!). It is not something they have to be taught. The innate desire to connect with nature is pre-wired from birth. It is thus drawing upon these inherent strengths of children to connect with the natural world that we then build upon and make use of as a therapeutic healing tool in play and expressive therapies.

DOI: 10.4324/9781003152767-2

In this growing field of nature-based therapies, mental health practitioners who work with children and families are discovering the therapeutic benefits of nature-based play and expressive therapies (Chown, 2014, 2018; Courtney, 2017, 2020; Courtney & Mills, 2016; Dhaese, 2011; Ellard & Parson, 2021; Langley, 2019; Mills & Crowley, 2014; Montgomery & Courtney, 2015; Rivkin, 2014; Shin & Swank, 2018; Swank & Shin, 2015; Swank et al., 2020). As mental health practitioners and play therapists adopt nature-based practices, there have been various titles given to this modality, including Nature-Based Play Therapy, Child-Centered Nature-Based Play Therapy, Outdoor Child-Centered Play Therapy, Eco-Play Therapy, Nature Play Therapy, and Outdoor Play Therapy (Langley, 2019). These nature-based expressive and play therapies can encompass various expressive arts as children's play often includes creative activities, movement, storytelling, and more. Whatever title is used, these nature-based play and expressive therapies fall underneath the umbrella of the growing field of Ecotherapy and Ecopsychology philosophy (Roszak et al., 1995), through which much exciting research is occurring about healing benefits of nature (Buzzell & Chalquist, 2009; Ellard & Parson, 2021). The beneficial use of nature is also flourishing in school curriculums and after school programs such as the Forest Schools in the United Kingdom (Knight, 2013, see also https://www.forestschools.com/), the Bush Kinder schools in Australia, or the Scandinavia concept of *udeskole,* meaning "outdoor school" (Bentsen, 2013; Broström, 1998).

Nature and Children: A Call to Action

One of the leading contributors to this bourgeoning interest in children's need for nature is credited to journalist Richard Louv, author of *Last Child in the Woods,* who coined the phrase "Nature Deficit Disorder" to describe the growing concern of children having reduced and low access to nature (Louv, 2008). While not a medical designation, this has been attributed as more of a "call to action." As such, it has led to an overall identification of concerns related to children's decline in physical and mental health including attention-deficit disorder, depression, anxiety, and others. Emerging research shows support for time in nature as emotionally beneficial, especially for children (Ellard & Parson, 2021; Swank & Shin, 2015). However, children and families are often more out-of-touch with nature than ever before.

In current society, children are often missing essential nature exploration. This can be attributed to various reasons such as technological distractions, schools cutting back on recess, lack of access, and even parental concerns for perceived harm of being outside (Courtney & Nowakowski-Sims, 2019; Louv, 2008). However, Louv advocates, "Every child needs nature. Not just the ones with parents who appreciate nature. Not only those of a certain economic class or culture or gender or sexual identity or set of abilities. *Every* child" (Louv, 2012a, para 1, sent. 1–4). It is only within the past 150 years, since the beginning of the industrial revolution, that we have slowly lost our visceral connection to nature and land. As humans we are part of nature and many people still feel a deep need to connect with the natural world. Many of today's children experience nature, not by direct contact but instead by classroom representations, internet exposure, video games, and so forth. A recent study by Michaelson et al. (2020) examined why "screen time" for adolescents reduces time in nature. The outcomes indicated that the teens perceived that being outside in nature was uncomfortable and was associated with a "loss of control" while being indoors was perceived as "comfortable and safe." The addictive component of screen time was also indicated as a barrier to getting outside (Michaelson et al., 2020). Furthermore, community land restrictions, fear of litigation, and growing safety concerns have all made their contribution to this ever-increasing disconnect between children and the natural world. Conn (1995) noted, "The most obvious effect of the industrial age is that much of what we touch in our everyday lives is far removed from its roots in the Earth" (p. 160).

Some professionals are exploring the possibility that many of the behavioral disorders observed in children might well be, in part, a consequence of this disconnect (Louv, 2008, 2012; Rivkin, 2014; Swank & Shin, 2015). Many therapists who work with children in a traditional playroom setting have, for the most part, neglected to include nature objects, such as plants, flowers, shells, and stones, and the wonderful and meaningful metaphors that they inspire, substituting instead a room of plastic objects. Most trainings in play and expressive therapies do not often include that a play space can also be conducted outdoors where the gifts of nature can be used as therapeutic materials.

Nature and the Therapeutic Powers of Play

When children play in nature outside, there is often an exuberance that accompanies this play. As they leave the constraints of being indoors, children are naturally and instinctively louder, faster, and even freer in their outdoor play. As Charles Schaefer, known affectionately as the "father of play therapy," is often quoted: "We are never more fully alive, more completely ourselves, or more deeply engrossed in anything than when we are playing" (Schaefer, 1994, p. 66). This is especially true when playing outside! It has been noted that Margaret Lowenfield, another play therapy pioneer, included an outdoor play garden area for her child clients (refer to, https://lowenfeld.org/). One can observe that even the most inattentive child can quickly become focused on watching a worm crawling on the ground, and an anxious teen can become calmer when looking for images made by clouds in the sky. Conducting therapeutic activities outside in nature can lead to more opportunities for messy play, risky mastery play, and unstructured free play—all of which are often in short supply for children, but so very needed for optimal emotional growth and development.

Play in and of itself, whether indoors or outside, provides curative factors for change. These were first identified as the therapeutic powers of play by Schaefer (1993, 1999). These curative powers were then expanded by Schaefer and Drewes (2014) to 20 specific agents of change encompassed within four overall categories that are often referred to as the cornerstones for play therapy practice (see Figure 1.1). In a recent journal article by Ellard and Parson (2021), they explored the current play therapy nature-based literature where they utilized the therapeutic powers of play as a frame of reference to assess each article within their review. The Association for Play Therapy (APT) defines play therapy as "the systematic use of a theoretical model to establish an interpersonal process wherein trained play therapists use the *therapeutic powers of play* to help clients prevent or resolve psychosocial difficulties and achieve optimal growth and development" (2020, para. 3; italics added). Figure 1.1 illustrates each category and the specific curative factors that fall within. The authors of this chapter recognize that all of the categories can be accessed within nature-based play whether in the playroom or outdoors.

These therapeutic powers of play are often explored within a traditional indoor playroom perspective. However, the agents of change are rarely considered when playing outdoors or with nature's "toys" such

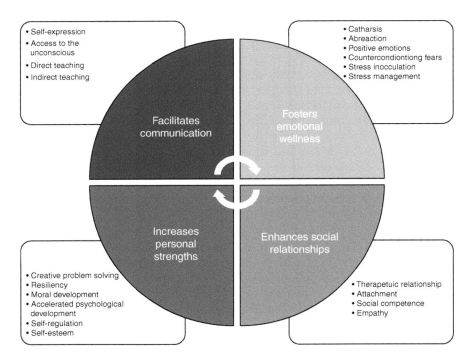

Figure 1.1 Therapeutic powers of play conceptualized by Schaefer and Drewes (2014).

Source: Used with permission from Judi Parson.

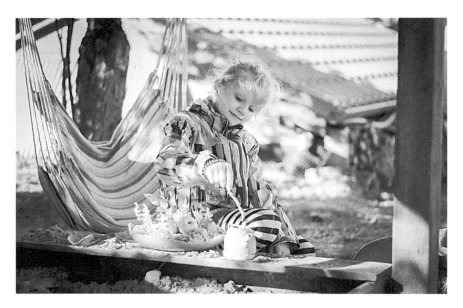

Figure 1.2 Girl creating in the sand in an outdoor play space.

Source: Can Stock Photo/KatarinaGondova.

as sticks, stones, and leaves. Nature's playground inspires all types of creative and resourceful play where something as simple as a stick can be imaginatively transformed into a sword to duel with, a broom to fly, a baton to twirl, a musical production to conduct, or a spoon to stir, and so much more. For those therapists who do not have the ability, experience, or comfort to take clients outside, these toys from nature can be brought inside to be utilized as far as the imagination can go (Langley, 2019).

Outdoor nature play areas can be naturally utilized with either directive therapies, where the therapist guides a more structured nature intervention, or a non-directive approach, where the child is able to freely make use of the nature items available, such as in Nature-Based Client-Centered Play Therapy (Swank & Shin, 2015, 2018). Even a small green space can provide opportunities for nature-based therapeutic activities. Some therapists are now designing outdoor areas for specific interests to incorporate nature more fully in their therapeutic practices. For example, some therapists are creating areas for outdoor kitchens, climbing areas, sand and mud spaces, movement areas, labyrinths, or places to build and create using pieces of wood and stone. (See Figure 1.2 for an example.)

Another incentive to including nature in play and expressive therapies is that even small amounts of time engaging nature can have positive emotional enhancements. One study found that spending as few as five minutes outdoors simply by sitting on a bench improved mood (Neill et al., 2019). This means that even therapists with limited time or access outdoors can help provide emotional benefits with nature-based interventions. This can also lead to helping parents and families become more comfortable in nature in small doses, titrating for longer periods of time to build a sense of security.

Aspects of nature-based play and expressive therapies can also be adapted to online applications such as over telemental health (Langley, in press). For example, a client can gather nature items such as pinecones, sticks, stones, and leaves, either prior to or during a telemental health session. These items can then be used in various ways depending upon the activity and shared over the screen. The therapeutic powers of play are applicable in nature-based play and expressive therapies whether they are conducted inside, outside, or even virtually. They become a therapeutic "dynamic duo" to further promote adaptive outcomes for clients. These positive correlations can be best summarized in the "12 Cs" (adapted from Courtney, 2017) of nature-based play and expressive therapies:

- **Empowers Concentration** – Time in nature has been proven to increase attention, focus and concentration (Faber Taylor & Kuo, 2009; Kuo & Faber Taylor, 2004). Often these improvements have occurred with simple outings and walks in nature. Since many childhood conditions such as attention deficit hyperactivity disorder (ADHD) have a component of poor concentration and focus, this nature time could be a more natural prescription for some of these conditions.

- **Boosts Cheerfulness** – Simply put, being in nature helps improve mood (Capaldi et al., 2014). Playful explorations in nature often evoke feelings of awe and wonder, which leads to the release of dopamine, the "pleasure chemical" in our brain. The more pleasure we feel, the happier or more cheerful we become.
- **Encourages Creativity** – Our creative problem-solving increases after being in nature, sometimes by as much as 50 percent! (Berman et al., 2008). In addition, nature lends itself to many "gifts" for expressive art materials for all types of creative art making.
- **Promotes Calming** – The "grounding" effect of nature elicits connection with the earth, and overall calming of our senses and even our brain (Berman et al., 2008). Trauma and other stressful images and memories are stored in the limbic systems of our brains. Nature can be a powerful intervention to help calm the nervous system to lower stress and increase emotional health.
- **Elicits Compassion** – As we spend time in the environment, it naturally grows a desire to take care of it and its inhabitants for future generations. As we help take care of nature, in turn, nature can help take care of us. This compassionate caring for the earth builds a sense of empathy for others and nature itself.
- **Improves Communication** – Families that play together communicate better! The added element of nature facilitates opportunities for enhanced communication—even among siblings and groups too.
- **Provides Catharsis** – Nature is naturally cathartic! By going outside, we get an immediate release from the indoors. Children's play becomes louder, freer, and more active—thus, providing a safe environment to discharge repressed feelings and emotions.
- **Enhances Connections** – Research indicates that children's connection to nature supports overall well-being and grows a sense of stewardship and responsibility to care for the environment (Salazar et al., 2020). As well, when children and families are outside enjoying nature activities together, it enriches the connection between them.
- **Builds Character** – Being in nature builds character! As children and teens are exposed to nature experiences, it builds a sense of consideration for the land and others and strengthens an overall respect and empathy that builds character. While children and teens can often be self-focused, nature experiences can broaden their awareness in novel ways to promote care for humanity, as well as looking out for nature.
- **Invites Cooperation** – Conducting nature-based activities outdoors provides opportunities for cooperative skill-building via taking turns, working together to complete a task, or creating a work of creative art together.
- **Inspires Confidence** – Playing in nature often involves assessing and taking risks. Risky play boosts confidence as new skills and tasks are performed and accomplished. Examples of risky play can be climbing on rocks, walking on a log, climbing a tree, or something as fun as rolling down a hill.
- **Welcomes Curiosity** – Children are naturally curious. As their exposure to nature increases, children will investigate their surroundings to learn more. They become more intrigued as they deepen these explorations. Interestingly, the root word of curiosity is "cure." While delving into nature, children are naturally generating a cure for the outer stressors of the world. This play on words takes on new meaning in a "wonder-full" way.

Research Benefits of Children's Connection to Nature

At an intuitive level, it makes sense that children's contact with nature has beneficial mental health consequences, as identified with the aforementioned "12 Cs." But what about the evidence to support that idea? For the most part we have the Children & Nature Network to thank. The organization has compiled a multidisciplinary group of experts to comprise their Scientific Advisory Council that focuses on curating a vast array of peer-reviewed research literature that supports the benefits of children and nature (See: https://research.childrenandnature.org/research-library/). At this point, the network has amassed around a 1000 research studies that highlights the benefits of contact with nature. Much of the research shows improved benefits in the areas of academic performance with enhanced memory and attention, positive social developmental interactions, behavioral changes, and an increase in children's cognitive and emotional mental health, including increased imagination and creativity. Diagnoses and problem areas that showed increased positivity include depression, decreased anxiety, impulse disorder, ADHD, and autism (Annerstedt & Währborg, 2011; Bratman et al., 2019; Faber Taylor & Kuo, 2009; Hummel & Randler, 2012; Kuo & Faber Taylor, 2004; Li et al., 2019; Mygind et al., 2019; Roberts et al., 2019; Sawitri, 2017; Stevenson et al., 2018; Vanaken & Danckaerts, 2018; Weeland et al., 2019; Wells, 2000; Yar & Kazemi, 2020, to name a few). Research specific to play therapy is emerging and Jacqueline M. Swank at the University of Florida, and colleagues have taken the lead in this area including examining the benefits of Nature-Based Client-Centered Play Therapy (Shin & Swank, 2018; Swank et al., 2017; Swank & Shin, 2015; Swank & Swank, 2013; Swank et al., 2020). See also Walker (2021) for research related to Outdoor Child-Centered Play Therapy and a good summary of other play therapy research conducted by Ellard and Parson (2021).

One of the first steps to understanding children's connections to nature is to find the right instruments of assessment. Salazar et al. (2020) compiled a comprehensive "Practitioner Guide to Assessing Connection to Nature" document. The following nature-based measures may be combined with other known child emotional and behavior scales to include perceptions related to nature. Rice & Torquati (2013) created the Children's Biophilia Interview scale that can be implemented using gender neutral puppets and is based upon Wilson's biophilia hypothesis (Wilson, 1984). This scale was validated with a diverse range of cultural populations and examines attitudes of the outdoors verses indoors. Another great measure for children is the Children's Environmental Perceptions Scale (CEPS) that was tested and validated among diverse populations (including African American, Hispanic, and non-Hispanic White) and it has a child-friendly Likert scale of a visual of thumbs up or down (Larson et al., 2011).

The Connectedness to Nature Scale for children (also has an adult version) assesses for children's emotional and experiential response to nature (Mayer & Frantz, 2004; Navarro et al., 2017. The Connection to Nature Index (CNI) was designed to assess for children's feelings in nature (Cheng & Monroe, 2012). This index can be used to predict children's interest in participating in nature-based activities. One study by Cheng and Monroe (2012) found that children who had previous experience of nature, who had a home near nature, and families that valued nature, were more likely to have a higher connection to nature as measured by the CNI. The Love and Care for Nature (LCN) instrument measures for children's sense of awe, wonder, feelings of love, responsibility, and emotional closeness to nature (Perkins, 2010). Another assessment tool is to have children draw their perceptions of nature such as, "Draw a picture of nature and nature around you" (Profice, 2018). Scoring rubrics can be implemented to analyze the drawings as completed by separate scorers using the rubric.

Nature Therapy Ethical and Safety Considerations

Looking to the ethics of competent practice and the growing number of specialized therapies aimed at working with children, there are few references to be located that address the specific concerns of working with children in outdoor environments. There are several factors that need to be considered regarding therapy in outdoor settings including the following:

- Confidentiality—This cannot be guaranteed in outdoor settings.
- Emotional safety—There may be clients who have encountered some difficult or traumatic experiences in nature that the practitioner needs to be aware.
- Physical safety—The outdoor environment potentially poses several safety hazards including bites from insects, or exposure to the elements like rain or sun.
- Medical conditions—such as asthma, or allergies to pollen and plants may preclude or limit the ability to be outdoors.

Therefore, a separate informed consent form specifically geared toward outdoor child and family sessions must be utilized by practitioners providing nature-based services. The authors of this chapter along with Jacqueline M. Swank, PhD worked together on formulating an outdoor child and family informed consent form that addresses the aforementioned issues among others (see Appendix B). This template is meant to serve as a springboard for practitioners to then create their own forms with the recommendation to seek legal consultation pertaining to the applicable laws and rules that may apply within an individual practitioner's state or country.

Another consideration for therapists who want to incorporate nature as part of therapeutic practice is for nature itself. One of the features of connecting with nature is becoming more aware of ways to protect it for current as well as future use. Nature is good for us, and we need to be good to nature. Most nature enthusiasts rely on nature ethics such as the concept of "Leave No Trace" which basically means to keep things as they were found. That said, clients can be encouraged to use nature items that have fallen to the ground, such as a leaf, thus the deep-rooted phrase: "Picking *UP* rather than picking." This concept can also be a way to teach children about having empathy for the earth environment—such as not taking all the acorns that could be a potential food source for animals. Another time-honored quote, attributed to various sources, states: "Take nothing but pictures, leave nothing but footprints." A more recent addition to this idea is, "Build nothing but memories." As an example, this phrase could discourage the practice of stacking stones, known as cairns, in the natural environment as they disrupt dwelling spaces for creatures, as well as interfere with trail markers. "Catch and release" is often a sustainable approach used for fishing and can be adapted for therapeutic activities as well. Hence, once children are done playing with nature's toys, they can then be "released" back into nature.

Closing Summary

This chapter has served to introduce the use of nature-based play and expressive therapies to set the stage for the chapters to follow. Throughout the chapters in this book, therapists will provide various applications of ways to include nature-based interventions from both directive and non-directive perspectives to include a wide range of topics within the traditional play therapy indoor settings as well as in outdoor environments. As you read through the chapters in this book, the authors have provided interventions and techniques from varied theoretical perspectives with supportive case vignettes or case studies to demonstrate the approaches presented.

Reflection Questions:

1   Discuss with a partner the concept of "nature deficit disorder" as coined by Louv, and share your thoughts or concerns related to this nonclinical disorder. Do you agree or disagree with this concept? Elaborate your opinion.
2   Review the 12 Cs in this chapter and with a partner discuss some examples of how you might have experienced each one of the 12 Cs related to nature within your life.
3   Look over the Nature Informed Consent form (Appendix B). Discuss with a partner the varied ethical considerations found on the form. Do you think the form is complete? Are there any other considerations that you think need to be addressed within the form? Explain your *answers*.

Appendix A

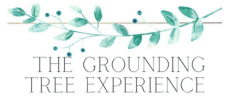

THE GROUNDING TREE EXPERIENCE

A Nature Play Therapy Intervention

Janet A. Courtney, PhD, RPT-S & Jamie Lynn Langley, LCSW, RPT-S

DESCRIPTION:

This intervention utilizes the availability of nearby nature, such as trees or other nature elements to use as an external regulator to assist the client to calm, focus, connect and be grounded.

RECOMMENDED SETTING:

Access to an outdoor environment with at least one tree to support a multi-sensory experience.

GOAL:

To provide connection to nature as a natural grounding resource.

INSTRUCTIONS:

Nature can play a role in assisting to regulate emotional states. Practitioners can facilitate clients to access a nearby tree for a grounding experience to calm and regulate. Once a client chooses "their tree," they are guided to first place their hands on the tree trunk and to focus on how their hands feel against the bark (e.g. warm, rough, cold). Next, have them pay attention to their breath and attune to the surrounding sounds and scents of nature. They are asked to feel the gentle support of the ground beneath their feet and to imagine that they have strong solid roots going deep into the earth. To expand this metaphorical nature connection, they can draw/paint or create out of clay an image of their tree grounding experience.

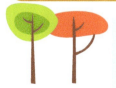

EXTRA FUN:

As an alternative, clients can be guided in a visualization to experience this tree grounding intervention.

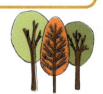

Appendix B. Informed Consent for Outdoor Therapy Services

I _____(parent/guardian) give consent for my child to receive individual, family and/or group therapy services outside of the office setting, a service offered through _____(name of provider). Outdoor services will be held in _____ location. (If this location changes, then a separate consent form will be provided.)

Services rendered outside the office include varied nature-based child counseling and play therapy interventions. Please share if the child has had any challenging exposure related to nature or the outdoors. This could include, hurricanes, tornados, car accidents, wasp stings, fear of water, or anything else that could be triggering to your child in a nature play therapy session.

_____

Although, every reasonable precaution will be used by this provider, I recognize that confidentiality for my child/family cannot be fully guaranteed in an outdoor environment. Therefore, I accept the possibility that other people may hear parts of my child/family's conversation, or see my child/family engaging in therapeutic activities with the therapist.

I recognize that outdoor environments have inherent risks such as exposure to the sun, weather, bugs and animals (such as, mosquitos or ants). Therefore, this provider recommends that the parent or guardian make available sunscreen, water, bug spray, and appropriate attire for outdoor play and weather conditions for your child's health and protection. Please list here any medical concerns for your child/family such as allergies that this provider should be aware of in providing therapy services in an outdoor space.

_____

I hereby affirm that my child/family does not have any conditions or concerns which would prevent or limit participation in outdoor therapy services. I acknowledge that my child/family's involvement in outdoor therapy services is purely voluntary and in no way required.

_____ In consideration of my child/family's participation in outdoor therapy services, I hereby release _____(name of provider) from any claims, demands, and/or causes of action as a result of my child/family's voluntary participation.

_____ I understand that the therapist will provide the rationale for the treatment.

_____ I can choose not to participate in outdoor therapy services, now or at any time in the future. I can also revoke my consent to any outdoor therapy services at any time.

I HEREBY AFFIRM THAT I HAVE READ AND FULLY UNDERSTAND THE ABOVE STATEMENTS.

_____

Client signature   Date

_____

Parent/Guardian signature   Date

_____

Therapist signature   Date

References

Annerstedt, M., & Währborg, P. (2011). Nature-assisted therapy: Systematic review of controlled and observational studies. *Scandinavian Journal of Public Health*, *39*, 371–388. https://doi.org/10.1177/1403494810396400

Association for Play Therapy (APT). (2020). *About APT*. https://www.a4pt.org/page/AboutAPT

Bentsen, P. (2013). *Udeskole in Scandinavia: Teaching and learning in natural places*. Retrieved February 9, 2021 from: https://www.childrenandnature.org/resources/udeskole-in-scandinavia-teaching-learning-in-natural-places/

Berman M. G., Jonides J., & Kaplan S. (2008). The cognitive benefits of interacting with nature. *Psychological Science*, *19*(12), 1207–1212. https://doi.org/10.1111/j.1467-9280.2008.02225.x

Bratman, G. N., Anderson, C. B., Berman, M. G., Cochran B., & de Vries, S. (2019). Nature and mental health: An ecosystem service perspective. *Science Advances*, *5*(7), eaax0903. https://doi.org/10.1126/sciadv.aax0903

Broström, S. (1998). Kindergarten in Denmark and the USA. *Scandinavian Journal of Educational Research*, *42*(2), 109–122. https://doi.org/10.1080/0031383980420201

Buzzell, L., & Chalquist, C. (Eds.) (2009). *Ecotherapy: Healing with nature in mind*. Counterpoint Publishing.

Capaldi C., Dopko R. L., & Zelenski J. (2014). The relationship between nature connectedness and happiness: A meta-analysis. *Frontiers in Psychology*. https://doi.org/10.3389/fpsyg.2014.00976

Cheng, J. C., & Monroe, M. C. (2012). Connection to nature: Children's affective attitude toward nature. *Environment and Behavior*, *44*, 31–49. https://doi.org/10.1177/0013916510385082

Chown, A. (2014). *Play therapy in the outdoors: Taking play therapy out of the playroom and into natural environments*. London, UK: Jessica Kingsley Publishers.

Chown, A. (2018). *A practical guide to play therapy in the outdoors*. New York, NY: Routledge.

Conn, S. A. (1995). When the earth hurts, who responds? In T. Roszak, M. E. Gomes, & A. D. Kanner (Eds.), *Ecopsychology: Restoring the Earth, healing the mind* (pp. 156–171). San Francisco, CA: Sierra Club Books.

Courtney, J. A. (2017). The art of utilizing the metaphorical elements of nature as "co-therapist" in ecopsychology play therapy. In A. Kopytin & M. Rugh (Eds.). *Environmental Expressive Therapies: Nature-Assisted Theory and Practice*, (pp. 100–122). New York, NY: Routledge.

Courtney, J. A. (2020). *Healing child and family trauma through expressive and play therapies: Art, nature, storytelling, body, mindfulness*. New York, NY: Norton & Co.

Courtney, J. A., & Mills, J. C. (2016). Utilizing the metaphor of nature as co-therapist in StoryPlay®. *Play Therapy*, *11*(1), 18–21.

Courtney, J. A., & Nowakowski-Sims, E. (2019). Technology's impact on the parent-infant attachment relationship: Intervening through FirstPlay® therapy. *International Journal of Play Therapy*, *28*(2), 57–68. https://doi.org/10.1037/pla0000090

Dhaese, M. J. (2011). Holistic expressive play therapy: An integrative approach to helping maltreated children. In A. A. Drews, S. C. Bratton, & C. E. Schaefer (Eds.), *Integrative play therapy* (pp. 75–93). Hoboken, NJ: John Wiley & Sons.

Ellard, M., & Parson, J. A. (2021) Playing in the field: Scoping the therapeutic powers of play for nature play therapy. *British Journal of Play Therapy*, *15*(Spring), 42–64.

Faber Taylor, A. F., & Kuo, F. E. (2009). Children with attention deficits concentrate better after walk in the park. *Journal of Attention Disorders*, *12*, 402–409. https://doi.org/10.1177/1087054708323000

Hummel, E., & Randler, C. (2012). Living animals in the classroom: A meta-analysis on learning outcome and a treatment-control study focusing on knowledge and motivation. *Journal of Science Education and Technology*, *21*(1), 95–105. https://doi.org/10.1007/s10956-011-9285-4

Kellert, S. R. (1993). Introduction. In S. R. Kellert & E. O. Wilson (Eds.), *The Biophilia hypothesis* (pp. 18–25). Washington, DC: Shearwater Books/Island Press.

Knight, S. (Ed.) (2013). *International perspectives on Forest School: Natural spaces to play and learn*. London: SAGE Publications Ltd. https://doi.org/10.4135/9781446288665

Kuo, F. E., & Faber Taylor, A. (2004). A potential natural treatment for attention-deficit/hyperactivity disorder: Evidence from a national study. *American Journal of Public Health*, *94*, 1580–1586. https://doi.org/10.2105/ajph.94.9.1580

Langley, J. L. (2019). Nature play therapy: When nature comes into play. *Playground* (Spring/Summer), 20–24. https://cacpt.com/wp-content/uploads/2019/04/Playground-Spring-2019.pdf

Langley, J. L. (In press). Nature play therapy and telehealth: How green time and screen time can play well together. In J. Stone (Ed.), *Telehealth and play therapy: Foundations, populations, and interventions*. Routledge.

Larson, L. R., Green, G. T., & Castleberry, S. B. (2011). Construction and validation of an instrument to measure environmental orientations in a diverse group of children. *Environment and Behavior*, *43*(1), 72–89. Retrieved January 2, 2021 from: https://eric.ed.gov/?id=EJ910770

Li, D., Larsen, L., Yang, Y., Wang, L., Zhai, Y., & Sullivan, W. C. (2019). Exposure to nature for children with autism spectrum disorder: Benefits, caveats, and barriers. *Health and Place*, *55*, 71–79. https://doi.org/10.1016/j.healthplace.2018.11.005

Louv, R. (2008). *Last child in the woods: Saving our children from nature-deficit disorder*. Chapel Hill, NC: Algonquin Books.

Louv, R. (2012a). Every child needs nature not just the ones whose parents appreciate nature (para. 1, sent. 1–4). http://richardlouv.com/blog/every-child-needs-nature-not-just-the-ones-with-parent-who-appreciate-natur/

Louv, R. (2012b). *The nature principle: Reconnecting with life in a virtual age*. Chapel Hill, NC: Algonquin Books.

Mayer, F. S., & Frantz, C. M. (2004). The connectedness to nature scale: A measure of individuals' feeling in community with nature. *Journal of Environmental Psychology, 24*(4), 503–515.

Michaelson, V., King, N., Janssen, I., Lawal, S., & Pickett, W. (2020). Electronic screening technology use and connection to nature in Canadian adolescents: A mixed methods study. *Canadian Journal of Public Health, 111*, 502–514.

Mills, J. C., & Crowley, R. J. (2014). *Therapeutic metaphors for children and the child within*. (2nd ed.). Philadelphia, PA: Brunner-Routledge.

Montgomery, C. S., & Courtney, J. A. (2015). The theoretical and therapeutic paradigm of botanical arranging. *Journal of Therapeutic Horticulture, XXV*(1), 16–26. Retrieved January 2, 2021 from: https://www.ahta.org/journal-of-therapeutic-horticulture-25-1---2015

Mygind, L., Kjeldsted, E., Hartmeyer, R., Mygind, E., Bølling, M., & Bents, P. (2019). Mental, physical and social health benefits of immersive nature-experiences for children and adolescents: A systematic review and quality assessment of the evidence. *Health & Place, 58*. https://doi.org/10.1016/j.healthplace.2019.05.014

Navarro, O., Olivos, P., & Fleury-Bahi, G. (2017). "Connectedness to nature scale": Validity and reliability in the French context. *Frontiers in Psychology, 8*, 2180. https://doi.org/10.3389/fpsyg.2017.02180

Neill, C., Gerard, J., & Arbuthnott, K. (2019) Nature contact and mood benefits: Contact duration and mood type. *The Journal of Positive Psychology, 14*(6), 756767. https://doi.org/10.1080/17439760.2018.1557242

Perkins, H. E. (2010). Measuring love and care for nature. *Journal of Environmental Psychology, 30*(4), 455–463. https://doi.org/10.1016/j.jenvp.2010.05.004

Profice, C. (2018). Nature as a living presence: Drawings by Tupinambá and New York Children. *PloS one, 13*(10), e0203870. https://doi.org/10.1371/journal.pone.0203870

Rice, C. S., & Torquati, J. C. (2013). Assessing connections between young children's affinity for nature and their experiences in natural outdoor settings in preschool. *Children, Youth and Environments, 23*(2), 78–102. Retrieved January 2, 2021 from: https://core.ac.uk/download/pdf/188140696.pdf

Rivkin, M. S. (2014). *The great outdoors: Advocating for natural spaces for young children* (rev. ed.). Washington, DC: National Association for the Education of Young Children.

Roberts, A., Hinds, J., & Camic, P. M. (2019). Nature activities and wellbeing in children and young people: A systematic literature review. *Journal of Adventure Education and Outdoor Learning*, 298–318. https://doi.org/10.1080/14729679.2019.1660195

Roszak, T., Gomes, M. E., & Kanner, A. D. (1995). *Ecopsychology: Restoring the earth healing the mind*. San Francisco, CA: Sierra Club Books.

Salazar, G., Kunkle, K., & Monroe, M. C. (2020). *Practitioner guide to assessing connection to nature*. Washington, DC: North American Association for Environmental Education. Retrieved December 1, 2020 from: https://www.aee.org/assets/assessing_connection_to_nature.5.11.20%201.pdf

Sawitri, D. R. (2017). Early childhood environmental education in tropical and coastal areas: A meta-analysis. IOP Conference Series: Earth and Environmental Science, 55. Retrieved January 2, 2021 from: https://iopscience.iop.org/article/10.1088/1755-1315/55/1/012050

Schaefer, C. E. (1993). *The therapeutic powers of play*. Aronson

Schaefer, C. E.(1999). Curative factors in play therapy. *The Journal for the Professional Counselor, 14* (1), 7–16

Schaefer, C. E., & Drewes, A. A. (2014). *The therapeutic powers of play: 20 core agents of change* (2nd ed.). Wiley

Schaefer, C. E. (1994). The nature of play. In C. Schaefer & H. Kaduson (Eds), *The quotable play therapist: 238 of the all-time best quotes on play and play therapy* (p. 66). Jason Aronson.

Shin, S., & Swank, J. M. (2018). Nature-based play therapy with pre-adolescents. In E. Green, J. Baggerly, & A. Myrick (Eds.), *Play therapy with pre-teens* (pp. 107–122). Lanham, MD: Rowman & Littlefield.

Stevenson, M., Schilhab T., & Bentsen, P. (2018). Attention Restoration Theory II: A systematic review to clarify attention processes affected by exposure to natural environments. *Journal of Toxicology and Environmental Health, Part B, 21*(4), 227–268. https://doi.org/10.1080/10937404.2018.1505571

Swank, J. M., Cheung, C., Prikhidko, A., & Su, Y. (2017). Nature-based child-centered group play therapy and behavioral concerns: A single-case design. *International Journal of Play Therapy, 26*, 47–57. https://doi.org/10.1037/pla0000031

Swank, J. M., & Shin, S. (2015). Nature-based child-centered play therapy: An innovative counseling approach. *International Journal of Play Therapy, 24*, 151–161. https://doi.org/10.1037/a0039127

Swank, J. M., & Swank, D. E. (2013). Student growth within the school garden: Addressing personal/social, academic, and career development. *Journal of School Counseling, 11*(21), 1–31. Retrieved January 2, 2021 from http://jsc.montana.edu/articles/v11n21.pdf

Swank, J. M., Walker, K. L. A., & Shin, S. M. (2020). Indoor nature-based play therapy: Taking the natural world inside. *International Journal of Play Therapy, 29*(3), 155–162. https://doi.org/10.1037/pla0000123

Vanaken, G.-J., & Danckaerts, M. (2018). Impact of green space exposure on children's and adolescents' mental health: A systematic review. *International Journal of Environmental Research and Public Health, 15*(12). https://doi.org/10.3390/ijerph15122668

Walker, K. (2021). Outdoor child-centered play therapy with attention and social-emotional competencies in children, dissertation, May 2021; Denton, Texas. (https://digital.library.unt.edu/ark:/67531/metadc1808455/: accessed July 5, 2021), University of North Texas Libraries, UNT Digital Library, https://digital.library.unt.edu

Weeland, J., Moens, M. A., Beute, F., Assink, M., Staaks, J. P. C., & Overbeek, G. (2019). A dose of nature: Two three-level meta-analyses of the beneficial effects of exposure to nature on children's self-regulation. *Journal of Environmental Psychology, 65.* https://doi.org/10.1016/j.jenvp.2019.101326.

Wells, N. M. (2000). At home with nature: Effects of "greenness" on children's cognitive functioning. *Environment and Behavior, 32,* 775–795. https://doi.org/10.1177/00139160021972793

Wilson, E. O. (1984). *Biophilia.* Cambridge, Massachusetts: Harvard University Press.

Wilson, E. (1993). Biophilia and the conservation ethic. In S. R. Kellert & E. O. Wilson (Eds.), *The biophilia hypothesis* (pp. 31–40). Washington, DC: Shearwater Books/Island Press.

Yar, M. A., & Kazemi, F. (2020). The role of dish gardens on the physical and neuropsychological improvement of hospitalized children. *Urban Forestry & Urban Greening, 53.* https://doi.org/10.1016/j.ufug.2020.126713

2 "Not Just a Walk in the Park: Complex Layers of Integrating Nature Into Play Therapy Practice"

Judi Parson and Megan Ellard

Introduction

Play provides access to the child's inner thoughts and feelings, and play therapy provides rich experiences, which may be offered across different spaces, to target and enhance the scope and strength of the therapeutic powers of play. When a child comes to play therapy, it is in the creation and maintenance of the therapeutic relationship that acts as the rudder to navigate the course of the intervention. Through the relationship, the therapist has access to the child's world: their sense of self; their relationships with others and the environment; their struggles, worries, and concerns; their beliefs, fantasies, and imaginations; and their position in the family, community, and their world. When a child also has additional needs such as children who are diagnosed with a neurobehavioral disorder associated with prenatal alcohol exposure (ND-PAE), for example, fetal alcohol syndrome (FAS) or fetal alcohol spectrum disorder (FASD), there is a need for the therapist to understand the disorder or diagnosis in the context of the child's world and their play ability in order to provide solid therapeutic matching and titrate sessions accordingly.

Seven-year-old Sharon was referred to play therapy because she had a complex family history, developmental delay, and many of the symptoms included in a ND-PAE diagnosis (Hagan et al., 2016). She loved smelling and touching everything, exploring objects, and manipulating them to try and figure out how things worked, and she really, really, really enjoyed messy play. She would always begin each session by enthusiastically scanning the room whilst providing fantastical accounts of her most recent events. At times she tried to stay on task but was often distracted and frequently jumped from one activity to another. Other times her play appeared frenzied, muddled, and confused. Initially, staying in the playroom was limited to about 30 minutes, with hindsight I wondered if she was telling me of her desire to be outside. I understood later that the outdoors environment provided her with a cognitive break from the intensity of indoor play therapy.

The therapeutic benefits of outdoor play are many, including its natural regulatory effect (Hanscom, 2016). For Sharon, the indoor play was fun but she often verbalized that it was hard or that she was tired. She expressed many moments of disappointment, frustration, anger, and dysregulation. To further understand Sharon's level of play ability, and to plan and titrate her sessions accordingly, an assessment called the Child Initiated Pretend Play Assessment (ChIPPA) (Stagnitti, 2007) was used as a baseline before and after the play therapy intervention.

This chapter aims to present Sharon's therapeutic story based on her play ability, personal choice in play activities and clinical reasoning at various points throughout this integrative nature-based Play Therapy intervention. Following a brief introduction to the therapeutic intervention and description of the ChIPPA, Sharon's case study will be presented to showcase how nature-based experiences were integrated into her play therapy.

Integrative Nature-Based, Humanistic Play Therapy

To meet the psychotherapeutic needs of Sharon, an integrative Play Therapy approach was used. This was based on the premise that "one size does not fit all" and by integrating both theoretical and practical biophilic elements, it was hypothesized that nature-based, learn to play, and humanistic play therapy would enhance therapeutic effectiveness.

DOI: 10.4324/9781003152767-3

Biophilic Benefits

It is important to firstly establish that being in nature has a range of therapeutic benefits in and of itself. Biophilia is a term, initially coined by social psychologist Eric Fromm (1964), and then biologist Edward Wilson (1984) popularized the term in his text titled "Biophilia." Biophilia has been defined as "the innate, genetically determined affiliation of human beings to nature and other living organisms" (International Living Future Institute (ILFI), 2018, p. 23). A range of disciplines and fields now apply biophilia concepts and principles to inform biophilic building designs and support the creation of spaces that positively impact the human psyche. Biophilic designs can help inform the play therapist to create and maintain therapeutic spaces that integrate the elements and associated attributes. The six biophilic design elements include (1) environmental features (e.g., water, air, sunlight, and animals); (2) natural shapes and forms (e.g., botanical and animal motifs, shells and spirals, and eggs and oval shapes); (3) natural patterns and processes (e.g., sensory, bounded spaces, and complementary contrasts); (4) light and space (e.g., natural light and inside–outside spaces); (5) place-based relationships (e.g., cultural connections to place, landscape orientation); and (6) evolved human–nature relationships (e.g., curiosity and enticement, security and protections, mastery, and control). For more detail, please see the ILFI (2018) *Biophilic Design Guidebook*. Examples of biophilic connections in the case example are identified later in this chapter.

What is important to play therapists is that the biophilic benefits of nature may inform and strengthen therapeutic integration. Van Wieren and Kellert (2013) reviewed the biophilic values of nature and found that being in nature led to the following benefits:

- Aesthetical appeal of nature led to curiosity, intellectual development, imagination, and creativity.
- Emotional attachment to nature led to bonding, nurturance, and cooperation.
- Avoidance of nature led to coping, security, protection, and awe.
- Control of nature led to mastery skills and self-confidence.
- Material use of nature led to comfort, security, and efficiency.
- Understanding of nature led to cognition, problem solving, and critical thinking.
- Connecting with nature led to meaning purpose, feeling of kinship, and relation.
- Representational expression of nature led to communication, language, and design (p. 245).

With such a wide range of benefits, it makes sense to combine therapeutic benefits of nature and play. By reviewing the aforementioned nature benefits, it is easy to identify synergies with the specific Therapeutic Powers of Play (TPoP) (see Figure 1.1 in Chapter 1) as identified by Schaefer and Drewes (2015). Ellard and Parson (2021) in their scoping review of the benefits of nature play identified 15 of the 20 TPoP in the 14 articles that met the inclusion criteria for the study. However, before integrating nature therapeutically, it is important to provide the foundational orientation and essential skills in the provision of play therapy.

Humanistic Play Therapy

Humanistic play therapy is built on the foundations of Carl Rogers' Person-Centered Therapy (Meador & Rogers, 1973) and adapted by Virginia Axline (1974) for use with children. Axline called her approach to play therapy as "nondirective, also referred to as child-centered play therapy (CCPT), highlighting the person-centered therapist attitudinal conditions of unconditional positive regard, empathic understanding, and congruence" (Ray & Jayne, 2016, p. 389). Humanistic play therapy approaches position the relationship between child client and the therapist as the "vehicle for dynamic growth and healing" (Bratton & Ray, 2002. p. 370).

As Sweeney and Landreth (2009) summarize:

> Child-centered play therapy is not a cloak the play therapist puts on when entering the playroom and takes off when leaving; rather it is a philosophy resulting in attitudes and behaviors for living

one's life in relationships with children. It is both a basic philosophy of the innate human capacity of the child to strive toward growth and maturity and an attitude of deep and abiding belief in the child's ability to be constructively self-directing. Child-centered play therapy is a complete therapeutic system, not just the application of a few rapport-building techniques. (p. 123)

Humanistic play therapy strongly focuses on the therapist's ability to facilitate a safe space and therapeutic relationship with their client, creating the right conditions for the child to grow and heal. As Axline wrote, "the therapist's role, though non-directive, is not a passive one, but one which requires alertness, sensitivity, and an ever-present appreciation of what the child is doing and saying. It calls for understanding and a genuine interest in the child" (Cochran et al., 2010, p. 49).

Rogers (1980, cited in Cochran et al., 2010, p. 55), stated that the "therapist is willing for the client to be whatever immediate feeling is going on—confusion, resentment, fear, anger, courage, love, or pride." Each child should feel valued and cared about by their therapist, no matter what they are expressing or how they present. As Cochran et al. (2010. p. 54) explains, empathy should not be "all about emotions" but rather, "deep empathy should be about a total shared experience, including all key elements of the child's experience in the moment."

Therapists should be present in the moment with the child, using skills such as tracking and empathic reflections to demonstrate their focused attention and understanding of the child and their journey within their play. Congruence, also known as genuineness, is the ability for the therapist to be truthful toward the client in a way that supports their shared experiences within the therapy. As Cochran et al. (2010. p. 55) wrote "a 'pretense' of empathy or unconditional positive regard is not therapeutic. Child clients have an uncanny ability for knowing, at some level, when you are faking it." Being genuine, or congruent, with the child client means therapists are open to the connection and relationship and must embrace the concept that the child can captain their own therapeutic journey.

Nature-Based Play Therapy

When considering nature-based play therapy literature, Chown (2014, 2018), Fearn (2014, 2021), and Courtney (2020) inform the theoretical lens and benefits of working with the natural environment by integrating natural resources into the playroom and by taking play therapy into nature. Chown (2014) explores the changing attitudes toward nature, the developmental context of childhood including sensory and body awareness, and the connection to nature required to facilitate nature play therapy. Courtney (2020) incorporates nature and natural items into the play therapy room. She proposes bringing nature-based items such as stones, clay, flowers, sea glass into the playroom. Similarly, products such as leaves, gumnuts, seeds, feathers, wood, and stones were incorporated into the playroom in the case study that follows. Furthermore, the case study also follows the trajectory as Chown (2014) describes by building the therapeutic relationship within the playroom before transitioning into the outdoor environment. Fearn (2014) focuses on the sensory experience of being in nature rather than the product or outcome. Chown (2018) integrates the beneficial therapeutic possibilities that nature can be brought into traditional play therapy for children with complex social, emotional, and behavioral needs as well as a range of learning needs which is applicable for the case study presented in this chapter. When including animals in the play therapy, considerations should be taken to assess risk to ensure safety of the client and the animals within the context of the clinical practice setting.

Play Therapy in Nature

Fearn (2014) writes "natural environments provide experiences of connection with other life forms, like insect, mammal, tree, wind, rock, soil, water, flower, light, the suns heat, the coolness of rain and shade" (p. 115). She goes on to position nature play therapy as an opportunity for bodily immersion within the natural world. Fearn states that being in nature, as a cofacilitator in the therapeutic partnership, recognizes the sensory benefits particularly when combatting traumatic experiences.

Encouraging a child to become absorbed in sensory play in nature can override defensive patterns, and restore a whole and integrated sensory pathway, enabling her to draw full benefits from a dynamic relationship with the natural environment, and to respond through symbolic play with natural and found materials.

(Fearn, 2014, p. 116)

Case Study: Sharon and the Secret Garden in Her Play World

Sharon recently relocated to a new home following a breakdown in her previous foster family placement. The referral detailed a long list of disruptive behaviors including being mean to animals, setting fire to things, getting "into trouble" at school and a range of other symptoms, which made her sound like she was the problem rather than focusing on the underlying circumstances and her early-life trauma and neuro- biological implications. Whilst the trauma was significant, protective factors were needed to be amplified to increase self-regulation and prosocial behaviors. Fortunately, she was placed with a family that really wanted her in their lives and in their home. Although the new foster parents had little detail of Sharon's very early-life, they were aware of her mother's intake of alcohol and other drugs being used throughout the pregnancy. It was due to this scant history that a diagnosis of FASD was difficult to make.

Fetal Alcohol Spectrum Disorder

FASD refers to the range of problems caused by prenatal exposure to alcohol during pregnancy. Recent research has recognized the range of neurodevelopmental delays that alcohol exposure can cause in a fetus, and how these carry on into infancy, childhood, and adulthood. "FASD is used as an 'umbrella' term to encompass the diagnostic categories of Fetal Alcohol Syndrome, partial Fetal Alcohol Syndrome, Alcohol-Related Neurodevelopmental Disorder and Alcohol-Related Birth Defects" (Bower & Elliott, 2016, p. 4). However, inclusion and exclusion criteria are still undergoing future studies and scrutiny to ascertain diagnosis in children. FASD is thought to be underdiagnosed, as health profes- sionals can be unaware of the diagnostic criteria. "For a diagnosis of FASD, an individual must have prenatal alcohol exposure and severe neurodevelopmental impairment in at least three of ten specified domains of central nervous system structure or function" (Bower & Elliott, 2016, p. 13). These domains are as follows: brain structure/neurology, motor skills, cognition, language, academic achievement, memory, attention, and executive function, including impulse control and hyperactivity, affect regula- tion, adaptive behavior, social skills, and social communication. The presence of three facial abnorm- alities may assist in diagnosis but is not required if it is known that the fetus was exposed to alcohol and has impairments in at least three of these areas. Sharon certainly had difficulty in all the above domains.

Family History

The family constellation included biological parents both of whom have had little contact with Sharon from the age of three when she was first placed in emergency foster care. She has seven known siblings, three older and four younger. Two siblings resided in the same geographical location and the other siblings live a significant distance away. The family were focused on facilitating opportunities to re- connect Sharon with at least some of her kin that lived in the local area. She had enrolled in school and additional funding was provided to the school to facilitate and support remedial learning.

Meeting Sharon

The first time I met Sharon she walked into the playroom waiting area following her foster parent. Her shoulders were slumped, with her arms hanging by her sides, as she walked slowly and lightly into the clinic. She did not make eye contact with me for some time, rather her blue eyes darted around the room. Her unruly hair was a light brown in color. Her ears were pierced with bluebird stud earrings in each ear. Finally, when she did make eye contact with me, she gave me a short sharp smile and turned away from me and her foster parent. I noticed her thin top lip line and smooth philtrum, two of the facial features for FASD.

Her foster parent was advised to come alone to discuss play therapy. It is usual to explore the client's history in privacy, to complete the intake and consent forms and for me to get a more complete picture of the child's world. So that plan went out the window because I needed to engage with Sharon straight away. I spoke directly with her and introduced myself and showed her where the bathroom was and then moved quickly into the playroom explaining that the waiting room would be where her foster parent will wait for her, but today they would both come into the playroom together. She went straight for the dry sand tray and scooped up some sand and she watched it slide through her fingers. From this point, she glanced around the room and dashed from one area to the next, briefly exploring some play resources as she went. In this very first session, she completed a "world" in the sand tray, which featured buried treasure and a wishing well. She rearranged toys and categorized them according to new or prehistoric elements.

Introducing Play Therapy to Sharon

During this first introductory session, I explained play therapy, the structure, expectations, and freedom as well as the two rules. "That she gets to be the boss of the play and that we keep each other and the toys safe." She left the play therapy clinic asking "Can I come back tomorrow?" I explained that we would see each other every Thursday at 10 am, for an hour, for the next 12 weeks and then the adults will have a meeting, and you will have a break for the school holidays and then we will have another 12 sessions. I showed Sharon her personalized calendar plan and shared that with each session she could choose a sticker or draw on the numbered section until we filled them all in. I gave her a special appointment card for her to keep, reminding her of our play session appointment time.

The first 12 sessions focused on building the therapeutic relationship, assessing Sharon's play ability, understanding her attachment behaviors and strategies, and building a sense of identity. Unlike traditional child-centered or non-directive play therapy approaches, where the child leads the play and self-initiates a range of play activities, Sharon could not stay on one task and found it very difficult to self-initiate any play sequences. The therapist hypothesized that Sharon had a significant play deficit. Therefore, an appropriate assessment was required to evaluate her current play skills and abilities. The Child-Initiated Pretend Play Assessment (ChIPPA) was chosen as the most appropriate assessment tool and is explained next.

The Child-Initiated Pretend Play Assessment

ChIPPA is a norm-referenced standardized assessment of a child's play ability (Stagnitti, 2007). It is used with children 3–7 years and 11 months of age. For children 3 years of age, the assessment takes 18 minutes to administer and for children 4–7 years and 11 months of age, like Sharon, it takes 30 minutes to administer. The ChIPPA includes two sets of play materials and the child is invited to play with both sets in a time limited way. The first set of conventional imaginative toys includes a set of specific play materials: such as a truck and trailer, farm animals, fences, a small adjustable spanner, and toy dolls; and the second set of symbolic toys includes a shoe box, cardboard cylinder, fabric material, stones, and a doll "thing" made from white colored cloth wrapped around pillow stuffing and drawn together with elastic bands. Both sets of toys are dependent on the child's age, with larger toys that are easily manipulated for younger children.

Setting up for the ChIPPA

The assessment is set up in a makeshift "cubby house" made from a flat bedsheet draped over the backs of two dining or similar chairs. During the assessment, the examiner sits beside the child and informs the child that they may play with the toys in the ways they would like to play with them. During the middle third of the assessment period, the examiner models specific play behaviors for each set of toys. The child will potentially imitate the play behavior as modeled by the assessor.

Measuring Play Ability

The ChIPPA measures three key skills, Percentage of Elaborate Pretend Play Actions (PEPA), Number of Object Substitutions (NOS), and Number of Imitated Actions (NIA). These skills are scored twice,

Table 2.1 Pre-play Therapy ChIPPA

Score Summary—Pre-play Therapy	Raw Score	Standard Score	
PEPA Conventional (Conventional imaginative play)	48	72.5	
PEPA Symbolic	13	67	
PEPA Combined (PEPA conventional = PEPA symbolic)	61	65	
Number of Object substitutions (NOS)	0		Percentile
NOS Symbolic	4	79	10–25th Percentile
NOS combined (NOS conventional = NOS Symbolic)	4	79	
NIA (Conventional Imaginative play)	0	0–0	50th Percentile
NIA Symbolic	0	0–1	
NIA (Combined NIA conventional = NIA symbolic)	0	0–1	

once for each set of toys, as well as a total score for the session. The scores can be compared to a norm score or percentile rank. There is also a clinical observations sheet, where the assessor observes whether items were performed as typical or atypical sequences of play. In the case of Sharon, the assessment was video recorded and peer-checked to assess her level of play ability. For more information and training about the ChIPPA, please visit https://www.learntoplayevents.com/for-therapists/

The following (Table 2.1) shows the scores for Sharon. The normal range for a seven-year-old is 85–115, indicating that Sharon is significantly below average in her play skills, and therefore required therapeutic matching to target development of play skills.

The ChIPPA baseline indicated that a more cofacilitated and directive approach with sequenced scaffolding of therapeutic play skills was warranted. Therefore, an adapted Learn to Play program (Stagnitti, 1998) was integrated within the humanistic play therapy approach. This required theoretical combination of Axline's (1974) humanistic principles to establish therapeutic presence with the addition of working in the child's "zone of proximal development" as proposed by Vygotsky (1934/1997, p. 187 as cited in Stagnitti, 2021). Sessions were structured so that child-initiated play included therapist-directed moments to cofacilitate and extend play sequences within the playroom and then transitioned to the outdoor spaces. However, it is important to describe the setting to conceptualize this unique integrative approach.

The Play Environment

The playroom space is set on a few acres of land. Inside clients walked into the waiting room first, which had a lounge to sit on, books, some toys, inviting pictures on the wall depicting nature scenes and local cultural art. There was a kitchenette for parents and carers to make tea/ coffee and a separate bathroom off to one side. The playroom also had an ensuite bathroom, a wet area to facilitate access to water play, two sandtrays (one wet, one dry), low wooden bookshelves with a range of miniatures, including shells, natural produces, wooden blocks and offcuts, flora and fauna miniatures, symbols, toys, and a range of expressive play materials. The puppet theater with a range of puppets and role play dress-ups was in another section of the playroom.

The biophilic elements included natural sunlight that streamed through two large windows with vertical blinds to direct light and provide privacy. The walls were painted in colors found in nature and complementary tones to match the wooden doors and skirting boards. Adjacent to the waiting room was a large undercover outdoor play space, which was bounded by a retaining wall and raised planter herb boxes.

Leading from the undercover area are several steps that lead onto the upper hidden garden known as the secret garden. This was because the entry was through a lemon-scented star jasmine archway that opened into a larger area with a pagoda with cushioned seating for relaxing and onto another area by crossing a little bridge over a fishpond to reveal the huge granite rock face with a flowing waterfall. From a biophilic perspective, the curved pathway and numerous plants and smells infused the visual, auditory, and olfactory senses. It felt so very peaceful.

Establishing Therapeutic Relationship

To commence the play therapy intervention, it was important to build rapport and establish a therapeutic relationship with clear structuring and boundaries. To do this, Sharon explored the room and the toys and play materials. She liked playing a game with a balloon Balzac ball and spent a long time passing it back and forth and chatting about her family and school. She was attracted to the miniatures and especially the animal figurine toys. She would sort the toys according to color or size but not family groups. She placed the dinosaurs and fantasy dragon toys in the sandtray and lined them up as the "prehistoric" group. The other toys, such as the toy elephant, giraffe, kangaroo, wombat, pigs, goats, cows, ducks, and rabbits, were semi-grouped together based on size in another sandtray. The distinguishing sorting factor was whether they were alive or dead. It was a binary stance in Sharon's world.

House, Tree, Person

In one session, I suggested that she may like to draw a picture of a house, a tree, and a person and it was easy to align her drawing with that of an earlier stage of development. Kellogg (1970) studied thousands of children's scribbles and drawings to find that children's drawings across cultures revealed a similar pattern in drawing and art development. This revealed to me that Sharon was drawing more closely to children aged three to four years compared to her chronological age. The person and the tree were faintly drawn scribbles and the house appeared to be a lopsided shape of a triangle.

Sensory Play

If art was going to be difficult for Sharon, I reasoned that more sensory play with finger paints, sand, and water play may help facilitate and target lower brain development. She enjoyed music making and we connected through drumming and copying beats and rhythms. I noticed that Sharon frequently put the toys and art-making material to her nose and would smell the objects and often tasted them too. This was a moment for me to facilitate more sensory art making. I reasoned that having access to edible paints would facilitate her sensory play, so I made paints with water, sugar, cornstarch, and food coloring. This was a great success. She used the new paint brushes and then moved onto painting with her fingers and hands and was completely free to make a mess. For the first time, she suggested that we take the easel and paints outside to play. Over the coming weeks, her fine and gross motor movements were exaggerated and encouraged. The edible paints were consumed weekly and enhanced with edible flavors and scents to provide a multisensory experience. Syringes were filled and squirted onto the large butchers' paper with delight and then Sharon would touch, smell, and lick her art pieces.

Creating New Memories

A memory jar was created and Sharon chose which colour of powder paint to add to the sand to make a vibrant selection of different colored layers, which were carefully funnelled into the jar (with some help to ensure that it did not tip over). Sharon was able to speak about the people and the places she could remember. Some life storying work was emerging through the creation of the layers in her memory jar. She was starting to gain a sense of identity and connectedness to her previous and new family, albeit with missing elements, but it was a start.

Transitioning

Integrating a humanistic stance with Learn to Play Therapy (Stagnitti, 2021) provided opportunities to demonstrate and extend play sequences for Sharon to imitate the therapist to develop her play skills. Show and tell me games emerged, which provided a concrete starting point to extend her pretend play skills. She expressed the desire to play more and more outside.

The two other areas that are important to Sharon's play therapy experience was the inclusion of the chook pen and two poddy calves in their paddock. The black poddy calves resided in the paddock adjacent to the playroom. There were synergies in the fact that these calves were no longer cared for by their biological mothers but being raised by another family. We would visit the calves and feed them allowing Sharon's fingers to be sucked by the rough texture of the calf's tongue. On her therapy days, she could choose to feed them their milk formula. She would laugh at the sensation of her hand in their mouth. The rhythmical sucking provided a regulatory effect and she was learning empathy and nurturing another animal when previously she harmed small animals.

The chicken coop, also called chook pen in Australia, was accessed via the poddy calves paddock. We walked around the pen and there were two gates to be opened to access the brown chooks and their eggs. The first gate protected the chooks from other animals entering the chook pen as well as inhibiting escape of the chooks into other areas on the acreage. We discussed the need to keep the chooks safe from animals such as foxes, birds, and dogs. When Sharon wanted to collect the eggs, she would carefully carry the two or three eggs in a basket back to the play room. For many visits to chook pen, she accidentally broke the eggs on the way back. As time passed, she was able to transfer them back safely to the play room and would then take the eggs home to her family. She was learning to develop empathy and increasing her personal strengths of self-esteem and self-regulation through these experiences.

Sharon was demonstrating self-initiation and expanding her play skills. It was time to review her pretend play abilities using the ChIPPA once more. As Table 2.2 states, Sharon's pretend play skills were growing and again a second scorer tallied the video-recorded assessment.

When compared to the pre play therapy ChIPPA (Table 2.1), Sharon demonstrated a dramatic increase in her play ability. She was able to self-initiate and engage in imaginative play her play scripts and narrative were extending in depth and for a longer duration. She could engage and sustain a full 60-minute play therapy session by incorporating nature and natural objects into the play therapy room and by taking play therapy outdoors into the natural setting surrounding the play therapy clinic. She extended her play skills with use of conventional toys as well as integrating natural objects which symbolically enhanced her story.

The ChIPPA PEPA combined raw score showed a significant shift from 61 to 116 (standard score 65–92.5). Whilst this score is still below the norm for her chronological age, it does provide evidence that the nature-based, Learn to Play, humanistic play therapy approach expanded Sharon's play ability. Her family reported that she no longer deliberately hurt small animals, which coincided with the last time she dropped the eggs on her return from the chook pen back to the playroom. At home, her foster parents were taking her outside to engage in more and more playground activities and swimming. The foster family then participated in filial therapy to support the ongoing play and psychosocial development with Sharon. The provision of Filial Therapy further strengthened the effectiveness of her play therapy experience. Over the course of four months, the foster family engaged in psychoeducation and Filial Therapy in the playroom, which then transitioned into the home environment. At the generalization

Table 2.2 Post-play Therapy ChIPPA

Score Summary—Post Play Therapy	Raw Score	Standard Score	
PEPA Conventional (Conventional imaginative play) .	71	98.3	−0.11
PEPA Symbolic	45	90.99	−0.63
PEPA Combined (PEPA conventional = PEPA symbolic) .	116	92.5	−0.5
Number of Object substitutions (NOS)	0	85	Percentile
NOS Symbolic .	5	80.5	25th
NOS combined (NOS conventional = NOS Symbolic) .	5	80.5	
NIA (Conventional Imaginative play)	2	01	10th
NIA Symbolic	1		
NIA (Combined NIA conventional = NIA symbolic)	3	1	

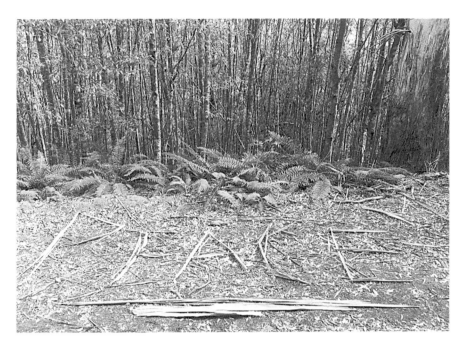

Figure 2.1 Saying goodbye and feeling at peace.

Source: Photo courtesy of author, Judi Parson.

section of the Filial Therapy, the therapist met with the family and together we walked through the treelined tracks and tossed the autumn leaves up in the air. This gave us a sense of freedom in healthy abandonment, which also marked the time as we said goodbye to each other. Saying goodbye in this place also facilitated an immersive experience in the natural world. After the family left, the therapist reflected on her own contribution to this therapeutic relationship, feeling a little sad, but also feeling calm and hopeful for Sharon. The word that came to mind was "peace" and so using the bark to spell out this word and then underlined—as sense of completion was felt (see Figure 2.1).

Conclusion

This chapter has highlighted evidence that supports integrating nature into the playroom as well as taking play therapy into the outdoors to provide immersive experiences in nature. Play therapists may incorporate the biophilic benefits of nature and may choose to incorporate biophilic designs into their indoor play therapy rooms. It is hoped that Sharon's story provides some guidance for play therapists wishing to utilize nature play therapy in their own practice. This case study has showcased how nature play therapy may move in and out of the traditional playroom, into the secret garden, cow paddock, and chook pen. Sharon and her therapist certainly shared a strong therapeutic relationship, with the experience of a unique integrative play therapy approach, ending with a therapeutic walk in the park.

Reflective questions and activities

1   When do you think that the sensory experience of integrating edible paints into the play experience could be useful?
2   How do you help the children treasure memories by using natural objects?
3   Walk outside and create your own nature mandala and reflect on the experience.
4   Next time you find yourself in a treelined track, use the leaves to create a word message for the next person to walk past.

Appendix A

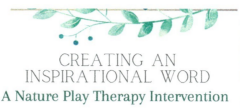

CREATING AN
INSPIRATIONAL WORD
A Nature Play Therapy Intervention

Judi Parson and Megan Ellard

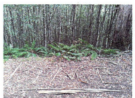

DESCRIPTION:

As you walk through nature, it can be easy at times to feel as though you are the only person in the world. By leaving a word or message on the ground, you leave inspiration for whoever next enters this space, as well as building a sense of connection with others.

SUPPLIES:

Rocks, bark, leaves, sticks, shells, flowers and/or other nature items that can be used to create words.

GOAL:
Leaving an inspirational word for others to find.

INSTRUCTIONS:
- Gather nature items such as rocks, bark, sticks and leaves and place them together in a pile.
- Choose a word or words you would like to write using the items, some suggestions are peace, kindness, love, flow, notice, found, inspire.
- Use the items you have gathered to create the word or words. If anyone walks by, you might like to invite them to create their own word, or you could leave extra items you gathered nearby so that others may later make their own word.
- Leave your word/message for anyone else who happens upon it to be inspired by.

EXTRA FUN:
As an alternative, you could meditate or engage in a visualization prior to creating your word, to find a word that speaks to you in that moment.

References

Arksey, H. & O'Malley, L. (2005). Scoping studies: Towards a methodological framework. *International Journal of Social Research Methodology*, 8(1), 19–32.

Axline, V. M. (1974). *Play Therapy*. Ballantine Books.

Berger, R. (2008b). Going on a journey: A case study of nature therapy with children with a learning difficulty. *Emotional & Behavioural Difficulties*, 13(4), 315–326. https://doi.org/10.1080/13632750802440361

Berger, R., & Lahad, M. (2010). A safe place: Ways in which nature, play and creativity can help children cope with stress and crisis - establishing the kindergarten as a safe haven where children can develop resiliency. *Early Child Development & Care*, 180(7), 889.

Berger, R., & McLeod, J. (2006). Incorporating nature into therapy: A framework for practice. *Journal of Systemic Therapies*, 25, 80–94.

Bratton, S. C., & Ray, D. (2002). Humanistic play therapy. In D. J. Cain (Ed.), Humanistic psychotherapies: Handbook of research and practice (pp. 369–402). American Psychological Association. https://doi.org/10.1037/10439-012

Bower, C., & Elliott, E. J. (2016). On behalf of the Steering Group. Report to the Australian Government Department of Health: *Australian Guide to the Diagnosis of Fetal Alcohol Spectrum Disorder (FASD)*. https://www.fasdhub.org.au/siteassets/pdfs/australian-guide-to-diagnosis-of-fasd_all-appendices.pdf

Chown, A. (2014). *Play Therapy in the Outdoors: Taking Play Therapy Out of the Playroom and into Natural Environments*. Jessica Kingsley Publishers.

Chown, A. (2018). *A Practical Guide to Play Therapy in the Outdoors: Working in Nature*. Routledge.

Cochran, N. H., Nordling, W. J., & Cochran, J. L. (2010). *Child-Centered Play Therapy: A Practical Guide to Developing Therapeutic Relationships with Children: A Practical Guide to Developing Therapeutic Relationships with Children*. John Wiley & Sons.

Drewes, A. A., & Schaefer, C. E. (Eds.). (2016). Play therapy in middle childhood. American Psychological Association. https://doi.org/10.1037/14776-000

Ellard, M. & Parson, J. A. (2021). Playing in the field: Scoping the therapeutic powers of play for nature play therapy. *British Journal of Play Therapy*, 15, 62–84.

Fearn, M. (2014). Working therapeutically with groups in the outdoors: A natural space for healing. In E. Prendiville & J. Howard (Eds.), *Play Therapy Today: Contemporary Practice with Individuals, Groups and Parents* (pp. 113–129). Routledge.

Fearn, M. (2021). Integrating the Therapeutic powers of play in nature-based settings. In E. Prendiville & J. A. Parson. (Eds.), *Clinical Applications of the Therapeutic Powers of Play: Case Studies in Child and Adolescent Psychotherapy* (pp. 46–55). Routledge.

Fromm, E. (1964). *The Heart of Man: Its Genius for Good and Evil*. Harper & Row.

Gill, T. (2014). The benefits of children's engagement with nature: A systematic literature review. *Children, Youth and Environments*, 24(2), 10–34. Retrieved 5/2/2021 from: http://www.jstor.org/action/showPublication?journalCode=chilyouteniv

Hagan, J. F., Balachova, T., Bertrand, J., Chasnoff, I., Dang, E., Fernandez-Baca, D., Kable, J., Kosofsky, B., Senturias, Y. N., Singh, N., Sloane, M., Weitzman, C., & Zubler, J. (2016). *On Behalf of Neurobehavioral Disorder Associated with Prenatal Alcohol Exposure Workgroup*. Elk Grove: IL: American Academy of Pediatrics. Neurobehavioral disorder associated with prenatal alcohol exposure. Pediatrics. September 27. https://doi.org/10.1542/peds.2015-1553

Hanscom. J. A. (2016). *Balanced and Barefoot: How Unrestricted Outdoor Play Makes for Strong, Confident, and Capable Children*. New Harbinger Publications.

International Living Future Institute™ (2018). *Biophilic Design Guidebook*. Retrieved 5/1/2021 from: https://living-future.org/wp-content/uploads/2018/06/18–0605_Biophilic-Design-Guidebook.pdf

Kable, J. A., O'Connor, M. J., Olson, H. C., Paley, B., Mattson, S. N., Anderson, S. M., & Riley, E. P. (2016). Neurobehavioral disorder associated with prenatal alcohol exposure (ND-PAE): Proposed DSM-5 Diagnosis. *Child Psychiatry Human Development*. Apr, 47(2), 335–346. https://doi.org/10.1007/s10578-015-0566-7.

Kellogg, R. (1970). *Analysing Children's Art*. National Press.

Liles, E. E., & Packman, J. (2009). Play therapy for children with fetal alcohol syndrome. *International Journal of Play Therapy*, 18(2), 192–206. https://doi.org/10.1037/a0015664

Meador, B. D., & Rogers, C. R. (1973). Client-centred therapey. In R. Corsini (Ed.), *Current Psychotherapies* (pp. 119–165). Peacock Publishers.

Parson, J., Stagnitti, K., Dooley. B., & Renshaw, K. (2020). Playability: Observing, engaging, and sequencing play skills for very young children. In Janet Courtney (Ed.), *Infant Play Therapy: Foundations, Models, Programs, and Practice*. Routledge.

Ray, D. C., & Jayne, K. M. (2016). Humanistic psychotherapy with children. In *Humanistic Psychotherapies: Handbook of Research and Practice* (2nd ed., pp. 387–417). American Psychological Association. https://doi-org.ezproxy-b.deakin.edu.au/10.1037/14775-013

Sarah, B., Parson, J., Renshaw, K., & Stagnitti, K. (2020). Can children's play themes be assessed to inform play therapy practice. *Clinical Child Psychology and Psychiatry*, 1–11. https://doi.org/10.1177/1359104520964510

Stagnitti, K. (1998). *Learn to play: A practical program to develop a child's imaginative play*. Co-ordinates Publications.

Stagnitti, K. (2007). *The child initiated pretend play assessment (ChIPPA) [kit]*. Co-ordinates Publications.

Stagnitti, K. (2021). *Learn to play therapy: Principles, process and practical activities* (2nd ed.). Learn to Play.

Sweeney, D., & Landreth, G. (2009). Child-centered play therapy. In K. O'Connor & L. Braverman (Eds.), *Play Therapy Theory and Practice: Comparing Theories and Techniques* (2nd ed., pp. 123–162). Wiley.

Van Wieren, G., & Kellert, S. R. (2013). The origins of aesthetic and spiritual values in children's experience of nature. *Journal for the Study of Religion, Nature & Culture*, 7(3), 243–264. https://doi.org/10.1558/jsrnc.v7i3.243

Wilson, E. O. (1984). *Biophilia*. Harvard University Press.

3 Creation of Safe Space for Transformation and Healing: The Chrysalis Model of Intentional Design for Healing Gardens

Angela M. Cavett

This chapter introduces the concept of creating therapeutic healing gardens. Specifically, it describes the development of four different healing gardens that were conceived at the Chrysalis Behavioral Health Services and Training Center in Fargo, North Dakota.

History of Healing Gardens

Using nature for healing is both ancient and a new approach to helping people heal. Egyptian physicians used walks in nature as part of their treatment for royalty as did physicians during biblical times (Lewis, 1976 as cited in Davis, 1998). Asclepius, the Greek God of Healing had temples built in nature, away from cities (Sternberg, 2009). European countries and the United States used gardens in the 1700s and 1800s as a safe healing environment (Davis, 1998). Nature was replaced for a time with an almost exclusive focus on the medical model. Scientific focus tended to be on factors such as medication, sterility, and technological advances in science. Sternberg noted "the hospital's physical space seemed meant to optimize care of the equipment rather than care of the patients....Hospital planning assumed that patients could adapt to the needs of technology, rather than the other way around" (pp. 3–4). This changed slightly following the publication of a scientific study of the healing quality of nature. Specifically, how well patients recovered, measured by physiological measures such as use of pain medication was impacted by access to views of nature (Ulrich, 1984). The study compared those with a view of nature compared to a standard hospital view. The results were profound in their support for the visual experience of nature in healing patients. Since that time, there has been a revived interest in the healing properties of nature.

Healing Garden: The Meaning of Relationship

There is a sacredness and depth within the gardens that needs to be experienced within a therapeutic relationship. The symbolism and design are evocative, which provides an environment pregnant with potential for processing. This is much like the profound depth seen when a patient uses the sandtray or a play therapy room. The role of the witness is necessary for the therapeutic experience. It is the "being seen" that is necessary for processing and integration.

At the heart of it all, designing and creating healing gardens are about relationship. Therapy is more than developing coping skills; it is a deeper, lived, and connected experience. The main purpose is for engagement in relationship between the patient and therapist. It becomes triadic in a healing garden with the relationship between the client, the therapist, and the garden. This can extend to family therapy with the patient and family members or group therapy with multiple patients and possibly therapeutically trained animals. A healing garden allows for connectedness and through connection that clients learn to co-regulate their emotions and process experiences.

Definitions Related to Healing Gardens

There are several definitions that will be helpful when considering creating a Healing Garden. "Horticulture Therapy is a treatment modality that uses plants and plant products to improve the social, cognitive, physical, psychological, and general health and well-being of its participants" (Simson & Straus, 1998, p. xxiii). "Horticulture therapy is a process through which plants, gardening activities, and

DOI: 10.4324/9781003152767-4

the innate closeness we all feel toward nature are used as vehicles in professionally conducted programs of therapy and rehabilitation" (Davis, 1998). Horticulture therapy has three main treatment foci: Recreational, Educational/Vocational and Therapeutic (Shapiro & Kaplan, 1998). Healing gardens are designed with therapeutic outcomes driving how the gardens are developed (Kavanagh, 1998, p. 296). Healing Gardens are a place designed to facilitate healing either actively or passively. An Enabling Garden is defined by the benefit of the therapeutic relationship in the context of a shared activity between the therapist and the client (Marcus & Sachs, 2014, p. 3). Therapists may use a directive or nondirective approach with children, adolescents, and families when utilizing these spaces. The environment is also healing in and of itself. This can be achieved by being intentional with each step of developing the gardens according to the purposes for which they are designed.

Practical Matters Related to Development of the Chrysalis Healing Gardens

A factor to consider is the size of the space. Chrysalis has two large lots with enough space for four garden rooms. The direction of the garden matters. The garden space that was found was on the south and east of the building, which provides protection from wind and excessive snow while allowing for adequate light. A six-foot privacy fence was put in around the gardens and to divide the four distinct "rooms." Electricity was put into each of the gardens for water features.

Beginners Mind is a Buddhist concept often taught in therapy along with mindfulness. Beginners Mind was and continues to be an important concept to creating the Healing Gardens. Professionals have been instrumental in the growing knowledge base needed to continue the evolving process of creating healing gardens. During the course of development, a horticultural and a general architect, a horticulture professor, master gardeners, labyrinth creators, and a county extension horticulturalist were all helpful sources of knowledge. The information shared can range from what parasitic threats were developing for fruit in a particular region to the measurements required for accessibility.

The type of soil that is present is an important factor for a healing garden. Consultation with professionals about the soil, zones, and climate can save time and help with planning. A balance of sunny and shady areas allows clients to find comfort on different days at different temperatures and based on personal needs and preferences. Seating is offered in each area with variation for contemplation alone to dyadic seating in a swing for a couple or a parent and a child. Many benches are mobile to allow for changes as the needs of those using the garden change. They are often in groups of two so the therapist can join in or easily move a bench from a different area to the distance appropriate for the work that is being done. Some of the seating is covered completely, such as the Hugglepods, some partially such as a dyadic swing and some are not covered.

Boundaries of Healing Gardens

Healing Gardens can be developed to facilitate outpatient therapy at a private clinic. Therapists could reserve the gardens for certain time periods during times in which they have a client scheduled. Therapeutic goals could be structured and met in a particular garden. Gardens would not be available for people to use outside of therapy unless a particular tour was scheduled outside of therapy times. This would allow the gardens to be used solely for therapeutic purposes, protecting confidentiality of the clients served. Being closed to the general public also allows for therapist and client safety. Many children and adults seen in therapy have trauma histories. Knowing that the Healing Gardens cannot be accessed by those other than therapists and those who accompany them is a necessary part of therapy. Boundaries also allow for safety for the public.

Overall Symbolism in the Healing Gardens

Throughout all four Healing Gardens, symbols such as a birdhouse can represent connection to birds throughout their life cycle, as well as shelter for children and adults. In play therapy within the gardens, children decorate birdhouses and talk about connection with family. This is often done with children who are adopted, in/out of foster care and those with family experiences that pull for discussion of familial safety and a home. Birdfeeders are also important for both experiencing eating and being able to feed another living thing, engaging clients in reflecting on topics related to eating as it pertains to positive and negative attachment experiences.

Within the Chrysalis Healing Gardens, there are many spaces that are named after other significant people in my life. The arbors are named after Dr. David Crenshaw and Phyllis Booth. Entrances provide for the feeling of going from one space to another space. Arbors seem to mark a transition to a world of possibility. They represent the shifting to a different place where you can be in or even imagine a safe world and from that new place, new possibilities can be created. The waterfall is named after Eliana Maria Gil. Water symbolizes transitions through the life cycle including a strong connection with birth and rebirth. Water can be seen as the life source of the therapist in terms of the source of the knowledge. The shed with both directive play therapy toys and gardening tools are named after Sueann Kenney Noziska. The circular path in the Sensory and Active Garden is named after Dr. Bruce Perry. The circle represents a "spirit and the cosmos" (Nozedar, 2010, p. 12).

Ritual

Ritual is an important component of the Healing Gardens. The work of Jim Clarke (Clarke, 2011) provides a guideline for creating rituals with clients to be individualized for each person's presenting issues, history and goals. A ritual allows for "embodied language" such as releasing emotions in a way beyond words. Ritual allows for seven things. First, ritual allows for expression of acceptable emotions. Second, it allows for a welcoming of "dark" or "negative" emotions. Ritual includes an expression to others about the experience. Ritual should be performed in a meaningful place. The Healing Gardens were created intentionally to provide a meaningful place for transformation and, therefore, is an ideal place for ritual. Ritual includes symbolic expression to allow for expression beyond words. Symbol allows for an honoring of expression of experiences. Ritual also allows for "dramatic embodied action that expresses emotion" (Clarke, 2011). Finally, ritual includes the presence of a witness as articulated in the quote by Stephen Jenkinson "You need witnesses for wonder." The ritual consists of three steps (van Geneep, 1960). First, we prepare for the ritual. Next the ritual occurs. Following the ritual, the person needs to be able to integrate the purpose of the transformation of ritual into the client's life.

Rituals Can Be Created for Any Number of Presenting Concerns Including the Following

- Divorce
- Illness and changes
- Impending death related to illness
- Grief
- Life cycle issues
- Developmental changes
- Reconciliation, forgiveness

Four Healing Garden "Rooms"

Four Healing Garden "rooms" were created at Chrysalis with intentional purposes including, (a) the Spiritual Garden, (b) the Sensory and Active Garden, (c) the Butterfly Garden, and (d) the Social Garden. Although each has a primary purpose, they each replicate the primary purposes of the others.

Spiritual Garden

Main Elements of the Spiritual Garden: Labyrinth benches for contemplation

Who Uses the Space: The Spiritual Garden is designed for older adolescents or adults.

Symbolism and Plants in the Spiritual Garden

The Spiritual Garden has five elements, Earth, Water, Fire, Air, and Metal. There is a Contemplation Bench that pulls for deep and solitary thought. Within the space, there are symbols of angels, crosses, and Native American directions. There are rocks, some with words and some plain. Rocks can be decorated with art supplies, without confidential information such as names being shared. These rocks can be taken or left for others. There is a cairn. This has been symbolized as a way to the next world for use after death. Cairns are often used in nature by hikers to communicate that the next people that they are on the right trail, a powerful therapeutic message. As spiritual and deeper topics processed in this space may have an element of the shadow, placing the Spiritual Garden in the darkest area of the gardens makes sense. This placement may also allow for this area to be cooler during warmer summer days. Considerations for this garden might be the fencing and sense of protection. Plants that pull for connection to spirituality might be included, such as sage and lavender.

Main Purposes of the Spiritual Garden

The Spiritual Garden includes a labyrinth. Walking the labyrinth provides a deepening of experience. It can be used across spiritual traditions and as a walking meditation. However, daily use of the labyrinth allows for a practice that facilitates slowing down and integration. An in-depth discussion of the labyrinth will follow later in the chapter. The Spiritual Garden is meant as a place of deep contemplation, prayer, and meditation. The labyrinth pulls for mindful walking. It is a space meant for being with another to witness the person's transition through grief. It is a place of rebirth and renewal.

Metaphors of the Spiritual Garden

Many of the Spiritual Garden metaphors relate to the labyrinth. The labyrinth can be seen as a metaphor for life as Mary Reynolds Thompson (2014) highlights: "Every spiritual journey is at its heart a quest for wholeness. We long to feel a part of the vast and unfolding mystery of life" (p. XIX).

Common Play Therapy or Therapy Interventions in the Spiritual Garden

* Labyrinth
* Walking Meditations
* Mindfulness Meditation yoga
* Prayer
* Rituals with symbols in the sandtray
* Contemplation
* Building compost piles
* Gathering pinecones

What Is a Labyrinth?

A labyrinth is an ancient archetype, a sacred symbol used across cultures for thousands of years. It is a type of mandala and like all mandalas the labyrinth represents wholeness.

A labyrinth is sometimes confused with a maze but they are quite different. A labyrinth has a unicursal route, meaning there is one way to the center and this same route is retraced to exit the labyrinth. Unlike a maze, in which one gets lost, in a labyrinth the walker cannot be lost and indeed many experience the labyrinth journey as being "found" and the walk as a reflection of their life's journey.

There are many reasons to use a labyrinth and for why a labyrinth can be supportive of therapeutic goals. Many have described the labyrinth as being an archetypal map for the journey taken to heal or restore. Within the labyrinth, the walker takes steps and turns that lead eventually to the center. As one walks, they are on the path to the center. This center can be of the literal labyrinth but often it is also of deeper selves or spiritual selves. Many like to walk the labyrinth when they feel stuck about an issue or for inspiration. Often as people walk, they find answers within themselves. Certain experiences such as grief/loss and illness are times when one may benefit from walking. The walking can be helpful when certain feelings are being experienced, especially when those feelings are overwhelming or creating difficulties. Often people may want to walk the labyrinth when they are sad, angry, depressed or isolated.

Walking the labyrinth allows for the experiencing of feelings that may have been blocked and for

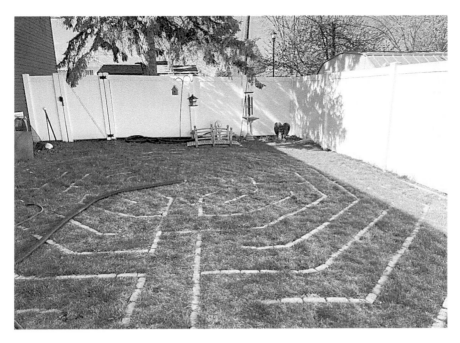

Figure 3.1 A brick labyrinth was built in the Spiritual Garden, which is used for mindfulness meditations that provides bilateral movement.

Source: Photo courtesy of author, Angela Cavett.

processing and integration of the feelings. Many feel that the labyrinth allows for deeper contemplation. This can be for prayer, meditation or for widening the range of possibilities in problem solving. Many find that during the walk, their intuition and creative problem-solving abilities are amplified. Walking the labyrinth can reduce stress. The walking typically slows their breathing, which stimulates the vagal nerve to reduce sympathetic nervous system (Sternberg, 2009). The labyrinth allows for internal focus, an opportunity to reflect on the feeling and knowing of the embodied self. The walking allows for a time focused on internal processing and reflection. Many feel that they access their inner creativity in the walking process. The labyrinth may be used therapeutically. The labyrinth is often used during times of transition such as pregnancy, marriage, divorce, menopause, job changes, after traumatic events, transitioning to college, and during periods of loss and grief. "The power to recognize, as the labyrinth shows, that in every end there is also a beginning" (Schaper & Camp, 2013, p. ix).

Therapeutically, the labyrinth might include a space for a small sandtray into which a symbol can be placed. During sandtray sessions, the therapist may suggest that the client could choose one or a few miniatures from their tray. These miniatures, symbolizing the content processed during recent sessions, might be placed in the small tray in the labyrinth. Walking the labyrinth then allows the client to focus on the miniatures and the emotional processing.

The following two vignettes provide clinical examples of how the labyrinth can be adapted to accommodate individual client needs. (See Appendix A for guidance on how to walk the Labyrinth.) (Figure 3.1).

Vignette of Markus, Age 17 years

Markus, a 17-year-old male fitting the criteria for bipolar disorder, was seen for individual therapy, which included talk, play, and art components. In session, he and his therapist had discussed the possibility of including a labyrinth walk. For a time, he had not brought up the labyrinth and neither had the therapist. At the end of a session where he had processed his feelings of hurt, isolation, and anger related to bully behaviors by peers, he asked if he could go the labyrinth for the remainder of the session.

He has been using the sandtray as he processed the bullying incident, which included behaviors by both himself and several peers. The therapist asked if he wanted to bring one of the miniatures with him to the labyrinth garden. He indicated that he wanted to bring three; a tornado, a zombie, and a mother/baby bear. When he arrived in the garden, he was reminded that there are ways one can use the labyrinth, but they are suggestions, and he can use it the way he feels he needs to. He decided to take off his shoes but did not want to wash his feet. He asked that the therapist to first walk the path to demonstrate the process.

When the therapist finished, he indicated that he wanted to walk it himself and he stepped to the sandtray within the labyrinth and placed each of the symbols. (At times people will chant, repeat a hymn, verse or saying during the labyrinth walk). He chose to walk in silence until he reached the center. When he got to the center, he indicated that he felt that his life had become like a tornado and was out of control. He indicated that at times he felt numb and that he felt he acted out with verbal aggression and mild physical aggression due to feeling a need for vengeance. The legitimacy of his anger with having many life challenges was processed and he seemed to accept that he can feel angry but also that he distances from it through a dissociative-like distancing while acting out.

Over the next several sessions, he would start with the labyrinth walk and he was able to express his anger in a safe therapeutic relationship. Over time he switched the zombie with a lion figure stating that he felt more in touch with his anger and that although he realized the anger was legitimate, he also knew he must not express it in ways that were damaging to others. He processed his feelings about the mother bear and cub figure and how he felt it reminded him of his relationship with his grandmother who protected and nurtured him. Over several sessions, he began to verbalize his thoughts at the beginning of the walk. He would place his miniatures in the sandtray, and often did it with silence or a mantra such as, "My anger can protect me, and I can show it without damaging others." The labyrinth sessions helped Marcus to find closure about the bullying.

Vignette of Sarah, Adoptive Mother

Sarah is a 34-year-old adoptive mother. Her daughter, Samantha, is the identified client with two sessions per week—one with Sarah and Samantha and the second with Sarah alone to process parenting a child with attachment concerns. Sarah had been given information about the Healing Gardens and what each could be used for in sessions. Sarah took off her shoes and washed her feet in preparation for her labyrinth walk. She asked to walk alone with a supportive witnessing by the therapist. She walked in silence. When she reached the center, she sighed and sat on the ground, wiggling her toes and focusing on her breath. When thoughts entered her mind, she allowed them to pass and to refocus on the breath. After a few minutes, she resumed her walk by following the path back out. When she exited the labyrinth and processed her experience, she reported a profound sense of purpose as a mother and a member of her faith.

Sensory and Active Garden

Main Elements of the Active/Sensory Garden

The Active/Sensory Garden includes the Butterfly Nursery, lilac "safe space," directive play therapy shed, rainbow garden, playground, and Sensory Garden.

Who Uses the Space: This space is used by children, adolescents, and families. It may be used with adults, especially if the Sensory Garden is needed to facilitate sensory mindfulness or while processing early experiences.

Sensory Experience

Research suggests that nature is beneficial to health outcomes even if the exposure is limited or uni-sensory, such as pictures of nature (Friedman & Kahn, 2004). However, there seems to be preliminary evidence that the "more" real the natural experience the more beneficial. There is improvement even with pictures of nature but increasing benefit the more realistic the exposure: "While pictures of nature are an important component of the environment of care, they cannot be a substitute for real nature views and therapeutic gardens" (Marcus & Sachs, 2014, p. 17). The neuroscientist Esther Sternberg suggests that part of nature's benefit is derived from the multitude of simultaneous positive sensory experiences (Sternberg, 2009).

The colors in each of the gardens was considered. Color can impact mood. Mood seems to respond to the wavelengths and intensity of light (Sternberg, 2009). Blue tends to calm people while reds and yellows stimulate. Not only colors but also light itself has healing property that is felt when using the healing gardens. "Besides lifting moods and changing stress hormones, full-spectrum sunlight can also change the heart rhythm of people with SAD—not the heart rate, but rather the time intervals between beats" (pp. 48). Studies of light in the hospital rooms of patients with depression show that those with sunnier rooms had shorter lengths of stay (Sternberg, 2009).

Sounds, including music, are known to impact mood. Smells impact mood. The aromas of certain plants have had healing properties known to people for thousands of years. Sternberg (2009) suggests that the oils that King David mentions in Psalms were likely referencing the healing and sacred properties of oils of such plants as chamomile, sandalwood, lavender, and geranium. Aromatherapies are the current therapies using scent to heal. Mood and sleep have been found to be changed through smell (2009). Smells are evocative of memories. The smells associated with traumas as well as connected to memory of safety and connection hold power in the healing process. Within the gardens of Chrysalis, medicinal plants are not used directly to "heal" patients but their presence has an evocative in their ancient pull towards healing.

To touch the ground allows for a powerful experience of grounding. Holding or digging in the soil while planting, weeding or playing in the mud, allows the person to experience touch. Not only is the sense of touch healing, the soil itself contains healing microbes. Studies of rats have shown that exposure to soil and the bacteria, mycobacterium vaccae, increases serotonin. The neurotransmitter serotonin is known to decrease depressive symptoms and improve cognitive functioning (Matthews & Jenks, 2010; Lowry et al., 2007).

The Active/Sensory Garden has a Butterfly Nursery. This space is filled with milkweed, the only plant eaten by Monarch larvae, caterpillars. This area provides living containment and safe space to children. It is created by lilacs and mock orange and has many evocative animal figures. Many of the animals including the turtles had tribal significance for families seen in this region. For many, the turtle often represents hiding and finding protection. There are also myths related to the turtle's body representing the world and the legs the four directions or four elements. Owls represent the Goddess of Wisdom and knowledge. The deer in the space are evocative in that they depict a vulnerable fawn and a protective doe. In mythology, the deer symbolizes the Hunter Goddess, fertility, and the Goddess of Learning. Foxes are included in this area and in mythology are often associated with deceitfulness and tricksters including the devil. Foxes are also associated with fertility. Lilacs are often evocative of early experiences for children in this region as they are grown on most farmsteads in the region. They were planted to symbolize grief from miscarriage or infant death. Their sweet, pleasant smell holds olfactory connections to many early experiences and those of the people who came before us. They were used to work through the struggles that are common across the generations. Mock orange symbolizes deceit. There is also a Rainbow Garden with several pots of each color of the rainbow. The Rainbow Garden is an extension of the Sensory Garden and contains sensory plants that allow for access to those who may be able to use the sidewalk but not walk on the pavers.

Plants in the Sensory and Active Gardens

There are numerous plants in the Active and Sensory Garden. The following is a partial list including, lilac, mock orange, rosemary, zinnias, echinacea, balloon flowers, pig squeak, grasses, strawberries, elderberries, raspberries, blueberries, tomatoes, dill, oregano, basil, mint, chamomile, succulents, lamb's ear, sage, thyme, roses, allium, mums, succulents, and cacti (Figure 3.2).

An Example of Metaphor in the Active/Sensory Gardens

After one client assisted in planting bulbs, they found that there was no shoot coming up. Digging into the soil it became evident that the bulb had been planted upside down. A sprout was growing

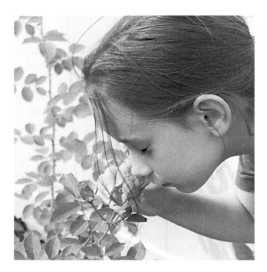

Figure 3.2 The Active and Sensory Garden provides opportunities for all senses, including tactile, auditory, visual, olfactory, gustatory, neuroception, interoception, proprioception, and vestibular.

Source: Photo courtesy of author, Angela Cavett.

slightly down but then turned up and grew towards the sun. It had to flip and reverse its direction, looking crooked and pale. To an observer it may have looked weaker and sick, but in truth, it was the strongest survivor amongst all of the new shoots. What a beautiful metaphor for personal growth in spite of trauma.

Main Purposes of the Active/Sensory Gardens

This area can provide a safe and natural space for the client to find rootedness and perform grounding exercises. The activities of gardening can provide outlets for anger, frustration, and sadness. The Active/Sensory Gardens provide connection to the life cycle during therapeutic experiences, such as grieving. The Active/Sensory Gardens allow clients to notice themselves providing nurturance not only for themselves but for other living beings. Being in the Healing Gardens allows for an active use of the body in the therapy, deepening interoception. This use of the body in the garden allows for embodied work in the therapeutic relationship. The Active/Sensory Gardens can allow for joy and pleasure within the dyad of the parent and child in therapy or with the client and therapist within a natural space of refuge and safety.

These Gardens can be used therapeutically to assist clients to express and process difficult emotions. When angry, a client might be encouraged to dig or push a heavy wheelbarrow full of plant materials or soil. When needing a mindful, repetitive task, another client might be directed to help weed. As a child assesses the need of each individual plant for hand watering, there may be direct or unspoken processing of the matching of "watering" one's own needs. Sweeping sidewalks might be done while discussing cleansing of the self from past hurts and experiences. These actions often happen simultaneously without directives by the therapist. It is as if the process is necessary, and the client needs an environment to allow for it and a therapist to bear witness to it.

The Sensory Garden brings to present awareness, self in relation to the environment. Mindfulness is about being in the present moment and the Sensory Garden allows for this optimally—through real-time engagement. It is not a place for observation with distance. Instead, it allows for immersion into the garden with the full self. The experience in the Sensory Garden allows the here-now experience that is sought in mindfulness meditations. Scripts or recordings for sensory mindfulness are commonly used in therapy but can be limited. The Sensory Garden is optimal for mindfulness. The following quote by Erwine describes how the fully lived sensory experience differs from one of only visual stimuli.

As Western culture has become a culture of the eye, the separation this creates between observer and that which is observed has contributed to the culture of the "I." As we stand back to see, we also remove ourselves from the world, and this taints our perspective of our place in it. We see ourselves, as users or stewards, not as fully immersed and active participants. This action disembodies us—from our own bodies and from the body of this living, changing planet. It emphasizes the distance from the cool, rational mind, not the messy interaction of the body immersed in place. Full sensory space, on the other hand, is an embodied place, a place of dwelling. Benedikt examines between vision-centric "exteriorist" design, which places us as observers outside the space, and sensory-rich "interiorism" which places us within an enveloping spatial experience.

(Erwine, 2017, p. 16)

The same could apply to the simple auditory mindfulness meditations often used in therapy. Other senses including proprioception, neuroception, and interoception are also considered in the Sensory Garden. The sensory garden space allows for this fully lived, "interiorism."

The Sensory Garden brings to present awareness, self in relation to the environment. The olfactory sense is stimulated by plants, including monarda, rosemary, lilac, thyme, sage, roses, allium, sage, and mints. One can smell the sweet smell of roses. Most enjoy the smell of the rose and breathe deeply and fully in a manner that enhances parasympathetic arousal of the nervous system. Smell evokes strong memories. The smell of produce such as tomatoes or onions can bring memories of earlier experiences. The visual sense is stimulated by each plant in the garden, including the lilies, zinnias, and echinacea. The auditory sense is stimulated by windchimes, grasses of different densities and heights, balloon flower, pig squeak, and musical instruments, including the drums, gong, and chimes. There are different things to walk on that make noise, including crunchy pebbles and bigger rocks. Rain and wind, insects and birds all contribute to the sounds of the garden. The visual sense is stimulated by fruits including raspberries, strawberries, elderberries, and blueberries as well as herbs, including dill, oregano, basil, mints, and chamomile. The sense of touch is stimulated by moss, succulents, lamb's ear, cacti, rocks, dirt, mud and pebbles, grass and moss, wind, snow, and rain. Rose petals and thorns are present for touch.

Within the gardens there are many plants that are connected to age-old healing or medicinal plants. Sage and sweetgrass are grown and Native American clients have used it to make smudge sticks. With most, they are present but not consumed. For instance, catmint can be helpful with menstruation and while it is present, it is not prescribed. Although it may be noted when directly impacting our clients, the process is not done or prescribed by therapists. What the presence of healing plants does allow, however, is the deep connection to our abilities to heal and be healed in communities with the wise and traditional methods of healing. Although not prescribed and used medicinally, there are edibles that are consumed. Herbs are used from the sensory garden in the Connections Kitchen, a therapeutic kitchen. Sage may be used by Native American clients for smudging. The fruits, such as apples, blueberries, raspberries, and strawberries, are mindfully tasted.

There are small rocks and art supplies for children to write on. They can write messages to others; words of hope and encouragement. They can write words or inspirational messages to themselves. Rocks hold great meaning across cultures as symbols of grounding. We have rocks that have meaning in traditions such as Wicca and rocks are considered a symbol of the power of God. For instance, children have stood on the larger rocks singing "He is my rock" in reference to Christ. "Lame Deer, the Sioux medicine man, said, "Every man needs a stone to help him…Deep inside you there must be an awareness of the rock power, of the spirits in them, otherwise you would not pick them up and fondle them as you do" (Table 3.1).

Butterfly Garden

Main Elements of the Butterfly Garden: Garden enclosed by plants, Arbor into the garden, Patio with rocking benches.

Who Uses the Space: The Butterfly Garden is a space that was initially conceptualized as a children's garden. However, as it was being created it had an energy that seemed to call for adult conversation in dyads or triads.

Table 3.1 Common Play Therapy Interventions in the Active and Sensory Garden

Active play	Hide and seek or seeking safety in the safe space	Directive play interventions such as feelings hopscotch or coping skills connect four	Repotting plants	Arranging flowers
Flower drying	Building and decorating birdhouses	Building and decorating birdfeeders	Growing herbs for the Connections Kitchen	Harvesting
Taking cuttings from annuals	Making sachets	Weaving nature art	Creating nature mandalas	Walking labyrinth

Symbolism in the Butterfly Garden

The space holds symbolism such as lilacs, which have been used by farm wives in the Midwest grieving a miscarriage or death of an infant. There is an open bird cage to symbolize freedom from abuse. A waterfall symbolizes renewal as does the insect the garden is named after. This space was created as an enclosed space. When the shrubs grow in the next few years, there will be a living barrier between the outside world and the small and intimate rocking benches that sit on the small patio, which is surrounded by plants that attract pollinators. In this space, there is a felt-sense of safety, connectedness to the other, and interpersonal transformation. The curving path in the Butterfly Garden is similar to the curving paths of ancient times that were thought to be preferable since evil could not follow them as easily as a straight one. The five elements; water, fire, air, earth and metal are all represented. There is a cairn, which may represent the flight to the heavens after death. It is also representative of stones piled along nature trails to let fellow hikers know they are on the right path.

The plants in the Butterfly Garden were selected for their attractiveness to pollinators. The plants of the Butterfly garden include many which many cultures have found symbolic or medicinal. The lilac represents grief due to miscarriage or death of a young child. Rosemary represents remembrance. Dill represents luck. The iris presents hope and faith. Lavender represents longevity and sage wisdom. Though far from an exhaustive list of the plants in the Butterfly Garden, the reader is pointed to literature related to the meaning and medicinal properties of plants in their zones (Figure 3.3).

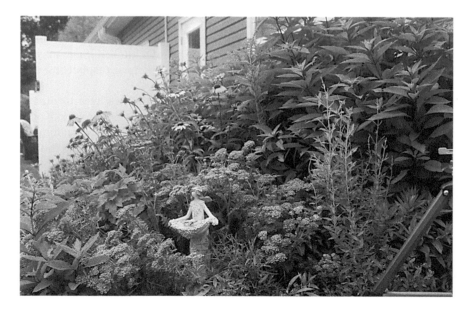

Figure 3.3 The Butterfly Garden has rocking benches surrounded by plants loved by pollinators, including Joe Pye Weed and Echinacea.

Source: Photo courtesy of author, Angela Cavett.

Purposes of the Butterfly Garden

The Butterfly Garden is a sacred place ideal for intimate conversations of passion and loss, intimacy, and desperation. It is a space created to process birth and death and the relationships that come between.

Plants in the Butterfly Garden

Recommended plants in the Butterfly Garden may include the following: echinacea, roses, sage, thyme, sedum, lavender, lilacs, rosemary, dill, salvia, mums, butterfly weed, allium, phlox, aster, geranium, Joe Pye weed, Russian sage, bee balm, hydrangea, and honeysuckle.

Metaphors in Butterfly Gardens

Constant nurturing is needed for these plants and bushes. Healing metaphors might focus on clients being attentive and giving just what is needed to each plant. Each individual type of plant has their own needs. Clients learn that they cannot grow a shade plant as if it is a plant meant for full sun; and that a particular plant needs more of an acidic or more alkaline soil. Sunshine, water, wind, and earth—all of these elements must be present in balance for the healthy plant (or person) to flourish.

Common Play Therapy or Therapy Interventions in Butterfly Gardens

• Dyadic or triadic processing of life cycle issues and challenges

Social Garden

Main Elements of the Social Garden: Fruit plants, circular seating area with fire, flower beds, and space for animals

Who Uses the Space: The Social Garden is intended for group therapy, family therapy, or animal-assisted play therapy. It was created to allow for seating for 12 in comfortable furniture. There are comfortable rocking chairs and loveseats (Figure 3.4).

Symbolism Including Plants in the Social Garden

This space includes two apple trees, named "Idunna" and "Isis" as well as blueberries. One of the apple trees was named "Isis" who was an Egyptian Mother Goddess (Nozedar, 2010). Mythology teaches that she taught men to heal and women to do tasks such as weaving. Idunna was a Norse Goddess of apples, spring, and rejuvenation. Gardens are intended for physiological and emotional nurturance and feeding. For instance, planting and providing blueberries can symbolize optimism and hope for the future. Possibly including Black-eyed Susans might represent encouragement and motivation. This space could also be designed for Animal Assisted Play Therapy or other therapeutic animal-assisted therapies. Room to run and play in these gardens would be optimal. Social Gardens could also include a large gong. Gongs have long been a symbol of transition and accomplishment. The gong can be used as a celebratory ritual for when clients meet their treatment goals. Providing fire symbols in the form of a hearth or fire pit in this space may represent connection and community, as well as destruction, transformation, and rebirth (Figure 3.5).

Purpose of the Social Garden

The primary purposes of the Social Garden are to have a place for relationships between humans, animals, and plants. This space allows for easy and comfortable connection to others. The intent is for this space to facilitate healing of the body, mind, and soul through social connection and support.

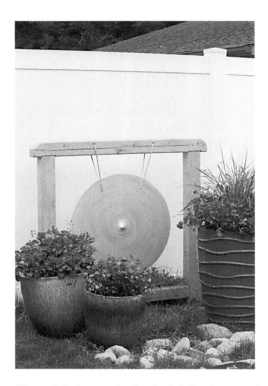

Figure 3.4 A gong in the Social Garden may be used to start and end meditation or rung after meeting a treatment goal.

Source: Photo courtesy of author, Angela Cavett.

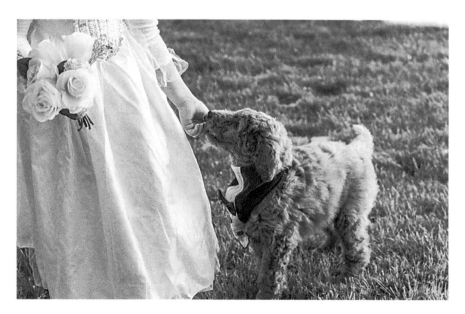

Figure 3.5 The Social Garden can be used for animal-assisted therapy.

Source: Photo courtesy of author, Angela Cavett.

Creation of Healing Gardens Summary

Healing Gardens were historically used and are currently becoming more common. The Healing Garden allows for relationship with nature and plants as well as the therapist–client. That relationship is the healing agent. Creating Healing Gardens must be intentional with the purpose guiding the process. If space allows, one may create different spaces or separate gardens for different purposes. Among the purposes, one may consider representing are spirituality, labyrinths, mindfulness spaces, including sensory mindfulness or walking meditation space, secluded areas or group spaces, and areas for active play. Practical issues such as soil types, size of the space, and climate must be considered. Often the planning requires consultation with experts across a range of disciplines from architects specializing in healing gardens, horticulturalists, and master gardeners. Choosing symbols can depend upon the clinical population one sees. Metaphors seem abundant in the gardens.

Reflective Questions

Taking on the role of the therapist, practice with a partner how you would engage the following:

A. Introduce and describe each garden's purpose.
B. Engage with the garden materials in each garden to enhance treatment goals.
C. Structure or help the parent set structure to help the client feel safe in the relationship.
D. Provide challenge within the garden to promote positive growth.
E. Enhance play/creativity in each garden to assist in therapeutic growth.

Appendix A

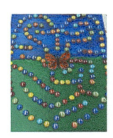

THE LABYRINTH JOURNEY

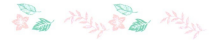

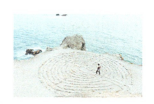

A Nature Play Therapy Intervention
Angela M. Cavett, PhD, RPT-S

DESCRIPTION:

This intervention invites the meditative practice of walking a labyrinth to reflect upon the journey inward. There is an added sandtray processing experience in the center of the labyrinth.

SUPPLIES NEEDED:

A labyrinth can be located or created.
A small sandtray and miniatures can be included.

GOAL:

To feel guidance during the walk, or a sense of purpose or new understanding as well as emotional processing.

INSTRUCTIONS:

First, a walking labyrinth can be located or created either indoors or outside. Then one prepares for the walk by clearing the mind and focusing on the breath. Socks and shoes can be removed as part of this process, and feet may be washed as a symbolic ritual of "letting go." The labyrinth at Chrysalis is built with bricks into the earth to allow for a breathtaking grounding experience and the walking of the labyrinth becomes a meditative process. Once the center is reached, a pause can ensue to reflect upon the journey inward. The labyrinth at Chrysalis contains a space built into it to hold a small sandtray into which an image or miniature can be placed to symbolize the journey and the content processed.

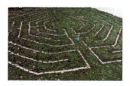

EXTRA MINDFULNESS:

One may focus on a prayer or mantra to enhance the walking mindfulness. CBT mantras such as "I am enough" or "I am filled with strength and courage" can be stated by the client while walking the labyrinth.

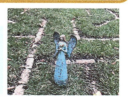

References

Clarke, J. (2011). *Creating rituals: A new way of healing for everyday life.* New York: Paulist Press.

Davis, S. (1998). Development of the professional of horticulture therapy. In: *Horticulture as therapy: Principles and practice.* Simson, S. P. & Straus, M.C. Eds. Boca Raton, FL: Taylor & Francis Group. pp. 3–20.

Deer, John (Fire) L. & Erdoes, R. (1972). *Lame Deer: Seeker of visions.* New York: Simon and Schuster. p. 113.

Erwine, Barbara. (2017). *Creating sensory spaces: The architecture of the invisible.* New York: Routledge.

Kavanagh, J. (1998). Outdoor space and adaptive gardening: Design, techniques, and tools. In: *Horticulture as therapy: Principles and practice.* Simson, S. P. & Straus, M.C. Eds. Boca Raton, FL: Taylor & Francis Group.

Lewis, C. (1976). Fourth annual meeting of the national council for therapy and rehabilitation through horticulture. September 6, Philadelphia, PA.

Marcus, C.C. & Sachs, N.A. (2014). *Therapeutic landscapes: An evidence-based approach to designing healing gardens and restorative outdoor spaces.* Hoboken, NJ: Wiley.

Matthews, D. , & Jenks, S. (2013). Ingestion of Mycobacterium vaccae decreases anxiety-related behavior and improves learning in mice. Behavioral Processes, 96. 10.1016/j.beproc.2013.02.007

Mortali, M. (2019). *Rewilding: Meditations, practices, and skills for awakening in nature.* Boulder, CO: Sounds True.

Nozedar, A. (2010). *The illustrated signs and symbols sourcebook: An A to Z compendium of over 1000 designs.* New York: Metro Books.

Shapiro, B.A. & Kaplan, M.J. (1998). Mental Illness and Horticulture Therapy Practice. In: *Horticulture as therapy: Principles and practice.* Simson, S. P. & Straus, M.C. Eds. Boca Raton, FL: Taylor & Francis Group. pp. 3–20.

Simson, S.P. & Straus, M.C. (1998). *Horticulture as therapy: Principles and practice.* Boca Raton, FL: Taylor & Francis Group, LLC.

Sternberg, E.M. (2009). *Healing spaces: The science of place and wellbeing.* Cambridge: Harvard University Press.

Thompson, M.R. (2014). Reclaiming the Wild Soul: How Earth's Landscapes Restore us to Wholeness. Wild Roots Press.

Ulrich, R.S. (1984). View through a window may influence recovery from surgery. *Science. 224,* 420–421.

PART II
Cultural Considerations

4 Let's Go Outside: Nature-Based Play Therapy Through the Lens of Cultural Humility

Meyleen Velasquez

Introduction: The Role of Nature in Child Counseling

Whether it is setting up a makeshift tent or drawing a landscape, given the opportunity, children will find a way to play in or to recreate nature. Nature can yield a connection to our most inner wisdom. Embedded deep into our hearts is a belief and a desire to thrive and grow. It is this desire that pushes us to seek a deeper connection with nature. Research on the benefits of nature demonstrates that spending time outdoors shows a positive correlation with decreased cortisol levels, regulation of the sympathetic nervous system, and even improved school performance (Strife & Downey, 2009; Williams, 2017). However, more and more, children are growing-up in nature-starved environments with little access to fresh air, trees, dirt, or sunshine.

Many Black and Brown children grow up in communities with limited access to green spaces and do not frequently visit public recreational areas such as community parks (Strife & Downey, 2009). This knowledge is vital as therapists work to increase awareness of environmental inequalities affecting historically marginalized communities. The potential reasons for the low use of public spaces have complex structural reasons ranging from cultural differences to a lack of transportation due to the unjust distribution of public green spaces (Borunda, 2020). A vital consideration for providers to keep in mind is that depending on our backgrounds and intersectional identities, playing outdoors can mean danger, including deadly police violence or deportation fears due to racial profiling (Rowland-Shea & Doshi, 2020; Scott, 2017). This danger is a reality for many families in the United States. Knowing the barriers that different communities face is one step toward providing competent care. This chapter explores how integrating cultural humility with nature-based techniques can support healing and emotional regulation.

Theoretical Framework

Cultural Humility

In the 1980s, Dr. Tervalon and Murray Garcia conceptualized cultural humility as a framework for working with clients through an anti-oppressive lens. Cultural humility calls professionals to take responsibility for challenging barriers that lead to social injustices by exploring personal attitudes toward diversity (Fisher-Borne et al., 2015; Tervalon & Murray-Garcia, 1998). Through this practice, therapists engage in critical self-reflection of their values, biases, and beliefs. This reflection remains continuous throughout the life of clinicians, supporting awareness of implicit biases. Therapists then critique their internalized beliefs and experiences against marginalized communities' experiences, increasing awareness of privilege (Fisher-Borne et al., 2015). Thus, therapists take responsibility for obtaining knowledge of historical oppression and systemic barriers. This knowledge is vital as most mental health providers in the United States are not members of groups with histories of social exclusions (Rosen et al., 2017).

Without critical self-reflection, intellectual knowledge without lived-experience can lead well-meaning providers to unintentionally harm and oppress clients (Rosen et al., 2017). A study conducted in 2016 by Hook et al. reported that over 80% of clients from ethnic and racial minority groups had experienced at least one racial microaggression by their therapists in counseling. "Microaggressions are brief, everyday exchanges that send denigrating messages to people of color because they belong to a racial minority

DOI: 10.4324/9781003152767-6

group" (Sue et al., 2007, p. 273). These subtle and indirect messages can have lasting effects on an individual's capacity to engage and complete counseling services.

Cultural humility fully recognizes that clients are the experts of their own lives, cultures, and intersectionalities. In sessions, therapists maintain awareness of feelings and thoughts that come up as they interact with the client. For example, before encouraging an increase in age-appropriate independence, a therapist working with a Latinx immigrant family might explore their own beliefs about child-rearing, independence, and family dynamics. Although Latin America encompasses many different countries and cultures, shared value systems promote the importance of family over the individual (Ayón et al., 2015). Familismo is a cultural orientation where Latinx families cultivate a sense of respect and interdependence among their children (Ayón et al., 2015). These value systems are different from dominant narratives, which prioritize independence among family members. Without understanding culture and internalized views, a provider might mistake these socialization practices as controlling instead of a vital part of healthy family functioning. A misinterpretation of family dynamics might lead therapists to commit microaggressions or to cause other harm. For instance, without humility, therapists might undermine parents by unintentionally implying that they should adjust to the dominant culture by suggesting recommendations like changes in curfews, allowances, or unsupervised time with peers.

A critically reflective practice can help providers increase awareness of internal and systemic biases regarding "best practices" for families. Through cultural humility, therapists also learn to recognize that most interventions have a dominant culture lens that is not fully applicable to most marginalized communities. In cultural humility models, this recognition is coupled with addressing injustices and inequalities that affect populations served (Fisher-Borne et al., 2015). An example might be advocating for services for a client who is undocumented or requesting that an agency provide psychotherapeutic services in the language most comfortable to the family so that all members benefit. In the latter example, a lack of providers who speak community members' languages indicates the need for systemic change.

Anti-racist and Anti-oppressive Practice

Most academic training programs and licensure bodies have requirements regarding working with individuals from marginalized communities. The framework that many educational programs take when it comes to diversity is cultural competence (Fisher-Borne et al., 2015). Recent criticisms of cultural competence posit that pedagogically based programs do not target intrinsic values, beliefs, and implicit biases that oppress clients and harm the psychotherapeutic relationship (Rosen et al., 2017). To balance power dynamics within the counseling relationship, therapists must be willing and able to examine patterns of internalized racism and biases present in white supremacist cultures. Further, the idea of competence can lead to the erroneous belief that one can be competent in someone else's experience.

Another criticism of cultural competence regards mastery of the "other." An example is where providers from dominant groups such as white, English-speaking individuals become comfortable with members of historically marginalized groups (Fisher-Borne et al., 2015). As the human experience is diverse and filled with complexities, it is a grave mistake for clinicians to consider themselves knowledgeable of someone else's culture because they attended a workshop (Tervalon & Murray-Garcia, 1998). Each complexity forms the basis of how individuals and families navigate the world. The theory of intersectionality provides the groundwork for understanding how different compounding identities face obstacles that increase risk (Crenshaw, 1989). When working with individuals, play therapists consider how identifying factors like physical abilities, gender, race, ethnicity, or religion intersect and impact how people navigate the world. This awareness sets the stage for child therapists to consider the role of cultural humility in working with diverse populations.

Building a Collaborative Relationship

Play therapy provides children with a developmentally appropriate space to explore challenging emotional and behavioral concerns. In most play therapy models, the containment and holding space happen within the context of the child–therapist relationship and the playroom (O'Connor et al., 2016). Now, what happens when a child pushes beyond the structure of a counseling room? When the call to play outdoors catches a clinician by surprise? Moreover, how do therapists navigate ethical decision-making and privacy concerns in the face of honoring the client's needs? When a child desires to play outdoors, cultural humility can support the therapists' decision-making skills in cocreating a therapeutic environment that meets diverse needs.

Therapists recognize that children can heal, given the right environment (Harper et al., 2019). As such, the container for the therapeutic growth becomes the child–therapist relationship beyond an office's confines. The therapists' capacity to tolerate changes can foster an environment for emotional transformation for the child client (Hicks & Bien, 2008). For the therapists, tolerating difficult emotions aligns with the critical self-reflection aspect of cultural humility. As therapists step outside of their comfort zone, they become better equipped to provide the openness necessary for appropriate cultural responsiveness (Sanchez, 2020). Receptivity to children's ideas begins to balance the power dynamics present in the client–therapist relationship where the therapists can move from expert to collaborator. In this way, nature becomes a catalyst for the therapeutic powers of play in action.

Nature as a Tool for transformation

The lack of a connection with nature affects long-term relationships with the outdoors (Strife & Downey, 2009). Therefore, encouraging the integration of nature-based therapies and tools into counseling goes beyond treating symptomatology. For many communities, access to nature was purposely taken away, whether through colonization or racist practices such as redlining, which to date remain present in the lives of marginalized groups (Borunda, 2020). Redlining is a form of segregation implemented by the federal government in the 1930s. The government rated neighborhoods on a scale from A to D to determine disbursement of property loans and other housing opportunities. The outcome was that "A" rated communities, predominantly white, received support, while "D" communities, mainly Black, were excluded. These practices directly contribute to the current wealth gap and environmental injustices such as limited park access (Borunda, 2020; Kibel, 2007).

Therapists must learn to navigate complex structures, such as racism, that might affect a child's relationship with the outdoors. Following the client's lead, assessing their comfort level, and supporting interactions with the earth can provide ports-of-entry to strengthen the child's connection with nature and their well-being. Swank and Shin (2015) reported that children engaging in outdoor activities demonstrate increased empathy, positive mood, and self-esteem. Consistent exposure to the outdoors during childhood might support interactions with nature in adulthood. In a way, the physiological benefits of nature act as a coregulator for distressing emotions, potentially increasing our capacity to tolerate stress. As therapists navigate the application of nature-based therapies, it is vital to recognize that these practices and ideas have been established traditions among many historically oppressed groups. This fact is especially true for indigenous communities whose land and practices were taken through colonization (Harper et al., 2019). This statement serves as a reminder that the road to cultural humility includes an intentional and focused reflection on history.

Child-Directed Play

Child-directed, nondirective, or child-centered play therapy is a modality that centers around the client and is appropriate for most emotional and behavioral concerns (Guerney, 2001; Schaefer & Drewes, 2014). Like Carl Rogers' person-centered approach to psychotherapy, therapists in a nondirective approach serve as facilitators for growth, providing space for the child to flow and express themselves (Ray & Landreth, 2019). In sessions, the child picks toys and chooses the direction of their time together with the therapist. This freedom means that at times the child can choose to engage with the therapist; other times, they can choose to play independently. However, what remains present is the observant, nonjudgmental, and accepting provider's presence (Guerney, 2001). Guerney (2001) discussed five tenets of nondirective play therapy:

- The child guides the session.
- The therapist does not address symptoms directly.
- The child's reality is entirely accepted, with limits only appearing for physical safety.
- Treatment remains child-centered.
- The therapist commits to avoid introducing other modalities.

Creating an environment where the child can express all aspects of themselves is vital for healing. The acceptance and unconditional positive regard that the therapists provide during a nondirective session creates an environment of empathy for that child client (Wilson & Ray, 2018). Parker et al. (2020) reported that two-thirds of children in the United States had been exposed to at least one traumatic incident. Considering these numbers, mental health providers must implement interventions to assess, treat, and prevent trauma-related symptoms from worsening.

A child who witnessed domestic violence may demonstrate externalizing symptoms at school, like defiance, leading to lower grades, visits to the principal, and limited healthy relationships with peers. A child experiencing recent migration to a new country might be experiencing multiple layers of trauma, including separation from family and friends, loss of belongings, loss of the familiar, adjustment to a new language, a new home, and multiple other acculturative stressors. Although more research is needed on child-centered therapy to treat trauma, a few studies have highlighted the intervention's benefits (Parker et al., 2020). These traumatic experiences might lead to different symptomatology, including depression and behavioral concerns. A systematic review of child-directed play therapy research demonstrated a statistically significant benefit of psychopathology symptoms (Parker et al., 2020; Wilson & Ray, 2018). Parker et al. (2020) reported that the most notable improvement in the research was with externalizing behaviors or emotional dysregulation, including aggression, hostility, and tantrums. Child-directed therapy honors the belief that children are the experts in their experience.

The Therapeutic Powers of Play

Schaefer and Drewes (2014) stated that "the therapeutic powers of play refer to the specific change agents in which play initiates, facilitates, or strengthens their therapeutic effect" (p. 2). Through this lens, play is the change agent, and nature provides the vehicle for healing. The integration of cultural humility supports the client in communicating needs and leading the therapeutic play (Sanchez, 2020). The therapists' capacity to apply the therapeutic powers of play within the framework of cultural humility allows them to reflect on the full experience of a child's life beyond the presenting problem. Fostering emotional wellness is a vital change agent that helps children process and manage the difficult emotions often associated with traumatic experiences (Schaefer & Drewes, 2014). Traumatic experiences change the developing brain's architecture, impacting socio-emotional development and potentially preventing the child from internalizing a sense of safety (De Bellis & Zisk, 2014). This lack of safety can manifest in significant emotional deficits that adults frequently conceptualize as behavioral problems. Providing a space for catharsis can allow the child to express emotional pains relieving symptoms that affect functioning (Schaefer & Drewes, 2014).

It is essential to mention that diverse viewpoints on catharsis' benefits exist within the child therapy field (Schaefer & Drewes, 2014; Schaefer & Mattei, 2005; Trotter et al., 2003). Trotter et al. (2003) posited that play therapy provides a space for understanding children and their feelings where they can "experiment, learn and rehearse" prosocial behaviors (p. 120). This chapter considers that for catharsis to be effective, emotional expression needs to be coupled with an increase in cognitive consciousness and useful strategies for managing big emotions (Schaefer & Drewes, 2014). Additionally, therapists support the safety of the intervention through setting appropriate limits (i.e., toys are not for breaking), providing materials conducive to big feeling expression (i.e., foam bat for hitting, playdough/clay/balled-up paper for throwing, or egg cartons for breaking), and managing safe outdoor space (e.g., a fenced outdoor space such as a school gym when conducting nature-based interventions).

Case Study: Jose, Age Eight Years

Repeated exposure to adversity places children at risk of developing emotional and behavioral problems (Parker et al., 2020). For many children, the sole focus of interventions becomes problematic behavior without attention for the traumatic experiences. For example, aggressive behaviors tend to be the most common marker for children referred to mental health services (Wilson & Ray, 2018). When trauma is not properly addressed, symptoms tend to worsen, affecting overall functioning and continuing their impact throughout adulthood (Wilson & Ray, 2018). In the following case, we see a young Latino boy exposed to a significant number of adversities and demonstrating marked behavioral concerns.

One kind of adversity addressed in the following vignette is migration-related family separation. Every year families across Latin America, particularly from Central America, decide to migrate to the United States due to wars, violence, and extreme poverty while leaving their children under the care of family members (Conway et al., 2020). When reunited with parents in a new country, children learn to navigate the complexities in the relationship with their caregivers, interacting systems, language, and multiple messy and big feelings.

The treatment provided in the vignette involves nature-based child-directed play through the lens of cultural humility. All identifying information in the vignette presented further is adapted to protect confidentiality.

Background and Presenting Problem

Jose was an eight-year-old Honduran child brought into counseling by his mother, Ms. Hernandez. Jose had been experiencing significant behavioral troubles at school, which led to frequent visits to the principal and failing grades. Ms. Hernandez reported that she left Jose in Honduras with her brother when he was about two-years old so that she could migrate to the United States to work and send money to support him. She expressed that the decision to leave was difficult but that she is happy to be back with her son. The dyad was reunited for three months. Jose did not attend school back when he was living with his uncle and spent most of his time playing with his friends. Ms. Hernandez mentioned that Jose could not write his name, although she said that she taught him how to hold a pencil for writing correctly a few weeks prior.

Jose reported having experienced physical abuse by various family members. His statements were corroborated by Ms. Hernandez, who said that Jose arrived with multiple marks and bruises on his arms and legs. Ms. Hernandez did not see Jose during the six years of separation but was able to talk with him on the phone several times throughout the year. At intake, Ms. Hernandez worked two jobs and noted that Jose spent most of his time indoors. She described her son as playful, strong-willed, and loving. The clinician observed that the neighborhood where the family resided had limited green spaces. Jose seemed connected to his mother, as evidenced by proximity seeking and calling out to her as he played. He seemed curious about me as he would look at my direction and smile from time to time. I could sense his playful nature as he moved about his house running and playing. I wondered about the immense amount of pain and confusion he must be carrying with him daily.

Jose's Treatment Plan

The following goals were set to support Jose:

1 Build skills to cope and positively express angry feelings.
2 Process and resolve trauma-related symptoms related to past physical abuse, separation from mother, and transition away from Honduras.
3 Build skills for strengthening social-emotional functioning.

Beginning Sessions With Jose

The first sessions with Jose were challenging for me as a novice clinician. He would run around his home throughout the meeting and seemed uninterested in engaging with me. Thus, the initial appointments were mainly with his mother. The fifth session took place in the school. The administration had given me a private space to conduct sessions, something no other school had provided. That day, Jose walked very slowly with me to the office as if he wished that we were heading to another place with each step. In this session, he chose to color and rip each drawing up and throw them on the floor.

His affect was flat during most of our time, although he made eye contact a few times. As we walked back to the classroom, I noticed that his classroom faced a large recess field. Seemingly out of nowhere, Jose said, "I want to play ball," and took off running into the field. I am embarrassed to admit this, but my first thought was, "How am I ever going to get this child back in his class?" Followed by, "I hope no one sees this!" as I ran behind him, trying to catch up. Once we caught up to each other, I noticed he was

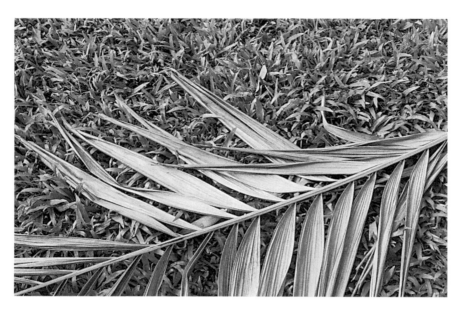

Figure 4.1 The author's cotherapist, the palm frond.
Source: 123RF, Dongli Zhang (123039692).

smiling brightly and had a sense of joy and accomplishment about him. I said to him, "You are really having fun," to which he reported, "I like to play outside." We smiled, took a deep breath after running, and I invited him to run back to the classroom.

A few sessions later, I picked him from his classroom, and he said to me, "let's go outside." I was concerned about privacy, comfort, and the Florida humidity, but I also recently learned about child-directed therapy and decided to follow his lead. We found a shaded area away from people who might hear our conversation. I sat on the grass with my play therapy materials and waited for him to choose an activity or toy. He began ripping pieces of grass off the ground and stomping on them with a mad face (Figure 4.1).

(*Excerpt from the session*)

Therapist:	You are stomping on the grass.
Jose:	(Went down on his knees, began punching the grass, then got up, ran, came back, and flopped down on the grass next to the therapist.)
Therapist:	*That was a lot you did! Then you ran back here and sat.*
Jose:	*I don't like it here.* (Began ripping pieces of grass one by one and holding them in his hand).
Therapist:	*You don't like being in school.*
Jose:	*I don't like any of this* (Referring to his adjustment to the U.S), *but I don't like it back home.*
Therapist:	*A lot happened back home.*
Jose:	(Begins kicking the ground)
Therapist:	*And things are different here.*
Jose:	*There's too many rules here, but I don't get into a lot of trouble with mom.*

The following week, I found Jose sitting at the main office as I entered the building. The guidance counselor informed me that he was throwing his pencil on the floor and would not listen to the teacher. Jose and I decided to meet outside in the field again. He was quiet, his arms crossed, and stomped as we walked. As we found our sitting place on the field, he remained quiet and began punching the ground.

Therapist:	*You are punching the ground. Seems like you had a tough day.*
Jose:	*I always get in trouble. The teacher has it out for me. Every day is something else.* (Grabbed a small rock and threw it.)

Therapist: *It's hard to be in class when we feel like we always get in trouble.*
Jose: (Got up and ran away from the therapist yelling), *"I don't like writing."* (Then he began punching and kicking the air.)
Therapist: *When we are mad, it can feel good to release it in a safe way.*
Jose: *I didn't want to write and the kids were looking at me and laughed.*
Therapist: *So you threw your pencil.*
Jose: (Grabbed a palm tree branch [palm frond] and began hitting the ground with it.)
Therapist: *You really didn't like it when the teacher asked you to write and the kids laughed*
Jose: (Made a loud noise with each banging of the frond.)
Therapist: *You are letting me know you were really mad.*
Jose: (Looked at therapist, nodded, and continued banging the palm frond.)

Subsequent Sessions

The following sessions held a similar frame. I tried to bring materials into our space that allowed a healthy expression of anger, giving Jose the space to lead our time together. In one session, he chose to hit a puppet with a stick multiple times. Thinking of his physical abuse survival, I provided reflections on how scared, sad, and mad the puppet must have been feeling. Jose repeated this for a few sessions before letting me know that the puppet was no longer in trouble. After that, our sessions involved creating houses for the puppet from pieces of stick, grass, and stones we found outside by the end of our therapeutic time together. His time in the outdoors allowed him to have full control of the session. Jose did not have many opportunities to control what happened to him throughout his life, but he learned to navigate making choices and hearing his voice acknowledged in our counseling. In the field, he could kick, run, and speak with a loud voice in a way that would have been difficult to recreate in an office environment. Jose intrinsically knew what he needed, using nature as his co-therapist.

Following our work outdoors in nature, Jose showed marked improvement in expressing his feelings in the classroom, a more positive relationship with his mother, as well as beginning to make friends. Additionally, with support from allied professionals/services, he started to understand his coursework demands.

Systems of Power and Advocacy

A culturally humble practice examines the systems of power present in a client's life. In Jose's case, several intersecting identities faced significant barriers to his well-being. He was a Person of Color, an immigrant, a child of a single parent, living in poverty, experiencing educational challenges, social-emotional concerns, and emotional and behavioral problems. His only language was Spanish, and although he received English as a Second Language (ESOL) instruction, the school was in English. As mental health professionals practicing from an anti-oppressive framework, our roles include advocating for appropriate services and intervening when injustices occur. The situations that arise when injustices take place can be difficult for therapists to navigate. When professionals from the dominant culture in leadership positions agree on unjust views against clients, it can feel impossible to voice concerns. The difficulties I experienced advocating for Jose stemmed from my identities and fears as I was an unlicensed, young, poor, brown immigrant provider navigating a new system. I was afraid of getting in trouble and compromising my job.

I noticed that nearly everyone I spoke to at the school perceived Jose as a "bad" child. During one visit, I was walking with Jose, and an individual unknown to me said, "*con el no se puede*" (roughly translating to "*this child is impossible to manage*"). I also noted that different professionals commented during meetings on Ms. Hernandez's unmarried status, her clothing, that Jose's father was not involved, and that he did not know how to write. These comments were judgmental, disrespectful, disregarded the client's needs, and spoke of their perception about their family. I found my voice through redirecting conversations and moving through my trepidation to ask, "what do you mean?" when judgmental material surfaced.

Advocacy also requires action. For me, at the time, this translated into connecting Jose and his mother with appropriate services, obtaining an evaluation from an occupational therapist, a tutor, aftercare so that his mother could work her jobs, and a full psychological evaluation to obtain an individualized educational (IEP) plan. Through cultural humility, providers learn to explore and challenge their internalized biases while also dismantling systemic barriers that oppress clients. Ultimately, Jose's mother chose to transfer him to a different school where he continued to thrive.

Therapist Reflection

A cultural humility practice entails engaging in the process of critical self-reflection. As I reflect on this case, I think about my ideas, at the time, regarding how children should behave in school, what the correct frame for counseling is, and the role of being a community-based therapist. When Jose requested meeting outdoors, my initial thoughts were regarding myself and my wellbeing. I was concerned about my comfort sitting outside. How could I justify a therapeutic intervention outdoors to the school administrators? I also remember my initial thoughts were that Jose did not want to "engage in therapy" and was defiant. These thoughts and concerns reflect my biases about his experience and internalization of the messages I gathered from other professionals working with the client.

When Jose indicated he wanted to be outside, I pathologized his request due to internalized stigmatizing messages about "oppositional behavior" instead of empathizing and recognizing that he was letting me know what he needed. As a Latina immigrant with proximity to whiteness, I also recognize that I must continuously increase awareness of implicit biases related to racism, colorism, and xenophobia. In this step, I examine messages received throughout my life regarding immigrants from other parts of Latin America. These racialized messages show up in interactions with clients from different backgrounds other than mine as implicit biases favor our ingroup (Ohio State University, 2016). An important recognition for providers to remember is that we can be members of marginalized communities and still contribute (consciously and unconsciously) to others' marginalization.

Implementing a Cultural Humility Practice

Practicing through a lens of cultural humility requires a life-long commitment to anti-racist and anti-oppressive practice. A continuous process means that practitioners approach learning and self-exploration with a sense of curiosity, recognizing that there will always be more room for knowledge and internal growth (Rosen et al., 2017). An open attitude to the idea that we do not hold all the answers prepares us to move toward humility. Humility also means that we accept that we will be wrong in our assumptions and look into the uncomfortable parts of ourselves, such as internalized racism, to limit further oppression. This section provides some reflective questions to support the reader's practice. However, as with learning any framework, best practice entails engaging in advanced training and clinical supervision with a specific lens of cultural humility with a provider of Color.

When we look to expand our knowledge of populations of which we are not a part, we need to seek supervision/consultation from members of that specific community. For example, if a cisgender therapist is looking to advance knowledge in supporting trans clients, they need to seek supervision and training from a trans provider. Practitioners may also benefit from engaging in their own psychotherapy to explore implicit biases, values, and belief systems around white supremacy, privilege, racism, and prejudices.

Questions for Reflection on Cultural Humility in Practice

- What power dynamics are present in this relationship and our interactions?
- What messages have I been exposed to regarding the client's background and experiences? How might those messages show up in the counseling space and my thoughts about the client?
- What hypothesis do I have regarding this client's experience?
- How are my hypotheses informed?
- How does the client perceive our interactions? How did I arrive at this conclusion?
- What steps can I take to help balance power dynamics in the counseling relationship?
- What are the systemic challenges present in this client's experience?
- What biases might they be facing from other providers?

- What systems do I navigate? How do I navigate them? What challenges do I experience? How do I manage those challenges? What privilege do I carry within those systems?
- What steps can I take to move systems of advocacy on behalf and in partnership with my client?

Closing Comments/Chapter Summary

Nature can be a powerful force of transformation in an individual's life. Through cultural humility, we learn to examine our interventions through our client's lens. As we engage in critical self-reflection, we explore the biases and belief systems that inform our thoughts, behaviors, and interventions (Rosen et al., 2017). In doing so, we can partner with clients recognizing that they are the experts in their experience. As a child explores nature in counseling, different emotions, experiences, and distress levels might appear. Therapists can support catharsis by providing a safe container for outdoor interactions based on child-directed principles.

Cultural humility also pushes us further than the therapeutic space, calling us to advocate for injustices and systemic oppressions present in our client's lives. In Jose's example, redirecting inappropriate conversations and connecting him to services provided powerful tools that promoted his well-being. Practicing cultural humility is a lifelong journey of learning, expanding our knowledge, and facing our biases. The more we do it, the better for our communities. Together, we can leave our world a little better than we found it. Si, se puede.

Reflective Questions

1   Reflecting on your knowledge of cultural competence, how does it differ from this chapter's representation of cultural humility?
2   Discuss with a group or colleague what you think might be possible reasons why Jose chose to play outside.
3   Reflect on a client you might be working with now or have provided services to in the past. What are some ways that you can integrate the outdoors into counseling sessions? How would you determine whether this was an appropriate course of treatment?

Appendix A

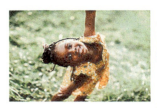

THE CULTURAL LENS

A Culturally Humble Nature-based Play Therapy Experience

Meyleen Velasquez, LCSW, RPT-S, PMH-C

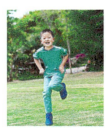

DESCRIPTION:

Cultural humility is a lifelong process that supports therapists in working with diverse populations by recognizing biases, power dynamics, and culture-specific needs in the therapist-client relationship. This framework supports therapists in integrating nature in a way that meets their client's unique needs.

RECOMMENDATIONS:

Critical self-awareness

Consultation with a BIPOC play therapist supervisor

A secure outdoor area

GOAL:

To engage in the lifelong process of cultural humility where play therapists can continuously challenge harmful belief systems and increase access to proper care while engaging in nature-based play therapy.

SELF-EXPLORATION:

- What power dynamics are present in this relationship and our interactions in this outdoor space?
- What messages have I been exposed to regarding the client's background and experiences? How might those messages show up in the counseling space and my thoughts about the client?
- What hypothesis do I have regarding this client's experience?
- How are my hypotheses informed?
- How does the client perceive our interactions? This nature-based experience? How did I arrive at this conclusion?
- What steps can I take to help balance power dynamics in the counseling relationship?
- What are the systemic challenges present in this client's experience?
- What biases might they be facing from other providers?
- What systems do I navigate? How do I navigate them? What challenges do I experience? How do I manage those challenges?
- What privilege do I carry within those systems?
- What steps can I take to move systems of advocacy on behalf and in partnership with my client?

References

Ayón, C., Williams, L. R., Marsiglia, F. F., Ayers, S., & Kiehne, E. (2015). A latent profile analysis of Latino parenting: The infusion of cultural values on family conflict. *Families in Society: The Journal of Contemporary Human Services, 96*(3), 203–210. https://doi.org/10.1606/1044-3894.2015.96.25

Borunda, A. (2020, July 29). How "nature deprived" neighborhoods impact the health of people of Color. *National Geographic.* https://www.nationalgeographic.com/science/2020/07/how-nature-deprived-neighborhoods-impact-health-people-of-color/

Conway, C. A., Roy, K., Hurtado Choque, G. A., & Lewin, A. (2020). Family separation and parent–child relationships among Latinx immigrant youth. *Journal of Latinx Psychology, 8*(4), 300–316. https://doi.org/10.1037/lat0000153

Crenshaw, K. (1989). Demarginalizing the intersection of race and sex: A Black feminist critique of anti-discrimination doctrine, feminist theory and antiracist politics. *University of Chicago Legal Forum, 1*(8), 139–167. https://chicagounbound.uchicago.edu/cgi/viewcontent.cgi?article=1052&context=uclf

De Bellis, M. D., & Zisk, A. (2014). The biological effects of childhood trauma. *Child and Adolescent Psychiatric Clinics of North America, 23*(2), 185–222. https://doi.org/10.1016/j.chc.2014.01.002

Fisher-Borne, M., Cain, J. M., & Martin, S. L. (2015). From mastery to accountability: Cultural humility as an alternative to cultural competence. *Social Work Education, 34*(2), 165–181. https://doi.org/10.1080/02615479.2014.977244

Guerney, L. (2001). Child-centered play therapy. *International Journal of Play Therapy, 10*(2), 13–31. https://doi.org/10.1037/h0089477

Harper, N. J., Rose, K., & Segal, D. (2019). *Nature-based therapy: A practitioner's guide to working with children, youth, and families.* New Society Publishing. https://amzn.to/2NtNmMd

Hick, S. T., & Bien, T. (Eds.). (2008). *Mindfulness and the therapeutic relationship.* The Guildford Press.

Hook, J. N., Farrell, J. E., Davis, D. E., DeBlaere, C., Van Tongeren, D. R., & Utsey, S. O. (2016). Cultural humility and racial microaggressions in counseling. *Journal of Counseling Psychology, 63*(3), 269–277. https://doi.org/10.1037/cou0000114

Kibel, S. P. (2007). Access to parkland: Environmental justice at East Bay Parks. *Golden Gate University School of Law.* http://digitalcommons.law.ggu.edu/eljc/2

O'Connor, K. J., Schaefer, C. E., & Braverman, L. D. (Eds). (2016). *Handbook of play therapy* (2nd ed.) John Wiley & Sons, Inc.

Ohio State University. (2016). State of the science: Implicit bias review 2016. *Kirwan Institute for the Study of Race and Ethnicity.* https://kirwaninstitute.osu.edu/research/2016-state-science-implicit-bias-review

Parker, M. M., Hergenrather, K., Smelser, Q., & Kelly, C. T. (2020). Exploring child-centered play therapy and trauma: A systematic review of literature. *International Journal of Play Therapy.* https://doi.org/10.1037/pla0000136.supp (Supplemental)

Ray, D., & Landreth, G. (2019). Child-centered play therapy. *Play Therapy, 14*(3), 18–19.

Rosen, D., McCall, J., & Goodkind, S. (2017). Teaching critical self-reflection through the lens of cultural humility: An assignment in a social work diversity course. *Social Work Education, 36*(3), 289–298. https://doi.org/10.1080/02615479.2017.1287260

Rowland-Shea, J., & Doshi, S. (2020, July 21). The nature gap: Confronting racial and economic disparities in the destruction and protection of nature in America. *American Progress.* https://www.americanprogress.org/issues/green/reports/2020/07/21/487787/the-nature-gap/

Sanchez, B. (2020). Cultural humility: A tool for social workers when working with diverse populations. *Reflections: Narratives of Professional Helping, 26*(2), 67–74.

Schaefer, C. E., & Drewes, A. A. (Eds.). (2014). *The therapeutic powers of play: 20 core agents of change* (2nd ed.). John Wiley & Sons, Inc.

Schaefer, C. E., & Mattei, D. (2005). Catharsis: Effectiveness in children's aggression. *International Journal of Play Therapy, 14*(2), 103–109. https://doi.org/10.1037/h008890

Scott, K. (2017, June 19). For children of Color playing outside is both dangerous and necessary. *HuffPost.* https://www.huffpost.com/entry/playing-outside-for-black-and-brown-kids-both-danger_b_5947e7f4e4b0940f84fe3077

Strife, S., & Downey, L. (2009). Childhood development and access to nature: A new direction for environmental inequality research. *Organization & Environment, 22*(1), 99–122. https://doi.org/10.1177/1086026609333340

Sue, D. W., Capodilupo, C. M., Torino, G. C., Bucceri, J. M., Holder, A. M. B., Nadal, K. L., & Esquilin, M. (2007). Racial microaggressions in everyday life: Implications for clinical practice. *American Psychologist, 62,* 271–286. https://doi.org/10.1037/0003-066X.62.4.271

Swank, J. M., & Shin, S. M. (2015). Nature-based child-centered play therapy: An innovative counseling approach. *International Journal of Play Therapy, 24*(3), 151–161. https://doi.org/10.1037/a0039127

Tervalon, M., & Murray-Garcia, J. (1998). Cultural humility versus cultural competence: A critical distinction in defining physician training outcomes in multicultural education. *Journal of Health Care for the Poor and Underserved, 9*(2),117–125. https://doi.org/10.1353/hpu.2010.0233

Trotter, K., Eshelman, D., & Landreth, G. (2003). A place for Bobo in play therapy. *International Journal of Play Therapy, 12*(1), 117–139. https://doi.org/10.1037/h0088875

Williams, F. (2017). The *nature fix: Why nature makes us happier, healthier, and more creative.* New York, NY: W.W. Norton & Company.

Wilson, B. J., & Ray, D. (2018). Child-centered play therapy: Aggression, empathy, and self-regulation. *Journal of Counseling & Development, 96*(4), 399–409. https://doi.org/10.1002/jcad.12222

5 Sacred Ground: The Cultural Implication of Nature-Based Therapy With Young Children and the Intersection of Culture

Harleen Hutchinson

Introduction

We live in a world in which one's race, culture, and ethnicity shape how one is viewed by society. Furthermore, society often lacks the ability to recognize the role of race in the green space movement. This lack of knowledge speak volumes regarding how society thinks, sees, and recognizes the environmental narrative of other races in the larger context. African Americans and other nondominant groups are often neglected and unrecognized as playing a significant role within the green space movement. Unfortunately, due to inequities and privileges that exist in our society, there seems to be cultural variations relating to access to green spaces. Finney (2014) contends that

> missing from the narrative is an African American perspective, a non-essentialized black environmental identity that is grounded in the legacy of African American experiences in the United States, mediated by privilege (both intellectual and material, influenced by race, gender, class, and other aspects of difference that can determine one's ability to access spaces of power and decision making), and informed by resistance to and/or acceptance of the dominant narrative. (p. 3)

Furthermore, as the educated and class gaps widen, the need to gain access narrows for racialized groups such as blacks and people of color. Historically, racism in housing practices and city planning has consistently shaped the socialization patterns in which blacks and people of color continue to reside in nature-deprived areas. As a generation of racist policies such as redlining, and neighborhood exclusion continues to perpetuate, the cycle of nature deprivation for blacks and people of color widens. According to Merchant (1989), symbols shape the experiences of African Americans and people of color, as it relates to their interaction with nature and trees. Unfortunately, the history of African Americans in green spaces is not elevated or acknowledged to solidify their experiences and narratives in mind. Finney (2014) asserts that less than 3 percent of outdoor magazines feature African Americans in advertising in green space.

Therefore, in order for African American young children to feel inclusive and embrace the outdoors, it is important that they see themselves reflected in others who look like them; in that way, they can give voice to their experience of the tragedy and triumph that they may be carrying with them through the genetic adaptation of their parents' traumatic experience to the outdoors. Therefore, relevancy, representation, triumph, tragedy, pain, and joy are emotions that one needs to acknowledge and grapple with, in order to recolor the outdoor space for African American young children and their families. It is in understanding their story and giving voice to their experiences that they are able to transform the green space movement to ensure equity and inclusion. According to Finney (2014), the trees in the woods are a reminder of the African American ancestral narratives. She further reported that in the song "Strange Fruit" by Billie Holiday, the southern tree became a symbol of violence done to black bodies which manifest as strange fruit hanging from poplar trees. Hence, legacies of internalized trauma regarding the outdoors are transmitted from the past into the present. This transgenerational adaptation is associated with past traumas of slavery, posttraumatic slave syndrome, or ongoing oppression and inequities, which often hinder African Americans' ability to interact with nature (DeGruy & Leary, 2005). Therefore, in order for true cultural transformation to occur, it is important to recognize the painful experiences of African Americans but also acknowledge how their resiliency in using the stars as their compass toward freedom during those terrifying moments in the woods provided them with the comfort

DOI: 10.4324/9781003152767-7

of the outdoors. The trauma residues of their past consistently shape their interactions to present day nature experiences, which are often transmitted to their children.

Research has consistently demonstrated the effects of a lack of nature exposure on children's psychological and behavioral functioning when they are deprived of a consistent level of environmental exposure in green spaces (Louv, 2018). When children are provided with the opportunity to be immersed in nature-based play, it stimulates a ripple effect within their five senses. This stimulation helps to form new connections in the brain, increasing skills such as curiosity, thinking, wondering, and self-regulation. When young children have time to move and play outside, they develop pathways to the brain and learn how to interpret sensory stimuli received from their environment. This allows the prefrontal cortex to integrate the information received from the outdoor environment in a higher cognitive format (Arvay, 2018; Siegel, 2012). Additionally, nature promotes self-regulation skills through activation of the parasympathetic nervous system, which allows the body to remain in a calm state. The mastering of self-regulation skills, for young children, is extremely important, especially for those who experience prematurity and suffer from reflux challenges. Therefore, it is important that children learn how to maintain a calm and alert state, to fully access the prefrontal cortex, in order to maximize their emotional, social, and cognitive potential.

Importance of Sensitivity to Culture

The needs of young children experiencing nature deficit must be addressed in the context of the family's cultural background, including practices within the child's community. When problems stem from a lack of exposure or fear of green space, these limitations not only affect the family, but also the child's psychological and social-emotional development. As we socialize young children into nature, through a socio-contextual lens, it is extremely important that we honor the family's experiences, in order to understand their narratives and help them connect the past to the present. This connection will aid in introducing children to a wide range of experiences that provides them with varied exposure to stimulate their overall sensory experience, thereby strengthening their immune system. Furthermore, when all African-American children and their families walk in diverse outdoor spaces and the diversity of nature is reflected by people who are in their green space, then will true equity and inclusion be realized. One framework that is often utilized as a tool to better understand the sociocultural and sociopolitical context of diverse culture is the Diversity Informed Tenets (Irving Harris Foundation, n.d). Here are the 10 central principles of the Diversity Informed Tenets:

1   Self-Awareness Leads to Better Services for Families
2   Champion Children's Rights Globally
3   Work to Acknowledge Privilege and Combat Discrimination
4   Recognize and Respect Non-Dominant Bodies of Knowledge
5   Honor Diverse Family Structures
6   Understand That Language Can Hurt or Heal
7   Support Families in Their Preferred Language
8   Allocate Resources to Systems Change
9   Make Space and Open Pathways
10   Advance Policy That Supports All Families

These Tenets were developed as a tool to promote full inclusion and equity in addressing the needs of all families. Its aim is to raise awareness about inequities, while deepening self-awareness and reflective capacity to create intentional action for change, to ensure equity and inclusion. The following is a case example in which nature-based intervention served as a key treatment for a preterm infant and his mother, with use of the diversity informed tenets during modes of engagement in self-observation and self-awareness to create an understanding of the lived experiences of oppression, and inequities.

Case Study: Aponi's Story: Past and Present

Aponi is a 28-year-old Kenyan Black female who loves the outdoors and would retreat to the outdoors whenever she felt stressed after a long day of work. However, after the traumatic birth of her son, Calian, around the 33 weeks of her pregnancy, Aponi's life changed. She reported that Calian was born weighing four pounds and remained in the NICU for 10 days. According to Aponi, due to challenges with her pregnancy, she was separated from Calian for five days, prior to being reunited with him. She expressed the pain she felt from not being able to hold Calian upon delivery and spoke about the separation, and grief she experienced. After Calian's was released from the hospital, she attempted to introduce the outdoors to him as a way of coping with his reflux issues and the stressors she experienced. However, she reported that during her well-baby visit, she disclosed to the social worker that she had been taking Calian outdoors to experience the calmness of nature, and reported that in her country of origin, it is not uncommon for babies to experience the outdoors after birth. The social worker became concerned and informed Aponi that, due to Calian's vulnerable state, introducing him to the outdoors was not appropriate and informed her that such practice could be considered medical neglect.

After Aponi left the clinic, she became concerned and reached out to a supportive friend, who provided her with reassurance and connected her with a culturally sensitive infant mental health clinician. Upon meeting Aponi in her home, she was very anxious and afraid of sharing her thoughts relating to the outdoors and the many challenges that she had experienced coping with Calian's issues of reflux and stress. The clinician introduced the idea of nature-based therapy as a means of coping with Calian's reflux and stressors. The clinician also explored with Aponi her cultural belief surrounding the environment and nature-based therapy. By introducing Aponi to the concept of nature-based therapy, this provided an opportunity for her and her baby to promote calm and strengthen Calian's immune system. As the clinician wondered, along with Aponi about her experiences, her fears and anxiety lessened as she began to speak more freely about the many challenges that she had experienced with Calian, such as the development of severe reflux and allergic issues after birth, which increased Aponi's fear of the outdoors.

After weeks of consulting with Aponi, to gain insights into her current emotional challenges and their connection to her cultural beliefs, the clinician began to initially integrate the use of therapeutic infant massage to help regulate Calian's reflux issues. During the course of the therapeutic massage, a holding environment was provided for Aponi to explore her fears of introducing Calian to nature, in order to help with his reflux and social-emotional challenges. Aponi shared her concerns regarding her fears of exposing Calian to the outdoors and her belief of not being "a good-enough mother."

The clinician began to provide Aponi and her 10-month-old son, Calian, with six sessions of mindfulness nature-based therapy. In each session, the clinician began with a transitional nature-based mindfulness activity to help calm and regulate Calian's emotions. During the first nature-based session, Aponi was very cautious and expressed concerns relating to her fears of being neglectful. The clinician helped Aponi to process her current fears by creating a safe holding environment to help make the cultural connection between her own cultural beliefs and her current cultural experiences in the United States. This allowed Aponi to intersect both cultures, while embracing and infusing her own cultural beliefs into the nature experience. She described her changing experiences of penalty and privilege when she emigrated from Kenya to the United States. She shared her immigration experience from a social context in which discrimination and privilege came, for no apparent reason.

As she reflected, she shared her experience and encounter of the social worker's privilege and use of power in a mindset that was defined by hierarchy and exclusion, related to the social worker's misguided belief about a specific race and culture. In practice with the Diversity-Informed Tenets, the clinician acknowledged privilege where it was held and used it strategically and responsibly to bring awareness to the fact that privilege may play a role in the therapeutic relationship. Aponi felt acknowledged, seen, and heard, and expressed her appreciation toward the clinician's authenticity in recognizing the importance of her past negative experiences and its impact on current relationships. As Aponi began to see the benefits of engaging in five minutes of daily nature-based mindfulness, the clinician and Aponi began to explore other nature-based activities that could be implemented in her back yard. While Aponi appreciated the outdoors, she had never practiced mindfulness with Calian. She indicated "I have never imagined the benefits of mindfulness Zen Yoga to have such tremendous benefits." The clinician reminded Aponi of the healing power of nature and reinforced the importance of her returning to her roots and reconnecting with nature (Figure 5.1).

"Nature inspires creativity in a child by demanding visualization and the full use of the senses" (Louv, 2018, p. 7). It is young children's deep innate connection with nature that contributes to the healing

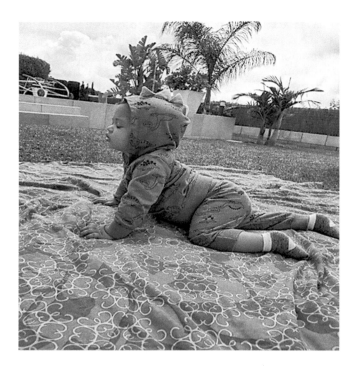

Figure 5.1 Baby Zen Yoga in the park.

Source: Photo courtesy of Harleen Hutchinson.

power of their relationship and development. Aponi became intrigued with mindfulness nature-based therapy as she witnessed Calani's resulting calmness (Roszak et al. (1995). She stated:

> It's as if my son has reclaimed this sacred earth and has become one with nature. What I am witnessing with my son is what I have experienced in my country in the great outdoors but coming to America has stifled my view of nature exposure with my baby.

Aponi's past interactions with people, in general, and those within various social constructs, reinforced reminders of distrust of mainstream institutions that did not acknowledge or understand her cultural beliefs. Although the clinician was Black, she did not belong to Aponi's Kenyan culture, nor shared the same Kenyan beliefs. The embracing and acknowledging of Aponi's racial stress reactions facilitated development of a healthy understanding within cross-racial relationships. However, the clinician's commitment to learning about the Kenyan culture, and the awareness of how sociocultural contextual factors can impact a person's sense of self, provided a vehicle to recognize and acknowledge how these intersects can affect the internalized biases we place on families when introducing them to environmental nature-based therapy with young children.

Nature-Based Mindfulness Zen Yoga: Five Minutes

Place your baby on his stomach, and position yourself on your stomach, next to your baby. Begin by breathing in, and exhaling out, as you push air out of your lungs.

Pay attention to your heart, and your senses, giving attention to the sensation of the air, the sound, and the smell of fresh air.

Continue to breathe in, and out, focusing on the sensation of the breath, your hands on the grass, and its connection to the earth.

As you continue to breathe in, focus on the energy you feel from being one with the earth. And as you breathe in, on the out breath, welcome gratitude to yourself and your baby.

Say, Mother earth, I reclaim your energy from this sacred soil to transform my mind, my spirit and my heart. Mother earth, I reclaim your energy from this sacred soil to bless my baby, calm his spirit and strengthen him.

As you breathe in, focus on the color of the grass, say thank you for sharing your presence with me and my baby, and on the outbreath, welcome kindness to you and your baby, as you come back to awareness of the breath, letting go of all your stress, you may open your eyes when you are ready.

As you transition to a standing position, feel the connection to the earth, notice how your foot feels on the ground as you embrace your baby. Focus on the rhythm of your steps, as you focus on your baby with a soft gaze.

Now continue to focus on his gaze as you whisper, thank you Mother earth for peace, blessings, health and the opportunity to share this sacred ground with you and my baby.

Reflections on the Therapeutic Process

The treatment of Aponi and her baby illustrates the importance of using a cultural lens to understand the symptoms of a mother and her baby, to reinforce the need to bridge cultural and nature-based experiences and interrupt the transmission of cultural biases related to green space treatment. The clinician blended different treatment modalities to help the mother understand how her maternal depression, and affect regulation were influencing her baby's social emotional functioning. The success of this intervention was based on the need to "promote conditions for adults to feel comfortable and motivated during the time spent outside. Adult's involvement will influence the type of experiences that children have access to and how they incorporate new knowledge" (Bento & Dias, 2017, p. 150).

Through this process, Aponi was able to witness the healing power of nature-based green space, in spite of her difficult circumstances. As treatment ended, the clinician was pleased to see that Aponi 's emotional commitment to her baby was free from contamination of cultural biases, providing hope that she can continue to embrace environmental nature space through her own cultural lens, to foster a positive green space experience for Calian. Attaining the mission of equitable access to green space for all African American young children and families demands anti-racist thinking and action. Kendi (2019) points out that we must be conscious of how race is used by white people to wield power that privileges them over people of color, especially in those unchartered territories, such as green spaces, spaces where African Americans are not recognized nor welcomed. We must recognize the dynamics of power and equity that reside in our relationships with families from diverse backgrounds in order to open authentic dialogue and build a trusting relationship that centers around equity and inclusion for all.

Reflective Questions:

1 How does understanding the cultural intersection between race and nature help guide clinical practice during the parent-child relationship?
2 How might the experience of Zen Yoga and nature play promote self-regulation of the child?
3 How might reflective supervision help a clinician to examine the thoughts and feelings that may arise due to issues of race, inequities, bias, and inclusion when providing nature-based interventions to promote the parent–child relationship? Role play with a partner a mock supervisor and supervisee session related to this question.

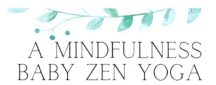

A MINDFULNESS
BABY ZEN YOGA

A Nature Play Therapy
Intervention
HARLEEN HUTCHINSON, PSY.D.

DESCRIPTION:

This activity is a guided meditation for mother and baby that helps them become calm, and be fully present with their bodies while in nature.

SUPPLIES NEEDED:

- Blanket to cover the ground to lie down upon.
- If possible, find a grassy area.

GOAL:

For parents to bring about a sense of mindfulness peace and connection to the earth and their baby.

INSTRUCTIONS:

Place your baby on their stomach and lie down next to them in the same position. Begin by breathing in and exhaling out, as you push air out of your lungs. Pay attention to your heart and your senses, giving attention to the sensation of the earth, surrounding sounds, and the smell of fresh air. Continue to breathe in, and out, focusing on the sensation of your breath, your hands touching the grass, and your connection to the earth. Focus on the energy you feel from being one with the earth and feel gratitude to yourself and your baby. Say, "Mother earth, I reclaim your energy from this sacred soil to transform my mind, my spirit and my heart. Mother earth, I reclaim your energy from this sacred soil to bless my baby, calm his spirt and strengthen him." As you breathe in, focus on the color of the grass and the surrounding area and say, "Thank you for sharing your presence with me and my baby." On the out breath, welcome kindness to you and your baby, as you come back to awareness of the breath and letting go of any unwanted stress and worry.

EXTRA FUN:

Embrace your baby in a standing position and begin to walk. Focus on the rhythm of your steps and breath in and out as you gaze and connect with your baby.
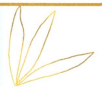

References

Arvay, C. G. (2018). *The healing code of nature: Discovering the new science of eco-psychometrics.* Boulder, CO: Sounds True Publishing.

Bento, C., & Dias, G. (2017). The importance of outdoor play for young children's healthy development. *Porto Biomedical Journal, 2*(5): 157–160. Elsevier, Espana.

DeGruy, Leary, J. (2005). *Post traumatic slave syndrome: America's legacy of enduring injury and healing.* Portland, Ore: Uptone Press.

Finney, C. (2014). *Black faces, white spaces: Reimaging the relationship of African Americans to the great outdoors.* Chapel Hill: University of North Carolina Press.

Glave, D. (2010). *Rooted in the earth: Reclaiming the African American environmental heritage.* Chicago: Lawrence Hill Books.

Irving Harris Foundation. (n.d.). Overview of the tenets. https://diversityinformedtenets.org/the-tenets/overview

Kendi, I. (2019). *How to be an antiracist.* Random House.

Louv, R. (2018). *The last child in the woods: Saving our children from nature-deficiency disorder.* Chapel Hill, NC: Algonquin Books.

Merchant, C. (1989). *Ecological revolutions: Nature, gender, and science in New England.* Chapel Hill: University of North Carolina Press.

Roszak, T., Gomes, M.E., & Kanner, A.D. (1995). *Ecopsychology restoring the earthhealing the mind.* San Francisco, CA, Sierra book club.

Siegel, D. J. (2012). *The developing mind: How relationships and the brain interact to share who we are* (2nd ed.). New York, NY: Guilford Press.

PART III

Healing Nature-Based Trauma Therapies

6 The Nature of TraumaPlay®: Incorporating Nature into the Seven Key Components

Paris Goodyear-Brown

TraumaPlay® is a flexibly sequential play therapy model for treating trauma and attachment disturbances with children, teens, and family systems. Synthesizing best practice standards and evidence-based trauma-focused therapy modalities, the seven key components of TraumaPlay® serve as an umbrella framework for trauma treatment. Ironically, the umbrella imagery embedded within the T of the TraumaPlay® logo is meant to evoke a sense of felt safety, a sense of being protected from the elements. While TraumaPlay® is an effective treatment for systems that have experienced a discrete traumatic event, it was created in a real-world laboratory with children who have experienced complex trauma, usually over a significant period. This model holds an understanding of the neurobiology of play and the neurobiology of trauma together and harnesses a multitude of pathways through play for one to heal the other. To this end, the play therapist's palette was created. It serves as a visual representation, for TraumaPlay® therapists, of the avenues available to therapists when a client becomes stuck in their trauma symptoms. Each paint splotch represents a mitigator that can be used in the approach to trauma content with clients. These are all ways to titrate the dose of exposure to hard things and nature holds a prime spot on the palette. (See Figure 6.1).

TraumaPlay® allows room for both nondirective and directive approaches to be employed and incorporates clinically sound elements of other evidence-based treatments such as child-centered play therapy, theraplay, and cognitive-behavioral play therapy, while offering original interventions that maximize therapeutic absorption through every play-based learning portal. Grounded in an integrative paradigm, this model translates evidence-informed trauma treatment with children into a sequence of play-based component modules. Each component represents an important dimension of trauma treatment and articulates both a specific treatment goal and accompanying interventions. The model differentiates between goals of trauma treatment that are best accomplished through nondirective methods and goals that are best served by cognitive-behavioral play therapy interventions, expressive therapy techniques, and dyadic treatment approaches. The key components include enhancing safety and security, assessing for and augmenting adaptive coping, soothing the physiology (which includes both enhancing self-regulation and expanding the role of Parents as Soothing Partners), increasing emotional literacy, play-based gradual exposure (this can take the form of posttraumatic play in a continuum of disclosure, experiential mastery play, or trauma narrative work), addressing the thought life, and making positive meaning of the post-trauma self. This chapter will offer examples of how the benefits of nature can be powerfully incorporated into each of these key components.

Enhancing Safety and Security

Nine-year-old Johnny was met with on a sunny day in the backyard of Nurture House. Johnny's parents are divorced, and he goes back and forth between homes. He spends much of his time in sessions processing the deeply different parenting philosophies, his parents' different beliefs about religion and faith and what this means for his relationship with God, and the conflicting feelings of protection and constraint he feels by the different boundaries set in each home. Several of the most recent sessions have involved Johnny and one or the other parent, and Johnny has pogoed around, bounced balls, and otherwise regulated his tension during difficult conversations with big body movement and engagement. This day, we were meeting individually. Johnny asked to go in the back yard, and then wandered about,

DOI: 10.4324/9781003152767-9

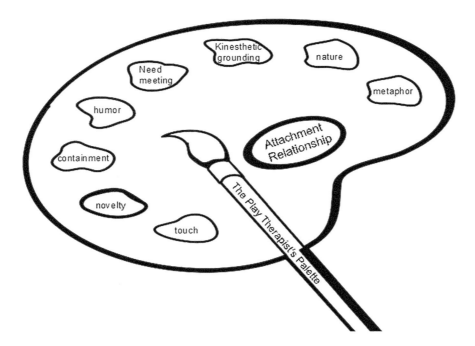

Figure 6.1 The play therapist's palette.

Source: Goodyear-Brown, 2019. Reproduced with permission.

touching each of the items mentioned earlier. He was very quiet, when he is normally talking a mile a minute. Commenting on the difference in his energy, he was reminded that this was his time, and he could use it however he wanted. He gravitated to the hanging daybed, which was directly in the line of the warming sun on a cold day, and laid down, curling into a ball. Pulling up a lounge chair, and then lying down near him, I eventually said, "sometimes we just need some time to rest." Johnny rocked himself in the daybed, noticed the ivy growing up the tree in the neighbor's yard that had grown higher than our seven-foot privacy fence, commented on the sound of the hanging chimes in the wind, and soothed his system. We often talk about allowing for silence in the playroom. It is just as important that we allow for silence in the natural environment. This permission to simply be quiet and still contributed to client's sense of felt safety in the session.

Felt safety is a precursor for healing. The neuroception of safety is sometimes tied to body temperature and, in some cases, a simple change of state triggers the reptilian brain stem into a "reset" for safety and focus. People who are experiencing extremely painful temperatures (they are freezing or uncomfortably hot) are unable to focus on the task at hand. This exteroception of temperature as a measure of safety is fascinating. We can exterocept other cues in auditory, visual, olfactory, tactile, and gustatory ways. We are fortunate to have a small pool in our outdoor space with a constantly running waterfall. The auditory encoding of this running water can quickly induce a shift in neurophysiological encodings of danger in the children we serve. Some clients have an immediate uptick in their sense of felt safety when they take in the ambient noise of the waterfall. It should not be lost on us that most of the sounds digitally recorded into a sound machine or a sleep app, with the primary intention of inducing physiological relaxation are nature sounds: the wind, the rain, the ocean.

Assessing Coping Strategies and Augmenting Adaptive Ones

A much-used intervention for assessing coping in TraumaPlay® is the Coping Tree (Goodyear-Brown, 2010, 2019). The clinician begins by drawing a fruit tree or fruit-bearing plant indigenous to the area and uses the fruit that falls on the ground and is left to rot as maladaptive coping and the fruit that ripens, is plucked, and used to make yummy food as a metaphor for adaptive coping. When therapists have access to actual fruit bearing plants, blackberry bushes, trees with unknown berries, and so on, this assessment activity can simply be focused around the actual, living plant.

If there are no fruit bearing plants available, container gardening can offer a similar metaphor. Before there was an easily accessible outdoor space in my therapeutic environment, a plant or two was kept in the office. One of these might be a kind of ivy or vine-like plant, the other would be a flowering plant of some kind. A personal favorite is the petunia, which has a mass of beautiful blossoms that then shrivel up. In order to keep the plant healthy, dead-heading must occur. That is, the shriveled blossoms need to be plucked, so that the plant has room and energy for new growth (you already hear the metaphor, right?). The plucking of dead pieces is itself a mindful activity and can become the touchpoint for identifying maladaptive coping strategies. It is explained to the client that when experiencing great distress, we figure out ways to cope to keep us safe through the hard thing. The coping we developed at the time the scary thing happened did a job for us at that time. Now that the child is safe, it may no longer be needed and may, in fact, be interfering with new growth. In some cases, we tape dead heads to a piece of paper as we write down the coping strategies that the client wants to let go of as we validated the adaptive coping currently in bloom in their life.

Another staple of TraumaPlay® is the activity named CopeCakes (Goodyear-Brown, 2010), in which the four ingredients that are combined to create healthy coping choices are played articulated, played with, and then made into CopeCakes. This can easily be translated to the natural environment, making mudcakes to represent each of healthy coping choices the client names. This allows the client to be fully engaged kinesthetically with dirt, water, and the resulting mud mixture.

Soothing the Child's Physiology

Mindfulness practice itself, such as Mindfulness-Based Stress Reduction (MBSR) (Kagan, 1990) helps develop enhanced interoceptive attention (what the inside of our bodies are telling us) (Farb et al., 2013), doing mindfulness work in nature can increase both the exteroceptive (how the body experiences the world around it) benefits as well (Van Gordon et al., 2018). Both forms of knowing are valuable aids in enhancing self-regulation, defined here as moving from either hyperarousal states or hypoarousal states back into an optimal arousal window (Siegel, 2010). In TraumaPlay®, a multitude of prop-based playful breath work options are offered and paired with focused attention tasks in the natural environment.

When one is staring at a blanketed snow-covered vista and one suddenly notices a cardinal perching on a branch, one's attention is captivated. This phenomenon has a name: involuntary attention. In the manifestation of a profound truth, when we cannot help ourselves from noticing a novel event in an otherwise typical landscape, we bring our full attention to the stimulus, whatever it might be. When children have experienced trauma, their hypervigilance can lead to their attention being involuntarily drawn to signals that have previously been associated with danger. For example, the child who was slapped across the face repeatedly by an angry and inebriated dad may have been removed from that home, experiencing physical safety in the present moment but not felt safety. In fact, this child likely scans the environment hypervigilantly for signals that danger is present. Any quick movement, even that of a bird flying or a leaf falling, may result in an involuntary focusing of attention. Attention restoration theory looks at methods for enhancing people's directed-attention abilities (Stevenson et al., 2018). One way to see this involuntary attention is that it exercises the lower-brain regions, as a novel or intriguing stimulus gently activates attention in bottom-up fashion, while giving top-down directed-attention abilities time to rest (Goodyear-Brown, 2019). Directed-attention is easier after these breaks. Therapists can help clients mitigate the effects of hours spent in online work or schooling by simply placing a bird feeder or potted plant within the sight line of their workspace.

TraumaPlay® clinicians employ stethoscopes, oximeters, and heart rate apps on cell phones to track heart rate in relation to upregulating and downregulating activities. Helping children understand the vagaries of their own autonomic nervous system responses requires at least three kinds of therapeutic work: psychoeducation, embodiment, and self-reflection. This author has found that much of what is experienced in nature to be helpful in explaining the hypoarousal and hyperarousal

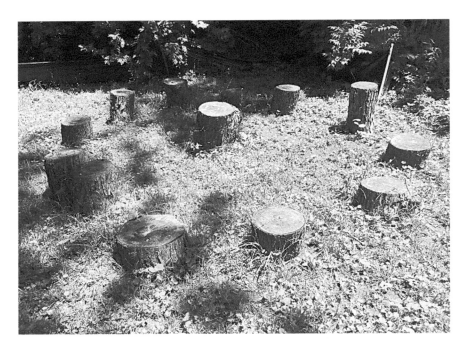

Figure 6.2 Circle of stumps with a life of their own.

Source: Goodyear-Brown.

states that are experienced multiple times a day. At one time, Nurture House had a circle of tree stumps in the back yard. Originally, this space was envisioned as a space for drum circles in the natural environment. Children would run to this farthest area of the backyard, stand up on one stump, and then strive to jump from stump to stump, completing the circle. Some of the jumps were easy and required no help from the therapist or the present parent, other stumps were so wobbly as they eroded or so far apart that they required an anchor-a helpful adult with a hand extended in the middle of the circle (see Figure 6.2).

When the child had completed the circle and was riding the high of this achievement, the therapist would often become curious about the whole "world" that lived under each stump. The ecology never disappointed, when a stump was overturned, there would be a myriad of bugs underneath some were grubs that could barely move and were bright white. Others were Roly Polys that would instantly curl into a ball and remain in that frozen state, and centipedes, who would speed away on their myriad legs. The contrast between the hyperarousal response of the centipedes, the death feigning/collapse response of the Roly Polys and the sloth-like response of the grubs who begin to wiggle but are not able to move quickly, depict all three states of arousal that occur when in a high state of alarm.

Interaction with birds, butterflies, insects, and other creatures that are found in nature can also elicit self-regulation practice all by themselves. Working with a client who tended to be unaware of himself in physical space, a session was conducted outdoors. He often barrels into things, utilizes more force than is necessary for a task and uses a very loud tone of voice in regular conversation. Once outside he had been bouncing on the Jumparoo and speaking loudly when he noticed a green lizard crawling on the cream-colored fence. We both became instantly still and agreed that we would try to get closer to it. We both understood that it would be scared by our big movements and skitter off, so we helped each other to move slowly and stealthily, with minimal noise, toward the fence. Although the lizard froze in its movement, we were rewarded by being able to get very close to it with our careful use of our proxemics. This child's full-body practice of self-regulation was motivated by both novelty in the environment and an understanding of how easily overwhelmed the lizard's system can become when quickness or bigness are perceived as threat. Powerful conversation about what feels "safe enough" both to the lizard and the little boy followed, all as an outgrowth of our sudden encounter with a lizard.

Bigness and Smallness in Space for Felt Safety

TraumaPlay® conceptualizes bigness and smallness of space as part of the way that the exteroception of safety is offered (Goodyear-Brown, 2021). The term "exteroception" refers to sensitivity to stimuli originating outside the body. Our felt sense of safety can be deeply affected by forms of exteroception-like the temperature in an air-conditioned play therapy room, the humidity and heat of a summer day, pelting rain, or intense wind. A baby who is wailing and inconsolable is taken outside and instantly distracted by some combination of a sudden change in temperature, humidity, and auditory input.

Proprioception refers to where your body is in space and includes balance, coordination, and agility. Our proprioception is informed by sensory neurons in our inner ear as well as stretch receptors located in the muscles and ligaments. A variety of swings meet the proprioceptive needs of children at Nurture House. The spinning swing (Figure 6.3), the magic carpet swing (Figure 6.4), and the huggle pod enclosed swing meet different needs for different children. In all cases, children are invited to explore the outdoor environment and therapist's triage the sensory needs based on the child's preferred play equipment.

Parents as Partners

From the time when cave people painted the walls of caves, humanity has dealt with the dangers of the external environment by sticking together. The need for someone to keep watch against intruders at night, to tend the fire while fending off wild animals, or as the Croods portrayed for us, join the sleep pile to provide warmth and safety against the physical elements has always enhanced connections between people. The phrase, "the enemy of mine enemy is my friend" is nowhere more profound than when we

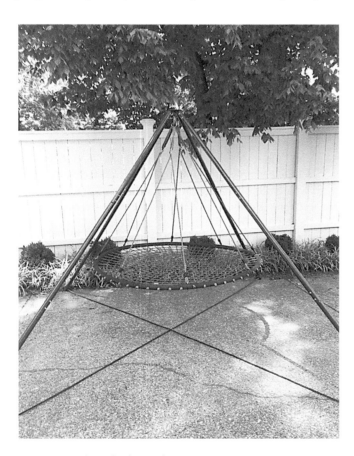

Figure 6.3 The spinning swing.
Source: Goodyear-Brown.

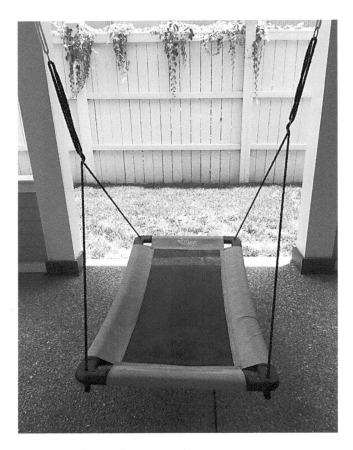

Figure 6.4 The magic carpet swing.

Source: Goodyear-Brown.

are facing brutal conditions in the natural environment. There is a wonderful song from Ceile Rain: "the big snow will make us brothers...in the big snow." While we can all think deep thoughts while ensconced in our cozy, protected nooks, the question of whom we would most rely on in moments of great danger is geared at eliciting our most ingrained attachment patterns. Parents are the first secure base, from which children explore the environment. As we grow in age and abilities, the circle of security that allows us to explore the world, separating both physically, emotionally, spiritually, and cognitively from our family members, expands. However, no matter your age, when environmental conditions threaten our sense of felt safety, we return to our haven, being welcomed back in our distress or neediness. Pretend play in the natural environment can promote attachment enhancement work. A multitude of scenarios that offer imaginal danger can help parent and child stick together more closely, experiencing themselves as a team. The imaginal threat of pirates attacking their ship pit the parent and child together against a pretend enemy. In some cases, the therapist plays the role of the enemy in these scenarios, offering an in-vivo experience of the dyad working together to defeat the foe, or to take back their territory.

Parts of the Nature Play area at Nurture House are intentionally built to invite opportunities for enhancing trust between children who have trouble trusting, either because of an early attachment wound or a more recent trauma. One of the ways that trust is expressed is in asking for help and many of the invitational challenges offered, like the slackline and the stump circle, are just on the growing edge of what a child can do on his or her own and what a child can do with a little help from an adult helper. Vygotsky & Cole (1978) calls this the zone of proximal development (Vygotsky), and we find it one of the primary ways to embody supported risk taking for children. The child who loves testing the proficiency of their physical body will often come into the backyard of Nurture House and run towards the slack line. They can get both their feet on top of it while holding onto the anchor beam, but as soon as they put one foot in front of the other, they find themselves in a very wobbly position. There have been times chosen to not offer a holding line above the tightrope, as this would allow children to create a competency surge independently.

When a core attachment wound, as is often seen in children adopted from institutions, with children who have experienced multiple caregiver disruptions, or children who are in foster care due to physical or sexual abuse or severe neglect, one of the primary treatment goals is helping these children expand their understanding of what a "Safe Boss" might be or look like. Each of these scenarios stems from a caregiver who was meant to protect and instead misused the power differential in the relationship or was unable to fulfill the roles of a Safe Boss for whatever reason. These children learn very early in life that no one really sees them, that there is no one they can truly rely on for help. Over time, this develops into an ingrained and deeply rooted belief: *I must control everything at all costs or I'll die.* Our first goal in these cases is to strengthen the attachment systems, to rewire the interpersonal neurobiology of at least on attachment relationship to embody a Safe Boss relationship (Goodyear-Brown, 2021). For this to happen, the competency surge that a specific child or teen feels needs to be paired with the help offered by another. When one thinks about the first steps that a baby takes, that joyous moment of independent movement is usually proceeded by multiple moments supported by their attachment figure. Figure 6.5 depicts a super athletic boy who experiences great surges of oxytocin when he conquers new challenges with his whole physical self. Once he had successfully crossed the entire slack-line with mom's help, he decided that planting his feet in one place, leaning heavily on mom, and jumping up and down would be much more fun than simply walking along the line. There is a duality of pain in these children from hard places: it is painful to do it on their own, whatever it is, and it can be equally painful to ask for help. In these cases, we are trying to mitigate the core fear that is triggered for these children whenever they must acknowledge the need for help with an immediate full-body experience of their power, in play, especially when this power is supported by a Safe Boss.

TraumaPlay® therapists often invite families on walks around the neighborhood. When they are curious together about the natural environment, attachment enhancement opportunities seem to present themselves endlessly. One such walk with six-year-old Billy, a highly dysregulated child and his mother occurred just after a hard rain. The earthworms were scuttling across the earth. Billy saw an earthworm and grabbed it up. His mom was asked to support her son's gentle holding of the earthworm and the

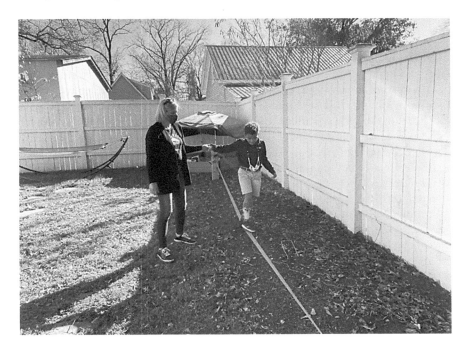

Figure 6.5 Risking help.

Source: Goodyear-Brown.

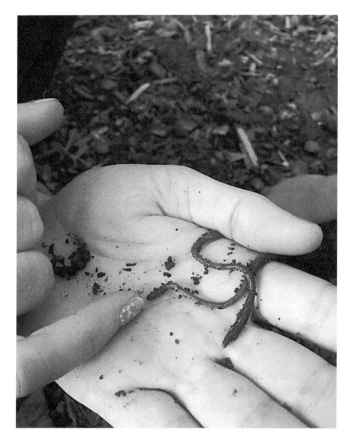

Figure 6.6 Worms and safe bosses.

Source: Goodyear-Brown.

therapist led a conversation about what earthworms need to live and grow, what they might be afraid of, and what could hurt them. The dyad agreed that the one earthworm on its own might feel afraid around these big humans. The hunt for a second worm began. Billy quickly found a much smaller worm and placed it next to the big one in mom's hand. Billy exclaimed, "I bet that's his mommy!" The therapist wondered out loud what it was like for the little earthworm to have the big one near, and Billy said, "It feels great" (see Figure 6.6.). The attachment enhancement provided through this moment was validating to both Billy and his mother, as he was reinforced in Safe Boss concepts and she was reinforced in providing comfort to him as a Safe Boss. They named the pair of earthworms the "Wiggly Ones." As treatment progressed, the dyad referenced these earthworms repeatedly as they grew in their ability to understand about sticking together through hard things.

Families who experience nature together seem to be more connected than those who do not (Izenstark & Ebata, 2016). To that end, another nature-based activity sometimes offered to families is a nature walk during which they gather berries and leaves, crush them up to make pigments, and then create art together, either using the pigments on the paper, or painting their own hands with the natural pigments and making handprints on stone instead of paper. One ancient way of making handprints involves a person putting their hand against the wall and then spitting from the mouth pigment that would outline the handprint. A TraumaPlay® therapist may fill up a water squirter with a mixture of water and pigments made from berries. The child places their hand on the cement walkway in the backyard (or on a piece of paper) and the parent squirts the mixture over the child's hand. This provides squeals of delight from the child. Although no one is insisting that the child keep their hand in place, the child wants to create a clear handprint and even when experiencing the startling effect of the water suddenly splashing over their hands, sensory defensive children bring more of their neocortex online to maintain self-control and stillness in order to finish the print. This stretches the window of tolerance for distress by pairing the work with a fun and novel outcome. To use the water squirter effectively while holding one hand still on paper requires the engagement of a second person, so when this activity is offered to a parent/child dyad they work cooperatively together, opening and closing circles of communication to create the handprint, as the therapist delights in the dyad and their joint efforts. If the roles are reversed, and the child wields the power of the squirter, another kind of self-control is practiced as the child waits for the parent's cue to squirt. This can be paired with social skills enhancement work, as therapist may prompt the child to check in with mom using the word, "Ready?" and wait for her response, "Ready!" before squirting. This same work of gathering berries, squishing them to release the pigment, and then painting with them can be done in individual work with a client as well.

Increasing Emotional Literacy

Nature's metaphors can help us explore, articulate, and play with a variety of human emotions. The basic elements: fire, air, earth, and water are a great starting place for this work. Each of these elements can show us the continuum of expression from helpful uses of the element, air for example, and extreme and dangerous expressions of elemental power. Air can offer us a gentle breeze on a warm day; it may be welcomed as it cools us down, but at its most intense, moving air becomes a tornado that can destroy all in its path, so goes anger. Water can be relaxing in the form of a shallow pool to dip our toes in or a babbling brook to rest beside. It can also become a dangerous deluge of rain while driving, or a tidal wave destroying all in its path.

In addition to the metaphoric exploration of nature for parallels with emotional expression, prop-based interventions can be offered that allow for emotions to be worked with in nature. While on nature walks, clients can be asked to pick up rocks, stones, or sticks of different shapes and sizes that can stand in for worries, frustrations, fears, or joys of various kinds. The Harpeth River is near the backyard. Therapists can walk with clients to the bridge or the water's edge and have them name worries out loud and then throw them into the river. Balloons can be provided for children to blow their anger into and then let them float them away on the surface of a small pool in the backyard of Nurture House.

Establishing Boundaries

TraumaPlay® is often used with children and teens who have been sexually abused or have problematic sexual behavior. The Tackling Touchy Subjects curriculum (Goodyear-Brown, 2013) is often adjunctive to TraumaPlay® and has a strong emphasis on examining boundaries, particularly within family systems and creating new boundaries in the wake of sexual violations. Boundary markers can be created with stones, sticks, trenches dug in the dirt, burms built above ground, and so on. Such work with children and adolescents who have been sexually abused can include creating markers in the natural environment that empower them in terms of the boundaries they want to clarify in other situations.

Trauma Narrative Case Example: Rainey, Age Five years

Rainey, a five-year-old female adopted from China, having already worked with her adoption story in LifeBook form with her therapist, was invited to augment her narrative knowing by working with her story in nature. She reflected an eagerness to continue her story work in addition to a curiosity and receptiveness to build her story in a new way. The client circled the backyard several times with her therapist by her side, who was offering reflections in response to her wonderings. Rainey appeared deep in thought as she touched, dug, and explored various parts of the backyard until she suddenly stopped and became intentionally focused on externalizing the world she found herself in.

Rainey took the therapist back to various snail shells she found in several garden beds and began collecting them in addition to giving therapist the prompt to do the same. She reported that "these are baby snails who don't have a Mom and Dad". She went on to say that "the babies need to be rescued by the Police and taken to an orphanage in China." She then said, "Their Mom put them out on purpose so that the police could take them to the adoption place." Client found a pail full of dirt and began using leaves, stones, sticks, and natural materials to create an "orphanage" for the abandoned snails. She was intentional about adding items to represent "safety, comfort, shelter and connection" such as a stiff magnolia leaf propped up on two sticks to create a shelter from rain, a flower to "make them feel happy", a small dish full of water and leaves for drinking and eating, a tiny purple button they could use as a toy, soft moss as a comfy place to sleep and a bird's nest as a place all the snails could go to be safe together. Rainey reflected much joy in her creation and eagerly brought all of the snail shells to it, carefully placing them within. She found an owl figure and placed it next to the orphanage. Client reported: "This is the police, but he's not supposed to be asleep." She identified a self-object and placed it in the orphanage putting a silver star sticker that she found next to it.

The client and therapist gently processed this creation together and Rainey spent several minutes playing with her creation, reflecting themes of play-based mastery and feeling empowered in relation to her adoption story, a place she did not appear to have any felt power in before. The experience of a nature-based narrative not only provided an additional form of containment for her externalized story, but it mitigated her approach to deeper, more emotional parts of her adoption story. Most importantly, she was able to be supported in experiencing the rescue of a traumatized self-object in a removed, safe way through the symbolic work of experiential mastery play and the coregulation of nature.

Addressing the Thought Life Through Messy Play

Many children with complex trauma come to treatment with a control foundation (Goodyear-Brown, 2021). Helping these children to tolerate the uncontrollable is often a treatment goal. Messy play provides gradual exposure to substances that cannot be fully controlled: mud, shaving cream, dirt, dried corn kernels, rice, beans, beads, sand, and so forth. The child whose physical system is constricted to tight, controlled movements, will often have similar cognitive rigidity patterns showing up in their play. The pairing of messy play with cognitive shifting work first begins with identifying the cognitive distortion or the negative self-talk, "I can't get it right! It's not perfect! I suck!" Fashioning cognitive replacement statements and offering a thought-stopping mechanism, and finally, practicing positive self-talk can off be accessed through and rehearsed in the midst of messy play.

Case Study: Bringing It All Together: Sally, Age Nine Years

TraumaPlay® therapists learn the components of the model individually, as well as specific interventions to support the pursuit of each goal, and then leave all the planning at the door, following the need of the child while being fully present all along the way. Narrating the events of just one session as an example of how the integration can look: Sally is a nine-year-old female adopted from the Ukraine at age three. During the assessment phase, Sally often responded to any new invitation with an automatic "no" followed by engagement in the task. She made it a point to say that she does not trust anyone. She had difficulty making eye contact, often demanded things instead of asking, and was fairly constricted in both her affect and her physical body. One day, the therapist mentioned that sometimes kids go on walks with their Safe Boss at Nurture House (Goodyear-Brown, 2019). Her ears perked up and she said, "I want to go on a walk!" It was explained that the therapist was looking forward to a time when they could go on a walk and explained the need for mutual trust between them in order to do so.

Therapeutic walking encourages many kinds of positive practice for children and teens: (1) asking with their asking words, (2) managing the transition from the building to the community and back again, (3) sharing power, and (4) exerting top-down brain abilities to choose direction (right or left, toward the park or downtown). Walks also encourage shared mindsight as therapist and client experience the natural environment together, making memories that are often novel and unique to the therapeutic dyad along the way. The next session, Sally asked to be in the backyard and the therapist read her *Mindful Monkey, Happy Panda* while she sat in the bouncy seat attached to the top of the climbing dome. When narrating the monkey's process of always thinking about the next thing while engaging in the current activity, she said, "That's like me!" When the book was finished, she asked if we could go on a walk. It was agreed that she was ready to let the therapist be her Safe Boss on a walk. She was introduced to the Mindful Meal exercise (see Figure 6.7). The client is given a paper plate with lines dividing the plate into at least five sections, or pie pieces. Each piece represents a different object found on the walk. Sally chose these categories: something rough, something smooth, something colorful, something curly, something crinkly, and something sparkly.

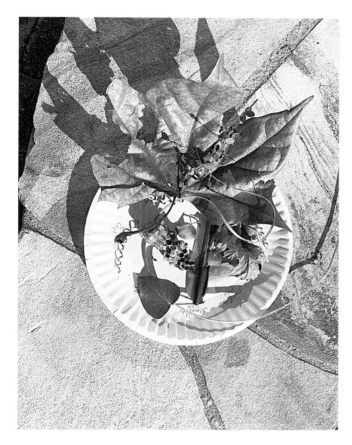

Figure 6.7 A mindful meal.

Source: Goodyear-Brown.

Sally chose to turn right, and began walking toward the river. She immediately found a rock that was rough, and very shortly after found a rock that was smooth. She had not considered that a rock could have either or both qualities and talked about show sometimes she was rough and other times kind. Once the railroad tracks were reached, the therapist stepped up on one rail and began balancing. Sally broke into a huge grin and exclaimed, "That's what I wanted to do!" Therapist invited her to balance on the other beam and we walked together for several lengths of rail in this way. We noticed what our shadows were doing and decided to try connecting through our shadows while balancing on our individual beams (see Figure 6.8).

As we walked, the therapist acknowledged, "I'm glad we could do this today." Sally responded, "Me too. I didn't trust you at first, but now I do, so I can go on a walk with you." Right at that moment, the train whistled in the distance. Sally squealed and I said, "We've got this. Let's stick together and get off the tracks!" Holding hands we quickly scrambled far away from the track. The train came barreling past us, and the engineer waved to us out the front window. Sally was incredibly excited, saying "I've never seen a train this way before!" It hurtled past at what felt like breakneck speed. Sally exclaimed, "This is scary!" Therapist responded, "It is kind of scary. Is it o.k. if I hold on a little tighter? I want to make sure you stay safe." Sally nodded, and my arm was placed around her shoulder. This action offered some containment and additional warmth in the wake of the draft being created by the rushing freight cars and allowed for an assessment for the level of rigidity in her body. Her heart rate slowly returned to normal and she began to point out the cars that carried graffiti and noticed more details of the train. She wanted to balance on the tracks again as soon as the train had safely passed and asked to have a picture taken to be able to show her mom (see Figure 6.9).

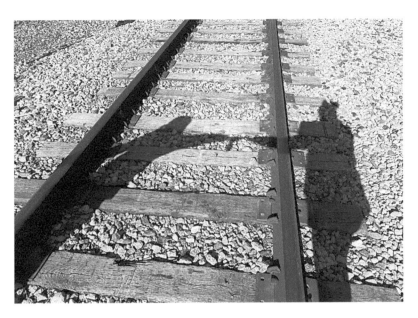

Figure 6.8 Shadows touching while balancing.
Source: Goodyear-Brown.

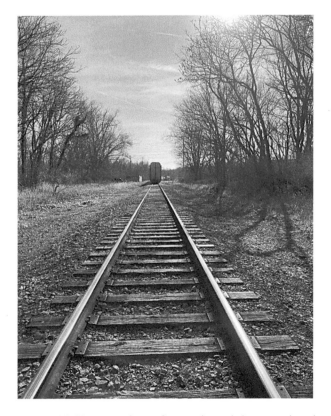

Figure 6.9 Neurocepting safety again and documenting the story.
Source: Goodyear-Brown.

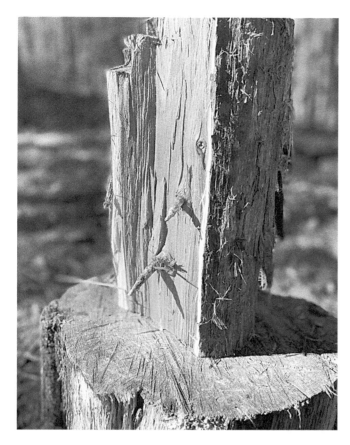

Figure 6.10 Strength stretching outward from within.

Source: Goodyear-Brown.

The excitement of this shared experience, paired with the mindfulness work of filling the Mindful Meal plate, met multiple therapeutic goals while further enforcing the Triad of Therapist Roles in TraumaPlay®: Safe Boss, Nurturer, and Storykeeper.

Conclusion

The benefits of nature are myriad and they can augment the therapeutic work being pursued in any of the key components of TraumaPlay®. This includes the belief that the individual and the family system can move toward health—toward integration of the trauma into a coherent narrative and a coherent sense of self, while leaching the emotional toxicity out of the events. Next is a picture of a log split during a wood mauling exercise. It is a remarkable metaphor for this work. As the log was split (causing some discomfort both to us and to the log), these branches, growing on the inside, were revealed. The new growth was happening under the surface. It is hoped that the Nature of TraumaPlay® offers a path toward unmasking the real child within the layers of trauma while inviting growth in their inborn resiliencies (see Figure 6.10).

Reflective Questions

1   Move into the natural environment. Notice the changes in your bodily responses as you move from the indoor environment (air conditioning or heat) into the natural environment. Move into direct sunlight and notice how your body responds to being warmed by the sun. Move into the shade and notice the cues that your body gives you in this shadow space. Pay attention to what your body is telling you (interception). Which environment gives you the strongest neuroception of safety?

2   Once in nature, find a spot where the trees grow close together. Spend some time noticing how your body feels in this "smallness of space." Find an open spot, for example, a field, and notice how your body feels in the "bigness of space." Reflect on which exteroception experience most strongly contributes to a neuroception of safety for you.

3   Go on a nature walk. Did you see anything novel? Anything that you were drawn to, that captured your full attention for a moment of time? How is this a form of mindfulness?

Appendix A

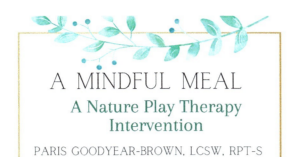

A MINDFUL MEAL

A Nature Play Therapy Intervention

PARIS GOODYEAR-BROWN, LCSW, RPT-S

DESCRIPTION:

The search for various natural objects that fulfill the categories on the plate invites children to hyper focus. Their deepening attention to the natural world enhances mindfulness.

SUPPLIES NEEDED:

Paper Plate

Marker

GOAL:

To bring about tactile grounding and sensory regulation, and exteroception.

INSTRUCTIONS:

Through s collaborative process the therapist and child decide on the kinds of objects to be found. A Paper Plate is then marked off into six sections, each one labeled with a category (For Example: Something Rough, Something Smooth, Something Colorful, Something Fuzzy, and Something Unexpected). The therapist and child work together to find an object in nature that fulfills each one of the categories.

EXTRA FUN:

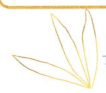
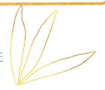

ONCE ALL THE OBJECTS ARE GATHERED, THE THERAPIST AND CHILD CAN USE THEM TO CREATE AN ART PIECE TOGETHER

References

Berman, M. G., Jonides, J., & Kaplan, S. (2008). The cognitive benefits of interacting with nature. *Psychological Science, 19*, 1207–1212.

Farb, N. A., Segal, Z. V., & Anderson, A. K. (2013). Mindfulness meditation training alters cortical representations of interoceptive attention. *Social Cognitive and Affective Neuroscience, 8*(1), 15–26.

Goodyear-Brown, P. (2009). *Play Therapy with Traumatized Children: A Prescriptive Approach.* Wiley and Sons.

Goodyear-Brown, P. (2010). *The Worry Wars.* www.nurturehouse.org

Goodyear-Brown, P. (2011). The worry wars: A protocol for treating childhood anxiety disorders. In C. Schaefer (Ed.), *Integrative Play Therapy.* Wiley and Sons.

Goodyear-Brown, P. (2013). *Tackling Touchy Subjects.* www.parisgoodyearbrown.com

Goodyear-Brown, P. (2019). *Trauma and Play Therapy: Helping Children Heal.* Routledge.

Goodyear-Brown, P. (2021). *Parents as Partners in Child Therapy: A Clinician's Guide.* Guilford Press.

Howell, A. J., Dopko, R. L., Passmore, H.-A., & Buro, K. (2011). Nature connectedness: Associations with well-being and mindfulness. *Personality and Individual Differences, 51*, 166–171.

Huynh, T., & Torquati, J. C. (2019). Examining connection to nature and mindfulness at promoting psychological well-being. *Journal of Environmental Psychology, 66*, 101370.

Izenstark, D., & Ebata, A. T. (2016). Theorizing family-based nature activities and family functioning: The integration of attention restoration theory with a family routines and rituals perspective. *Journal of Family Theory & Review, 8*(2), 137–153.

Moran, D. (2019). Back to nature? Attention restoration theory and the restorative effects of nature contact in prison. *Health & Place, 57*, 35–43.

Stevenson, Matt P., Schilhab, T., & Bentsen, P. (2018). Attention Restoration Theory II: A systematic review to clarify attention processes affected by exposure to natural environments. *Journal of Toxicology and Environmental Health, Part B, 21*(4), 227–268. https://doi.org/10.1080/10937404.2018.1505571

Siegel, D. J. (2010). *Mindsight: The New Science of Personal Transformation.* Bantam.

Stevenson, M. P., Schilhab, T., & Bentsen, P. (2018). Attention Restoration Theory II: A systematic review to clarify attention processes affected by exposure to natural environments. *Journal of Toxicology and Environmental Health, Part B, 21*(4), 227–268.

Van Gordon, W., Shonin, E., & Richardson, M. (2018). Mindfulness and nature. *Mindfulness, 9*(5), 1655–1658.

Vygotsky, L., & Cole, M. (1978). *Mind in Society: The Development of Higher Psychological Processes.* Harvard University Press.

7 Using Nature to Create Safety for Medical Trauma Integration

Rose LaPiere and Lisa Dion

To protect confidentiality, the names in this chapter have been changed. The masked case vignettes are based on stories and interactions that the therapists have experienced over their years of working with children and families.

Introduction

Safety is at the core of treatment when working with children or families to support the healing of trauma. Without safety, the ability to integrate trauma can be quite challenging. One of the ways we can create safety for our child clients is through the use of nature. Nature can help us create varied experiences of emotional safety for children and families that is often hard to access in trauma work. Nature isn't just a backdrop to help children heal, but is healing in and of itself. This concept will be reflected throughout this chapter as we examine how to use nature to create emotional and relational safety after a traumatic experience. For the purposes of this chapter, the examples used will focus on medical trauma; however, the application of nature can be used for any experience that our clients perceive as traumatic.

Neuroception of Safety and Polyvagal Theory

The following vignette of Shante' case briefly illustrates the importance of introducing how trauma can impact a child's body and how the disruptive behavior seen in a child is an indicator of the body's response to stress. Treatment interventions utilized in this case will be further explored in detail later in this chapter.

The Case of Shante': Creating Safety in Nature

The therapist first met Shante', a five-year-old child who experienced medical trauma. Shante's mother, Marjorie, wasn't sure how play therapy would help, but she was overwhelmed with Shante behavior at home and in school. The mother advised that Shante's received two shots during a wellness visit a few months ago, she was described as irritable, and having a hard time being soothed. Marjorie explained how she and a nurse had to hold Shante' as she screamed and cried, refusing to get the shots. Shante' also had a remarkable history of medical procedures early in life. Shante' often had aggressive outbursts in both settings. At school, when in a situation that required transition, she would roll on the floor, refuse to move, and scream at her teachers. At home when it was time for bed, Shante' would throw her books and toys on the floor, screaming. The parents and her school were confused as to why her behavior has drastically changed.

As it can be seen from this vignette, medical trauma can be hard to detect. Shante's misbehavior was confusing for her caregivers and teachers. Later in this chapter we will explore this case further to understand how her aggressive behaviors represented her body's response to the stress and overwhelm from her medical experiences and how nature was utilized as an external regulator to create safety.

As we explore how nature can help create safety and mitigate the potential impact of a medical situation on a child's nervous system, it is important to first define trauma. On the National Child Traumatic Stress Network website, they describe trauma as, "a frightening, dangerous or violent event

DOI: 10.4324/9781003152767-10

that poses a threat to a child's life or bodily integrity" (1st para., 1st sent). Similarly, on the website of the American Psychological Association, it highlights trauma as an "*emotionalr*" response to a terrible event like an accident, rape or natural disaste(1st para., 1st sent). A simple way of understanding what constitutes a situation registering as traumatic is that the brain perceives whatever is happening in life as overwhelming, or what Dion (2018) refers to as "too much." To understand this further, as a child perceives a threat or challenge and their autonomic nervous system becomes activated in a flight/fight/immobilization response, the child attempts to function within its own window of tolerance (Badenoch, 2017). The window of tolerance is described as the optimal state of arousal for integration (Ogden et al., 2006; Siegel, 2020). When an individual, or in this case, a child, experiences something that is *too much*, emotional flooding occurs moving the child outside of their window of tolerance. In these moments, integration of the experience becomes impaired. Depending on the degree and impact of this emotional flooding, the nervous system then potentially stores it as a trauma (Badenoch, 2017). The result is an activated defense response as seen in the case with Shante'. The trauma of her ongoing medical experiences were at the core of her challenging behaviors.

Polyvagal theory, developed by Stephen Porges, introduces the term "neuroception" to describe the process by which the neural circuits distinguish whether or not there is a threat in the environment. This process happens without our conscious awareness (Porges, 2011). What we understand from Polyvagal theory and what is needed for integration comes down to two words: safety and connection. Children must feel safe enough and connected enough to move toward the challenging thoughts, feelings, and body sensations that registered outside of their window of tolerance and were thus not integrated (Dion, 2018). In order to do this, children must be able to access their regulatory system. Porges (2011) explains that the autonomic nervous system not only has fight/flight/immobilization responses for danger but also has a social engagement/regulatory response that is activated when a person feels safe. When a child is feeling safe and his or her social engagement system is activated, he or she can communicate, play, relax, and learn (Delahooke, 2019). It is important to note that being safe and feeling safe are not the same. The felt sense of safety is accessed through the activation of the ventral vagus nerve. The introduction of the ventral vagal system in polyvagal theory sheds light for clinicians to begin to understand the significance of supporting and strengthening an individual's ability to activate this response (Porges, 2011). It is the ventral vagal response that allows individuals to "put the brakes" on the activation of the flight/fight/immobilization response. It helps engage higher centers of brain functioning, regulate through the intensity of activation, move back into the window of tolerance, and ultimately help an individual feel connected to themselves and to others (Badenoch, 2017; Dana, 2018; Dion, 2018; Porges, 2011).

As in the case with Shante', her nervous system was so overwhelmed and scared that it was registering as *too much*, her system was not able to access the ventral vagal response, and she was not able to regulate well. This could be either because Shante' never really learned how to regulate, or the situation is so far outside her window of tolerance that the ability to access this regulatory system is too challenging. In either case, she needs an external regulator for coregulation. The more a child becomes dysregulated, the ability to self-govern and integrate diminishes. When an attuned adult steps in and offers a mindful presence and a regulated nervous system, coregulation begins (Badenoch, 2017; Dion, 2018). Coregulation is a crucial element to engaging the ventral vagal system creating connection and safety (Badenoch, 2017). As the child and the adult interact, the child borrows the adult's regulatory capacity, which helps the child regulate through the challenging emotions (Dion, 2018; Schore, 2019).

The following section will explore how nature can be utilized as an external regulator to create safety for trauma integration.

Nature as an External Regulator for Trauma Integration

Think for a moment about your own experience in nature. Imagine the smell of flowers, visualize ocean waves, hear the sound of birds chirping, touch the bark on a tree, or feel your feet in the sand. What happens in your body as you imagine these different sensory experiences? Often we can become more aware and connected to our bodies and the natural world around us transforms as more vibrant. Nature awakens our nervous system through the sensory experience helping to create connection and awareness. Weber and Heuberger (2008) found in their research that taking in the smell of nature's plants when outdoors (i.e., garden) improved calmness, alertness, and mood. In a study by Gould van Praag et al. (2017), they found that listening to nature sounds decreases the stress response system (fight /flight/immobilization) and increases the ventral vagus response of the nervous system. In fact, the participants in their research who were the most stressed had the most significant gains in relaxation. In another study, nature was found to decrease anxiety, rumination, and help maintain a positive affect (Bratman et al., 2015). The act of touching nature items also opens a pathway that can have a direct connection to our own emotions, body sensations, and inner thoughts (Berger, 2017). Furthermore, listening to pleasant nature sounds after a stressful task was found to decrease the fight/flight response (Alvarsson et al., 2010). Bringing nature into a therapy practice, whether going outside or bringing nature elements inside, can help children work through their trauma in a way that brings safety to the nervous system and helps in the child's healing process. Nature, in and of itself, is an external regulator.

The body stores the energy of trauma in its tissues until it can be released (Van der Kolk, 2015). Nature can naturally provide a multisensory experience allowing access into the body where the trauma is stored. It creates a whole-body experience helping healing to deepen into the body. Whether a child is actively smelling the air or feeling the bark on a tree or passively sitting surrounded by nature's sights, smells, and sounds, nature safely engages the entire body in the therapeutic process. For children who are experiencing heightened states of arousal in their nervous systems, the additional support of an external regulator, such as nature, is necessary in order to help them be present with their internal experiences. Nature can offer a safe entryway into their bodies where the trauma is stored. It is able to hold a space for children to begin to notice the sensations, thoughts, and emotions inside of them, as well as feel more connected to their environment. There are many ways to integrate nature as an external regulator. Some interventions can be developed in the moment as the therapist and child are exploring nature. Other nature interventions can be planned and those ideas will be explored in the next section.

Getting Started with Nature Interventions

It is important for practitioners to consider how to facilitate the use of nature in the therapeutic process. Berger and McLeod (2006) described the client–therapist-nature concept as the "relationship triad," with nature considered as being a "co-therapist" (p. 87). When nature is considered as the cotherapist, it can take on a role in the therapeutic process in two ways: First, nature can take an active role to help the child work through trauma—such as a breeze taking away the hard feelings. The other way is by allowing nature to be experienced as a holding space in the background—such as sitting by a river and talking about hard feelings while listening to the water. It is important to note that in one session a therapist may go back and forth with nature taking an active role and nature creating a holding space in the background. It is up to the therapist to use their best clinical judgment and trust their intuition as to which way would be best for the client in the moment. In both situations, nature is a facilitator for healing and an external regulator.

A great way to begin integrating nature is by exploring questions with the family related to their nature experiences. Becoming curious about what the family already enjoys in nature is helpful for two reasons: First, it begins an introduction to nature-based play therapy, and second, it helps the therapist understand how to use nature to create safety for a particular family. Although nature is a powerful intervention for trauma work, it is crucial that the therapist knows if there have been any experiences in outdoor environments that were also traumatic for the child and family. For example, this could even include a car accident, or even a tree falling on someone's house from a storm. Having this knowledge helps the therapist further understand how to incorporate nature for emotional and relational safety. As the therapist explores and discusses nature experiences with the child and family, the therapist is also simultaneously scaffolding upon the inner resources of nature connections within the child. For example, knowing that the child enjoys gardening, the therapist may have a container of dirt, plants, and flowers as the "cotherapist" for the child to explore since that is already known to bring delight. This provides the child with opportunities to feel safe and grounded as the issues are explored further.

The following questions can be asked during the first three family sessions.

1   How often do you go outside? What keeps you from going out more?
2   What is your favorite place in nature?

3   What is a favorite memory you have in nature? (explore sight, sound, smell, taste, or tactile sensations)
4   Is there a tree (plant, flower, bird, or animal) that holds a special memory for you?
5   For parents, when you were a child, what were places in nature that you explored?
6   Have you or your child had any negative or traumatic experiences in nature? Are there things in nature that you do not like? (Consider giving examples of types of nature experiences that may be traumatic such as storms, floods, trees falling, etc.)

Nature Interventions for Creating Safety Inside the Office Playroom

If a practitioner does not have the ability to go outside with a client, nature can still be brought inside and used to create safety as trauma is explored. As well, some practitioners may choose not to go outside due to not having access to a safe location or green space, or the therapist may not feel comfortable in an outdoor setting. They may also be fearful that the child could get injured. Therefore, practitioners will need to explore these concerns before deciding to transition to having a play therapy session in nature. Here are some creative nature interventions that can be used indoors.

Building a Safe Space Nature Hut

Children love building forts and creating places to hide, seek refuge, and feel protected. Therapists often use tents or cozy corners to create this experience for children, but nature is able to offer its own version (see Figure 7.1). Using objects in nature such as sticks, flowers, and leaves, the therapist and child can

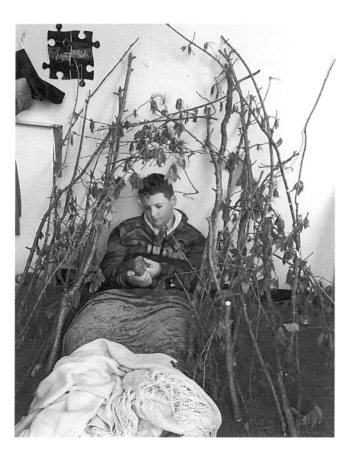

Figure 7.1 Lucas, age 10, sitting under a tent shaped from sticks with leaves, looking at a rock inside office playroom.
Source: Rose LaPiere.

build a nature hut together creating a safe space in real-time that a child can sit inside. The nature hut provides anchoring, while holding the child in a way that feels safe as the child revisits traumatic memories. While inside the hut, the child's senses can also be accessed by feeling the various nature objects used to create it. Touching nature is a way to become connected to your sensations, emotions, and the world around you (Berger & McLeod, 2006) (see Appendix A).

The following vignette of Lemont will show how the nature hut is able to be utilized as a safe space.

The Case of Lemont: Nature Hut as an External Regulator

Eight-year-old Lemont, with celiacs disease, had experienced a variety of medical procedures such as endoscopy, colonoscopy, and a series of blood tests. In a particular session, Lemont didn't want the therapist to look directly at him and the nature hut intervention helped create a safe way for them to be together without the intensity of the eye contact. As Lemont sat inside the hut, he was able to feel safe and his nervous system was able to begin to relax. In order to help hold the space for Lemont's overwhelming feelings the therapist sat to the side of the hut so eye contact could be avoided. Together, the therapist and the nature hut were able to cofacilitate and coregulate Lemont. The experience of the nature hut was so comforting to him that he asked to take home the items they had collected to make the nature hut so he could recreate it in his home. His mom reported that he would go into his nature hut whenever he felt upset or frustrated, helping him stay in his window of tolerance.

This vignette demonstrates the use of a nature hut to help a child feel safe while exploring the traumatic memory. Lemont benefited from having access to the nature hut at home because when he needed to feel anchored it was available to help support him.

Nature Pictures

Creating a regulated state can be fostered by using nature pictures, metaphor, and journaling. In the next vignette of Janice, we will explore how nature can offer ways for the child to connect to herself.

The Case of Janice: Reconnecting to Self Through Nature Pictures

Janice, age 12, had difficulty sleeping and talking about her feelings following an asthma attack incident that resulted in an ambulance taking her to the hospital in the middle of the night. During one session, Janice and her therapist spent time creating a journal filled with a collection of nature pictures. They used cardboard for the front and back covers and the pages in the middle were blank. The therapist and Janice worked on discovering what pictures and images she found in nature that helped bring a sense of peace, happiness, joy, excitement, or calm inside of her body and mind. Her collection included beautiful photos from images online to photographs she found around her community. One of the strategies to help her fall asleep better was to spend time going through her nature picture journal at bedtime. Sometimes, she would just spend time looking through the book and other times she drew more nature pictures.

Nature pictures had helped Janice to explore her traumatic memories and develop resources. Janice was able to look at her photos and recall the positive feelings that nature elicited, which helped her during the times she could not fall asleep. In the next section, we will observe Janice in therapy in an outdoor setting (see Appendix B).

Nature Interventions for Creating Safety in an Outdoor Setting

When practitioners think about integrating nature in play and expressive therapies, there can be several benefits to going outside. Spending time outside has significant health and wellness benefits, such as the reduced risk of stress and improved physical health (Gould van Praag et al., 2017; Maller et al., 2009; Twohig-Bennett & Jones, 2018). Some children also have a preference for being outside, which is important to consider. In the case of Janice described in the previous section, we can observe therapy with her now in an outdoor setting using an adapted Gestalt dialoguing technique with nature.

Case of Janice Continued: Nature Metaphors and Gestalt Dialoguing

During subsequent therapy sessions, Janice asked her therapist to spend some moments outside, bringing along the picture nature journal and some colored pencils. During one session, they chose to sit near a tree and the therapist then used a nature metaphor to help deepen Janice's connection to nature. The therapist talked about how trees help support each other with nutrition and send messages to each other when there is danger, like if an animal is eating their leaves. The therapist also shared that trees grow well together and rely on each other to grow and feel safe (Wohlleben, 2019). By sharing this nature metaphor, the therapist was not only creating an emotional connection to the trees, but also in an indirect way teaching Janice about herself. The therapist used the book Can You Hear The Trees Talking *(Wohlleben, 2019) to deepen the understanding about trees and human similarities. This book is also lovely for the therapist and child to read together.*

The therapist then encouraged Janice to write one of her worries to the tree in her journal, then pause, take a breath, and then write the tree's response. What emerged was a back and forth conversation between herself and the tree in her nature journal. Some of the writing was about her medical trauma and other writings were related to friendships and family life. These adapted Gestalt dialoguing (Oaklander, 2007) conversations served as an external regulator, creating a safe way for her to explore her challenging feelings. Once finished, the therapist helped deepen and further integrate the process by asking questions such as: What was that experience like for you? What do you notice now about how you feel about the problem? What was the message the tree gave you? What did you notice in your body as you were having the conversation with the tree? To continue the work, the therapist asked Janice if there was a tree at her home that she could continue dialoguing with.

In her journal writings to the tree the therapist was able to facilitate her expression of feelings. These nature interventions facilitated her ability to communicate her feelings and feel safe in her body (see Appendix C).

Symbolic Play in Nature

As children process their traumatic memories, they often recreate through play symbolic representations of the challenges they are exploring. As they explore nature, they are able to project their thoughts and feelings outside of themselves onto nature itself. The beauty of this is that nature safely can become whatever the child wants or needs it to be. The following vignette of Matt is an example of symbolic play nature.

The Case of Matt: Metaphors in Nature

Matt lost his dad when he was four years old during a heart operation. Matt, who was five when he started play therapy, was incredibly angry. He blamed the doctor and hospital staff for "not saving my daddy." He also refused to talk about his feelings to anyone. He would simply say, "I am so mad" and then end the discussion. Knowing this, the therapist decided to take Matt outside where there was a small little creek next to the office. They sat on a log quietly next to the flowing water, allowing nature to begin to regulate Matt. As he sat there, Matt began to find small rocks around him and then threw them into the creek. The therapist noticed he was beginning to throw them harder and harder. Matt's play had begun. As he threw them, the therapist began to name what he was doing and the emotions that were beginning to surface. Together, the therapist and nature cofacilitated and coregulated Matt as his anger began to pour out. The next session, Matt wanted to go back out to the creek. This time he asked the therapist to help him collect a pile of small rocks and leaves. He then began to separate them telling the therapist that she could have the leaves, and he would have the rocks as they were about to go to war against each other. In the grass by the creek, Matt set up a war scene using the objects he found in nature. In the end, all the rocks and leaves "died" and "it just wasn't fair." The therapist and Matt spent many sessions creating stories that allowed him to express his feelings.

In this vignette, the therapist and nature helped Matt create the symbolic play he needed to begin to explore the trauma of losing his father during a medical procedure, instead of having him talk about it.

Case Study: Putting It All Together: Creating Safety in Nature for Shante' in Both an Indoor and Outdoor Setting

Earlier in this chapter, the case of Shante' was mentioned and will now be further explored.

Background and Treatment

As shared earlier in this chapter, both parents were very concerned about Shante's aggressive behavior at home and in school. They also felt their connection to her had grown more strained as she was challenging to connect with, often refusing nurturing. The therapist learned that Shante' had a congenital heart defect when she was an infant, which required surgery and a few days stay in the neonatal intensive care unit (NICU). Even though Shante' had a scar on her body, the family never discussed with her why it was there. However, a few months prior to Shante' beginning play therapy, she stumbled across pictures of herself as a baby in the NICU on her aunt's phone. This discovery prompted the beginning of her learning about her medical procedures early in her life.

Shante's situation is common for many families that are not offered guidance from medical professionals on the importance of talking to their child as they get older about their medical procedures. As a result, families are often left uneducated about the potential impact of medical trauma as well as how to talk to their child about their experience. The first intervention for Shante' was to learn as much about her medical story as possible, as well as educating her parents on how trauma is stored and expressed in the body. The therapist helped her parents understand that much of Shante's sympathetic fight/flight activation was connected to her body's defense system and was still alert from the various medical procedures she had experienced. The therapist also helped her parents understand that it was going to be important to help create a sense of safety for Shante' in therapy so that she could move towards the stored trauma and ultimately integrate it. As well, during intake, the therapist explored Shante's experience of nature with her mom, as well as prepping the mother for "Talk Time" (Higgins-Klein, 2013), which is an opening session check-in, as shown in the following section.

First Session

In her first session, Shante' came into the playroom and hid behind her mom as the therapist bent down to say hello. With wide open eyes, she peeked out from behind her mom, quietly watching the therapist. Mom stayed in the play therapy session as the therapy was also focused on their relationship and connection. The therapist, Shante', and mom sat in a circle for 10 minutes of Talk Time. Mom shared that she loved when she and Shante' snuggled at night reading a book and Shante' watched her and smiled shyly. When her mom shared that recently Shante' had learned about her heart surgery as a baby, Shante' yelled, "no, stop it, stop talking." The therapist then said out loud, "Wow, mom, this is too much to talk about, let's take a breath, and we can visit this story another time." Shante' then began to explore the playroom and discovered some heart-shaped stones that the therapist had collected on a nature walk. The therapist told her that sometimes children like to make designs on the stones and sometimes they don't. Shante' grabbed a marker and held the stone in one hand as she drew a circle on it. Next, from the bottom to the top of the circle, she forcefully drew a vertical line. She repeated this on some of the other heart stones that she had found until it was time to leave.

Therapist Impressions of First Session

As the therapist reflected on the session, she understood that visiting the medical trauma story directly did not feel safe and was outside of Shante's window of tolerance. Therefore, the therapist will be using the imaginary world of play and nature to help her work through her difficulties so that healing can occur. Ultimately, it will be important in future sessions for the therapist to help Shante' integrate her medical trauma story with a safe external regulator—nature.

Middle Phase

Over the next few weeks, several nature interventions were introduced to help Shante' begin to move toward the challenging feelings she held inside. Shante' continued drawing the circle with the line on the remaining heart stones and began a process of burying them deep in the wet sand tray. On one occasion, she used her fist and pushed down on top of the sand that was covering the heart stones trapping the hearts underneath. The therapist reflected back to her that the heart stones were trapped and couldn't move. Once finished, she crossed the room and picked up a one-inch tree trunk slice that was stacked by the art supplies and then began to paint it. As she painted, the therapist shared that trees are similar to people. She explained that just like a person's heart pumps blood throughout the body, trees have to pump water from their roots to their top. Shante' listened to this nature story while painting the tree slice. The therapist chose to begin to use the metaphor of the tree pumping water to help Shante' begin to connect to the workings of her own heart and continued using it throughout their sessions. As Shante' painted, the paints mixed together and the painting began to turn cloudy and dark. When she looked at what she had created, she frowned, and the therapist reflected to Shante', "I see your frown looking at the colors that were mixed to cloudy and dark." Shante' did not respond and the session time was finished. She left the playroom and the tree slice behind.

At the beginning of the next session, her mom mentioned that Shante' had started to go outside at home looking for heart stones. Following Shante's connection with nature and the heart stones, the therapist suggested they go outside the office to hunt for more. As they walked around looking for heart stones, Shante' began to get sad as wherever they searched, no heart stones were found. To help Shante' regulate, the therapist named the sadness of not being able to find the hearts. Shante' sat down in the grass while saying, "A big angry storm came and washed them away." The therapist and her mom sat down with her and Shante' began quietly touching the grass and playing with the dandelions. As the therapist noticed this, she helped Shante' to begin to tune into her senses of touch/feel, smell, sound, and sight by inviting her to notice her experiences.

As nature and the therapist worked together to coregulate Shante', the therapist then wondered out loud the different feelings the heart stones may have had being washed away by the angry storm. Shante' continued to play with the grass and the dandelions as she listened. She then took an exhale sigh and laid back on the grass for further support as she thought about it. Noticing that Shante' was actively regulating herself and thus activating her ventral system allowing her to be with the challenging thoughts, feelings and sensations that were arising, the therapist asked Shante' if it was okay for mom to tell a small part of the story from when she was a baby needing her heart surgery. Shante' nodded yes and listened. As mom shared, Shante' continued to lay on the grass feeling the grass and dandelions in her hand allowing nature to help regulate her.

Later Phases

The next few sessions were also outside. Sometimes Shante', her mom and the therapist would take a walk together, sometimes they would take the art supplies outside and paint something they found in nature and sometimes they would sit on the grass and play with the flowers. In each session outside, when the therapist would take a moment and ask her if they could visit the story from when she was a baby, nature supported Shante'. During each sharing, Shante's window of tolerance expanded allowing for more parts of her story to be heard. Her mom also began to report less anger outbursts at home and at school. She also noticed that Shante's ability to tolerate transitions was easier on days the family spent time outside. Most importantly, her mom shared that Shante' had begun asking questions about her heart surgery and teaching her friends that trees have a heart to pump water.

Final Sessions

On her third to last session, Shante' began to hide the heart stones that she had drawn on around the room and then telling her mom she had to find them. Shante' announced that the angry storm had taken the heart stones and trapped them around the room. As mom looked for the heart stones, she found some trapped under pillows, some trapped under toys, and some trapped under the sand in the sandtray. As she found them, she untrapped them while telling them how special and important they were and how they were now safe. Each time one was discovered and freed, Shante' would smile.

In her final session, Shante' asked if she could paint on the tree trunk slices again. As she painted, the colors once again turned cloudy and stormy, but this time instead of frowning, she had an idea and smiled as she finished her nature art. Shante' had painted a bright beautiful rainbow on top of the dark colors and right in the middle, she had glued one of her heart stones with the circle and the line. The therapist reflected what she saw in the picture aloud and noticed Shante's smile. Throughout the final session, they shared stories about their adventures in therapy together with what they liked, what they will miss and what was hard. In the last 10 minutes of the session, Shante' quickly painted another tree slice and glued on another heart stone with a line on it. When completed, Shante' gave the second tree slice and heart drawing to the therapist. The session time was done and they walked out smiling together.

Case Reflection

Shante's therapeutic process takes us on a journey through the use of nature to facilitate the integration of her traumatic medical experience. Discovered underneath Shante's aggressive behaviors were frightening medical experiences that registered as overwhelming to her nervous system. The therapist and "cotherapist" nature became the external regulator to help Shante' move from a state of chaos in her nervous system to regulation, which helped her integrate the traumatic medical experience. Shante's behavior at school improved and she began to ask for help from her teacher when frustrated. Shante's parents were grateful to have more moments of connection with their daughter and be a part of her therapy journey. The parents were also relieved to understand the root of the problem and felt confident in the tools they developed in therapy to help Shante'. They continued to make sure as a family they had nature experiences throughout the week as that became essential in Shante's healing process.

Chapter Summary

Creating experiences for emotional and relational safety is an integral part of trauma integration. Without a felt sense of safety, children have a much harder time approaching the uncomfortable thoughts, feelings, and body sensations that are held inside. Nature has the remarkable ability to create safety for trauma integration as it can be both an external regulator for a child's activated nervous system and safely access the stored trauma in the child's body. Whether nature is incorporated into the playroom or outside in a play therapy session, nature can also offer therapists a range of creative interventions from which to work from. This chapter explored the use of nature in a variety of ways to help regulate children and their families as they processed the traumatic experiences they had been through. A specific focus on medical trauma was used in the examples as medical trauma is often overlooked. In each example, nature became an integral part of the treatment process as it held, supported, rocked, and ultimately created the safety needed for deep integration and healing.

Reflective Questions

As this chapter discusses the healing power of nature and its extraordinary ability to create safety and become an external regulator for trauma integration, it is important that practitioners take the time to reflect on their own experiences of nature. Taking the time to mindfully reflect and experience the therapeutic power of nature itself allows practitioners to open up new possibilities of how it may be used in play sessions. Much like any other tool or intervention, a practitioner would bring into a play therapy session (art, sandtray, puppets, etc.), if the practitioner does not know what the intervention can do or what it has the potential of eliciting inside the child, the therapist has a higher probability of not using the intervention effectively or at minimum not using it at its full potential. For these reasons, therapists are encouraged to try the following interventions from the Nature Interventions for Creating Safety sections and then reflect on the following.

1   Nature Photographs. Find a few nature photographs that elicit a feeling of groundedness, connection, and regulation for you. As you look at these photographs, notice what happens inside of your body. At a later time when your fight/flight/immobilization is activated, look at the nature photographs that you have found. Once again notice what happens inside of your body as you take in the nature imagery, allowing the nature photographs to become your external regulator. Make sure to take time to reflect on the power the nature photographs had on the activation of your autonomic nervous system and how they may create emotional safety for you (see Appendix B).

2   Gestalt Nature Dialogue. With something to write, find a comfortable place outside. As you look around, find something in nature that you feel drawn to. Start with writing what you would like to say to your nature object and then imagine its response back to you. Write it down. Continue this dialogue until you feel complete with this activity. Once complete, take time to reflect on the following questions: What was the experience like for you? What was the message the nature object gave you? What did your body feel like as you were having the dialogue? Once again notice, how nature was able to create safety and regulation for you (see Appendix C).

3   Nature Sounds. Find a time to sit quietly and explore various nature sounds. As you listen to different sounds, allow yourself to get curious about how each sound affects you emotionally and where you feel the sounds in your body. Experiment with listening to sounds outside in nature, as well as recorded nature sounds inside. When inside, also explore wearing headphones. As you engage in these activities, reflect on how the sounds can create safety and regulation for you (see Appendix D).

Appendix A

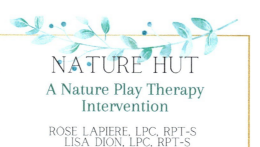

NATURE HUT
A Nature Play Therapy Intervention

ROSE LAPIERE, LPC, RPT-S
LISA DION, LPC, RPT-S

DESCRIPTION:

Children love building forts and creating places to hide, seek refuge, and feel protected.

SUPPLIES NEEDED:

Identify a part of a wall inside the playroom that can be used for the sticks to lean on
Sticks a few feet longer than the child's height
Smaller branches, flowers, leaves, and pinecones
Blanket, pillows, or cushion

GOAL:

Provides anchoring and safety as child visits traumatic memories.

INSTRUCTIONS:

The therapist and child collect the nature items together (the preferred way for this intervention), or the therapist can have the nature items prepared in advance. Once all the items have been collected the therapist helps the child lay a blanket down where the hut will be created. The larger branches are propped up against the wall creating an "A" shape. Next, the smaller branches are leaned on the larger branches creating the hut. For the final step, cover the frame with flowers, leaves, or pinecones. If outside is an option this can also be created against a tree. The therapist can ask the child to tune into their senses. Some questions might include: What does it smell like inside the nature hut? What is the temperature like inside the nature hut? Is there anything that you can touch while inside the hut? What does it feel like? What do you notice in your body as you sit inside?

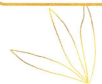

EXTRA FUN:

Pick a stuffed animal or figure that could be used to help explore the nature hut as an invitation for the child to do the same.

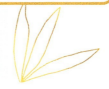

Appendix B

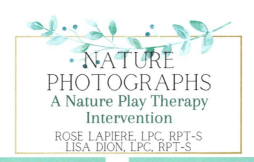

NATURE PHOTOGRAPHS
A Nature Play Therapy Intervention
ROSE LAPIERE, LPC, RPT-S
LISA DION, LPC, RPT-S

DESCRIPTION:

Viewing nature photographs can provide a grounding experience and help a client to become regulated.

SUPPLIES NEEDED:

Nature photographs

GOAL:

Nature as an external regulator, and grounding

INSTRUCTIONS:

Find a few nature photographs that elicit a feeling of groundedness, connection, and regulation. As you look at these photographs, notice what happens inside of your body. At a later time when your fight/flight/immobilization is activated, look at the nature photographs that you have found. Once again notice what happens inside of your body as you take in the nature imagery, allowing the nature photographs to become your external regulator. Make sure to take time to reflect on the power the nature photographs had on the activation of your autonomic nervous system and how they may create emotional safety for you.

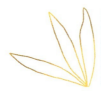

EXTRA FUN:
Try to find a nature setting that looks like your favorite photo. Notice what it feels like in your body to immerse yourself in that setting. Take photos to remember that feeling.

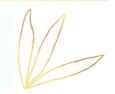

Appendix C

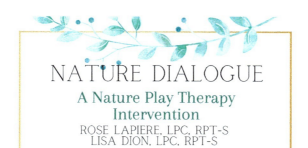

NATURE DIALOGUE
A Nature Play Therapy Intervention
ROSE LAPIERE, LPC, RPT-S
LISA DION, LPC, RPT-S

DESCRIPTION:

Gestalt Dialoguing with nature allows connection between nature and the client. The dialoguing helps with expression of feelings, awareness of possibilities on how to view a problem and a offers nature as the external regulator.

SUPPLIES NEEDED:

Pen/marker

Paper / notebook

A blanket or yoga mat

Pick a spot outside by a tree or flowers

GOAL:

Express feelings, nature as an external regulator

INSTRUCTIONS:

With something to write with, find a comfortable place outside. As you look around, find something in nature that you feel drawn to. Start with writing what you would like to say to your nature object and then imagine its response back to you. Write it down. Continue this dialogue until you feel complete with this activity. Once complete, take time to reflect on the following questions: What was the experience like for you? What was the message the nature object gave you? and What did your body feel like as you were having the dialogue? Once again notice, how nature was able to create safety and regulation for you.

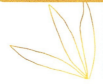

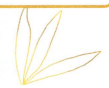

EXTRA PROCESSING:

When writing to your nature item chose a problem to ask for help. Notice what emerges as you reflect back when complete.

Appendix D

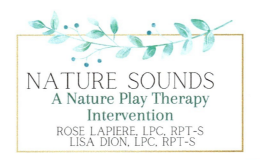

NATURE SOUNDS
A Nature Play Therapy Intervention
ROSE LAPIERE, LPC, RPT-S
LISA DION, LPC, RPT-S

DESCRIPTION:

Soothing nature sounds are a wonderful way to help clients regulate their nervous system. Explore a a variety of nature sounds that can be utilized during times of stress.

SUPPLIES NEEDED:

Headphones (optional)

Electronic device with the ability to access a variety of at least 10 different nature sounds

Paper and Pens

GOAL:
To increase a sense of safety and understand states of arousal

INSTRUCTIONS:

Have access to at least 10 nature sounds. The sounds can be pre-recorded directly from nature or accessed from music apps. Locations to search for nature sounds include https://www.naturesoundmap.com which has nature sounds recorded from all over the world. For younger children, create a playlist of soothing nature sounds and play it in the background of their play therapy sessions. For teens, listening to specific nature sounds while working through their trauma can be incredibly impactful. In both situations, the nature sounds help hold the space for the child to approach the uncomfortable thoughts, feelings, and sensations they have inside.

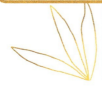
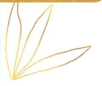

EXTRA FUN:
If comfortable, invite the child to close their eyes and feel as though they are in that nature environment.

References

Alvarsson, J. J., Wiens, S., & Nilsson, M. E. (2010). Stress recovery during exposure to nature sound and environmental noise. *International Journal of Environmental Research and Public Health*, 7(3), 1036–1046. https://doi.org/10.3390/ijerph7031036

American Psychological Association. (n.d.). Trauma and shock. Retrieved on February 14, 2021, from https://www.apa.org/topics/trauma.

Badenoch, B. (2017). *The Heart of Trauma: Healing the Embodied Brain in the Context of Relationships (Norton Series on Interpersonal Neurobiology)* (1st ed.). W. W. Norton & Company.

Berger, R. (2017). Nature therapy: Incorporating nature into arts therapy. *Journal of Humanistic Psychology*, 60(2), 244–257. https://doi.org/10.1177/0022167817696828

Berger, R., & McLeod, J. (2006). Incorporating nature into therapy: A framework for practice. *Journal of Systemic Therapies*, 25(2), 80–94. https://doi.org/10.1521/jsyt.2006.25.2.80

Bratman, G. N., Daily, G. C., Levy, B. J., & Gross, J. J. (2015). The benefits of nature experience: Improved affect and cognition. *Landscape and Urban Planning*, 138, 41–50. https://doi.org/10.1016/j.landurbplan.2015.02.005

Dana, D. (2018). *The Polyvagal Theory in Therapy: Engaging the Rhythm of Regulation*. W. W. Norton & Company.

Delahooke, M. (2019). *Beyond Behaviors: Using Brain Science and Compassion to Understand and Solve Children's Behavioral Challenges* (1st ed.). PESI Publishing.

Dion, L. (2018). *Aggression in Play Therapy: A Neurobiological Approach for Integrating Intensity* (1st ed.). W. W. Norton & Company.

Gould van Praag, C. D., Garfinkel, S. N., Sparasci, O., Mees, A., Philippides, A. O., Ware, M., Ottaviani, C., & Critchley, H. D. (2017). Mind-wandering and alterations to default mode network connectivity when listening to naturalistic versus artificial sounds. *Scientific Reports*, 7(1), 1–12. https://doi.org/10.1038/srep45273

Higgins-Klein, D. (2013). *Mindfulness-Based Play-family: Theory and Practice*. W.W. Norton & Company.

Maller, C. J., Henderson-Wilson, C., & Townsend, M. (2009). Rediscovering nature in everyday settings: Or how to create healthy environments and healthy people. *EcoHealth*, 6(4), 553–556. https://doi.org/10.1007/s10393-010-0282-5

National Child Traumatic Stress Network. (n.d.). Trauma types. Retrieved December 1, 2020, from https://www.nctsn.org/what-is-child-trauma/about-child-trauma.

Oaklander, V. (2007). *Windows to Our Children*. The Gestalt Journal Press.

Ogden, P., Minton, K., & Pain, C. (2006). *Trauma and the Body: A Sensorimotor Approach to Psychotherapy*. W.W. Norton & Company, Inc.

Porges, S. W. (2011). *The Polyvagal Theory: Neurophysiological Foundations of Emotions, Attachment, Communication, and Self-regulation (Norton Series on Interpersonal Neurobiology)* (Illustrated ed.). W. W. Norton & Company.

Schore, A. N. (2019). *Right Brain Psychotherapy*. New York, NY: Norton

Siegel, D. J. (2020). *The Developing Mind: How Relationships and the Brain Interact to Shape Who We Are* (3rd ed.). New York, NY: Guilford Press.

Twohig-Bennett, C., & Jones, A. (2018). The health benefits of the great outdoors: A systematic review and meta-analysis of greenspace exposure and health outcomes. *Environmental Research*, 166, 628–637. https://doi.org/10.1016/j.envres.2018.06.030

Van der Kolk, B. (2015). *The Body Keeps the Score: Brain, Mind, and Body in the Healing of Trauma* (Illustrated ed.). Penguin Books.

Weber, S. T., & Heuberger, E. (2008). The impact of natural odors on affective states in humans. *Chemical Senses*, 33(5), 441–447. https://doi.org/10.1093/chemse/bjn011

Wohlleben, P. (2019). *Can You Hear the Trees Talking?: Discovering the Hidden Life of the Forest* (Illustrated ed.). Greystone Kids.

8 The Integration of Nature-Based Play and EMDR Therapies in the Aftermath of Trauma

Jackie Flynn

Introduction

Playing in nature offers a natural balance of the nervous system when one experiences dysregulation from trauma, much like how the earth acts as an external regulator when excess electricity needs a grounded space to travel to prevent dangerous electrical overloads. Trauma changes how the brain functions and develops. Since the brain does not reach full maturity until around the age of 25, it is important for child and adolescent trauma therapists to use therapies that are not exclusively reliant on words, since development of language and speech are still in the works. Since nature-based play and expressive therapies do not require higher-level thinking or insightful moments, it can increase the positive effects of EMDR therapy. Play therapy facilitates communication, fosters emotional wellness, enhances social relationships, and increases personal strengths (Schaefer & Drewes, 2014). This can especially occur in natural environments.

Trauma also influences how children and adolescents approach their world. An array of emotional and behavioral challenges for the client, as well as their family system, may stem from their trauma if left unprocessed. Through the integration of EMDR and nature-based play therapy, clients' trauma can sometimes be resolved relatively quickly, varying from person to person. The practical play-based applications of the therapeutic use of natural elements with children and adolescents will be explored in this chapter through the integration of nature-based play and EMDR therapies. This integrative approach allows mental health therapists to support children and adolescent clients through the reprocessing of traumatic events that could otherwise leave them feeling emotionally stuck for years, impacting the way they approach their world.

It is important to note that people, regardless of age, have varying levels of stress resilience. What traumatizes one person may only be a difficult experience without any lasting effects for another. Regardless of the severity of experienced trauma, EMDR and nature-based play therapy can support adaptive resolution through reprocessing the distressing circumstances and traumatic memories.

EMDR Therapy and Trauma

Eye Movement Desensitization and Reprocessing (EMDR) Therapy is an eight-phase trauma treatment approach: History Taking, Preparation, Assessment, Desensitization, Reprocessing, Body Scan, Closure, and Re-evaluation. In 1987, Francine Shapiro, Ph.D., developed EMDR therapy after she experienced a reduction of distress associated with walking and eye movements following the realization of a disturbing circumstance in her life (Shapiro, 2017). Since that time, EMDR therapy has grown and evolved from primarily treating veterans into an internationally delivered therapy used to treat a range of issues troubling children and adults. Essentially, EMDR reduces emotionality and sensory intensity associated in the aftermath of trauma, therefore allowing people to live more fully.

A hallmark of EMDR therapy is the Adaptive Information Processing (AIP) model. The AIP model posits that maladaptively stored traumatic memories can limit one's capacity to attain adaptive resolve (Shapiro, 2017). In other words, the aftermath of trauma can negatively impact one's life. Through EMDR therapy, clients of all ages often attain adaptive resolution of their distressing memories, even ones from as early as development in the womb, through its eight phases. Often adaptive resolution can occur rapidly.

DOI: 10.4324/9781003152767-11

Distressing and disturbing events, also referred to as trauma, can especially affect children and adolescents. Traumatized children and teens often present their unprocessed trauma emotionally, cognitively, physically, and relationally. These may present as tantrums, school refusal, promiscuity, self-harming behavior, drug use, bullying, disordered eating, and other life-limiting maladaptive behaviors. Family systems especially experience disruptions, as trauma can greatly impact close relationships through a narrowing of the window of tolerance and reluctance to be vulnerable.

Since emotional memories can begin in utero, cognitive awareness of the touchstone traumatic event(s) or originating circumstances is not always accessible. Arthur Janov's book *Imprints* (1984) postulates that preverbal trauma is held in the nervous system into adulthood. By design, EMDR is a directive approach that requires the integration of nondirective elements to support practical application with children. This the "bottom-up" benefits of nature and play is ideal. For the purpose of this chapter, the term bottom-up processing is used to describe a focus on helping children and adolescents experience a "neuroception of safety", a phrase coined by Stephen Porges to describe the felt sense of safety without conscious awareness (Dana & Porges, 2018). Without a felt sense of safety, clients' progress can be greatly reduced, or in some cases, nonexistent, especially when it comes to working with children and adolescents.

Increasing Stabilization Through Nature-Based Play and Expressive Therapies

Nature-based play and expressive therapies provide a seemingly limitless amount of sensory-rich experiential opportunities. The outdoor environment is abundant with sounds, sight, smells, textures, and sometimes tastes. Grounding through the senses naturally supports stabilization as many traumatized children and adolescents experience a sense of disconnect and sometimes symptoms of dissociation. When a child creates a fort out of branches and palm fronds to keep out the "bad guys" while confidently climbing a tree, he or she experiences a sense of control and safety as he or she plays out his or her traumatic experience of feeling powerless and vulnerable. Through this type of nature-based play, children can be dually aware as they simultaneously remain present through the tangible sensation of the natural elements. EMDR processing, by design, supports a dual focus of attention as they remain in the present while processing trauma from the past or perceived future (Parnell, 2007).

Kinesthetic touch, perhaps the most functional method to stabilize, is especially helpful when it comes to healing from trauma. Touch is directly connected to the central nervous system and is considered our primary sense of experience (Courtney, 2020). When a child explores their natural world through play, organic emotional stabilization can occur. Stabilization is a key component of EMDR therapy, especially with children. In the history taking and preparation phases of EMDR, clinicians determine if the client is ready to proceed through an assessment of adequate affect regulation skills & resources to remain stable.

Nature offers stabilization and safety, which is essential throughout the EMDR Therapy process. Through an abundance of sensory rich experiences that are accessible in natural environments, traumatized children may struggle to move quickly toward adaptive resolution in an effort to make sense of their distressing memories due to their limited life experiences. Without a sense of stability and safety, such as what nature has to offer, trauma work can quickly cause great amounts of distress. Grounding child and teen clients by facilitating a connection with the earth through the safety of play as part of the therapeutic process, whether in real-time or through visualization, greatly supports attainment of emotional equilibrium in an otherwise dysregulated state.

Nature-based play helps children clients expand their window of tolerance as they reprocess their trauma(s) in a developmentally appropriate way. Playing in nature or with natural elements of nature supports their capacity to stabilize through the anchoring elements of sensory intake. It is important to realize that nature-based play therapy can occur individually and in groups. Research findings revealed that group nature-based play therapy increased participants' on-task behaviors and decreased total problems as measured in the study (Swank & Shin, 2015).

Play and nature combined support dual awareness, which is basically the capacity to be present with current safety and the distressing memories simultaneously. Nature can provide a sense of grounding to contain intense feelings, overwhelming body sensations, and thoughts. Natural environments reduce the parasympathetic nervous system, therefore decreasing stress and an overall feeling of well-being (Ewert et al., 2016). In this author's experience, EMDR sessions conducted outdoors tend to reduce the occurrence of abreactions, a strong level of emotional disturbance during EMDR reprocessing, since nature-based play offers a high level of stability through an abundance of resource development opportunities. For example, as a child playfully climbs atop a large rock to play out the role of a ship captain venturing upon a new land curious about the unknown with a sense of power and control, he or she may also feel the fear of the unknown. This is coupled with the release of somatically stored material in his or her body as he or she is metaphorically expressing a recent residential move where they left much loved family and friends to venture into the unknown circumstances of a new environment through play.

Traumatized children tend to initially approach nature much differently than children who have not experienced trauma. For these clients, gradually introducing nature elements into the sessions can be helpful. There are some exceptions, but for the most part many traumatized children and adolescents present with a dysregulated state at first. They will often relax overtime as the natural elements support a greater sense of well-being. Many clients experience a state change after they have been outdoors for a short duration. Play in nature naturally supports a state change as it offers children many opportunities to test physical and emotional limits from trauma, while it increases their capacity for emotional and physical expression. Increasing the capacity to change states is important, especially while experiencing EMDR therapy.

It is crucial for clinicians to respect the clients' wishes when it comes to going outdoors. Assertively demanding the integration of nature into a child's therapeutic work when the client is resistant to the idea of going outside could potentially strain or rupture the valuable therapeutic relationship. Maintaining the therapeutic relationship is essential. Empathic responses to clients' communication of felt danger creates a neuroception of safety that can ultimately cultivate trust. Another consideration for clinicians is to ensure privacy and confidentiality as much as possible, as implementing nature-based play and expressive therapy sessions in outdoor spaces could result in being seen by others.

Integrating EMDR With Nature-Based Play and Expressive Therapies

EMDR integrates quite well with other therapies, especially with nature-based play and expressive therapies. These nature-based therapies can occur outside, with the client and therapist physically immersed in the natural outdoor environment, as well as indoors through art and playful activities involving elements of nature such as leaves, stones, twigs, sand, and such.

As part of EMDR therapy, clinicians support clients with the reprocessing of traumatic memories that come with associations, such as memories, images, emotions, body sensations, and cognitions. EMDR therapists are trained to adequately prepare clients for therapy through the development and strengthening of resources to support the reprocessing of distressing material (Shapiro, 2017). Nature is abundant in resources both metaphorically and literally strengthening positive cognitions. For example, climbing on and hiding under a fallen tree can represent "I can handle this" and "I am safe." Mindfully exploring little ants as they create a mound can represent "I can do difficult things" or "I am strong." Creating the face of a nurturing figure with sticks, acorns, and leaves can support the "I am lovable" or "I am worthy" cognitions.

EMDR is an ideal treatment approach for children, especially as it integrates so well with nature-based play and expressive therapies. Children are not miniature adults and can greatly benefit from developmentally appropriate therapeutic approaches incorporating nature. Nature-based play and expressive therapies provide a seemingly unlimited number of options that far surpass the preparation phase of EMDR. Children can express memories, images, and emotions through nature-based play to greatly support the assessment phase of EMDR. This has included drawing pictures in the sand on the beach to illustrate an image that represents the worst part of a memory, choosing an element of nature to represent a positive thought about themselves such as "I'm like a tree because I can stand tall even when it storms", or measuring their level of disturbance associated with a memory by stacking rocks and pebbles up to show "how big it feels right now."

Wide-open natural spaces can also provide a plethora of opportunities for healing movement in therapy, which is necessary especially when working with children suffering from trauma related to immobilization. Through movement, stored energy from the trauma is naturally released (Levine, 1997). EMDR clinicians therapeutically use movement intentionally in therapy to engage children in bilateral stimulation. While many adults tend to remain in the same spot during EMDR sessions, child and teen clients may run, stop, or hop for their bilateral stimulation experience. The bilateral stimulation conducted rapidly is used to desensitize and reprocess identified targets throughout the therapy sessions. In the desensitization and reprocessing phases of EMDR therapy, both hemispheres of the brain are stimulated to support the integration of somatically stored materials. This may be accomplished through visual, tactile, or auditory means, which are known as the mechanisms of action (Shapiro, 2017). Clients may organically engage in bilateral stimulation in natural environments through their innate playful movements that involve scanning of their eyes while watching as they hop from one object to the next, by running and climbing through the movement of their arms and legs alternately, as well as other means that naturally occur while playing outside in wide open spaces. Playing in nature offers a seemingly limitless number of opportunities for children and teens to engage in bilateral stimulation spontaneously.

Creative, unstructured play, whether outside or inside using natural elements, allows for the expansion of clients' capacity for emotional expression while experiencing the grounding effects that nature has to offer. Emotional expression is a vital component of reprocessing trauma in therapy. Nature offers such a wide range of options when it comes to expression via art, movement, and more. Children create images with natural elements, playout disturbing memories such as tucking under a large rock to feel safe, move their bodies, and express themselves loudly and messily if necessary.

Playing in nature raises sensory awareness and supports immersion into the present moment, which can lead to feelings of aliveness (Cornell, 2018). Traumatized children and teens often struggle with presence. In other words, they may appear to be preoccupied and disconnected from their surroundings. Trauma may lead to intense hypervigilance, excessive worry, and limited capacity to connect. The outdoor natural environment is stocked with an unlimited amount of potential expressive arts materials such as leaves, twigs, bark, stones, sand, and more. In nature-based play and expressive therapy sessions, children and adolescents can become immersed in the present moment while experiencing somatic activation from their trauma(s), which is conducive to regulation, as well as connectedness to self and others. Nature can serve as an external regulator to support their capacity to move back into their window of tolerance.

When a child experiences a neuroception of safety, he or she tends to be more adaptable to change, open to learning new things, connected to others and naturally curious. The phrase "neuroception of safety", coined by Porges in regard to the polyvagal theory, refers to inner feelings of safety without conscious awareness (Dana & Porges, 2018). When working with children and adolescents in therapy, it is especially important for clinicians to provide as many cues of safety as possible, such as predictability, presence, gentle tones, and playfulness. This is especially the case for predictability, as the unknown can feel unsafe, resulting in a neuroception of danger. Natural environments are ideal for creating a neuroception of safety, especially in children. Responding to the innate need for connection to natural spaces through outside play organically creates cues of safety as healing from trauma, to reduce the rigidity and hypervigilance that is often experienced by traumatized children and teens.

The therapeutic relationship that can develop between a child and their therapist in play therapy treatment can provide a deep level of healing that is not reliant on words. Play and expressive therapies often surpass the limitation of words. There are several benefits of playing, especially in the aftermath of trauma. Schaefer and Drewes (2014) categorized the therapeutic powers of play in four major areas as: facilitating communication, fostering wellness, enhancing personal relationships, and increasing personal strengths. Whether conducted inside or outside, these therapeutic benefits of play are abundant. Outdoor nature-based play and expressive therapy sessions, however, offer additional benefits such as groundedness, (also referred to as earthing), enhanced dual awareness and increased mental clarity through the senses. This author has experienced that traumatized children especially benefit from playing in natural environments as they are able to move around more freely and connect with nature. Even a brief amount of time spent outside, whether directive with a specific activity or indirective as free play, can greatly support therapeutic goals.

There are additional areas where nature may assist presentations of trauma-related symptomatology. Since children and adolescents' brains are not fully developed, some may only complain of body-related symptoms. Somatically stored material through the felt sense of emotions in the body from the trauma can greatly affect how some may feel emotionally and physically. Common phrases such as "my tummy hurts," "my head hurts,' "I feel sick," and other verbal expressions relating to distressing body sensations can occur. Often, unknowing parents and caregivers may attempt to avoid the task at hand, such as going to school, playing in a sport, and such, to relieve the physical symptom. However, the child may actually be experiencing one of the many facets of trauma. For this reason, many clinicians educate parents and caregivers on the effects of trauma, as well as recommend that parents play with their children outside as a way to support a change of state for their child and teen clients.

Indoor sessions may limit movement due to the confinement of walls. Nature-based play therapy sessions that occur outdoors allow children to run, climb, and jump in natural spaces that incorporate needed movement. Somatic releases of traumatically stored material in the body occur as children playfully explore natural elements outside such as lifting rocks, climbing over things, running as they play games or acting out imaginative experiences. This physical movement while playing outdoors in therapy can greatly support the processing of trauma, as one of the biggest struggles that children and adolescents experience in the aftermath of trauma is feeling trapped or stuck in their arousal states. Often the movement that nature-based therapy facilitates supports the reprocessing as it releases the associated stored energy in the body. Their adaptability, openness, and ability to handle stress narrows as they remain stuck over time. Often, trauma is at the root of intense behaviors described by parents as irritable, panicky, and anxious characteristics without the ability to calm while struggling with deep despair, expressing inner resistance, and experiencing a neuroception of danger without the capacity to muster the energy nor the motivation to get things done. Sometimes traumatized children and adolescents alternate between these two states quickly and erratically. EMDR therapy delivered in natural spaces outdoors can support movement back into the window of tolerance to support optimal functioning.

Another important element of EMDR therapy is the closing playful movement can substantially support state changes of the body (Beckley-Forest & Monaco, 2020). EMDR clinicians mindfully close out therapy sessions with child and teen clients to intentionally orient them back to the present to facilitate stability. In this author's experience, the EMDR reprocessing is often much more effective when delivered outdoors in nature than in an indoor play therapy space.

Case Study

(Identifying details have been changed to respect client confidentiality.)

Narrative Background

Grace, a 13-year-old female, was scheduled for EMDR therapy for symptoms of social anxiety seemingly stemming from early childhood traumatic experiences following the finalization of her adoption. Her parents reported frequent intense emotional tantrums and school refusals that have occurred as early as three weeks of moving into the family home. The parents further described Grace's struggles in crowded social situations with a presentation of panic and disconnect, sometimes accompanied by nausea, vomiting, and stated feelings of light-headedness. Grace recently began refusing to attend school after her math teacher called on her to answer questions in front of the class, in which she burst into tears and ran out of the classroom to call her parents seeking early release from school.

Beginning EMDR Treatment Phases

In the initial EMDR sessions, a thorough history was taken during sessions with and without Grace present to gain a thorough conceptualization of her case. A list of potential areas to address, also known as a Target Sequence Plan, was developed and presented to the parents during a parent consultation session. Determination of the suitability for Grace to proceed with EMDR therapy was made during a participative discussion with parents as a thorough exploration of other events occurring in her life, her capacity to emotionally regulate and any pertinent resources to help her remain stable. The therapist and parents discussed how the integration of nature-based play therapy and EMDR could provide a sense of safety and equilibrium throughout the process. The parents agreed to pursue her treatment.

During the preparation phase of EMDR, Grace and her therapist spent approximately 15 minutes outside behind the office. Reciprocally, both Grace and the therapist playfully noticed elements in nature through the five senses while engaging in a mindfulness activity. As the activity progressed, a noticeable state change occurred as evidenced in Grace's body posture and movement. She appeared to be more relaxed as shown by the fluidity of her movements. In the following two sessions, Grace and her therapist progressively spent longer amounts of time outside tossing an emotional thumb ball back and forth, creating mandalas in an outdoor sandbox, and blowing bubbles. One of her initial sessions occurred during a rainy day so Grace showed interest in the natural elements (stones, sticks, and leaves) when directed to create a calm place. Her calm place was a beach scene. She mindfully explored elements of her beach scene through a sensory focused visualization of it as she described accompanying sounds, sights, textures, tastes, and smells. In the same indoor session, she also created a container with natural clay as a space for her to visualize putting her worries and thoughts in until she was ready to work through them. All the while, the therapeutic relationship between Grace and her therapist strengthened as she increasingly initiated communication with her therapist and presented with eagerness to attend sessions.

It was at this point that the therapist determined that Grace was indeed able to proceed with reprocessing the targets identified on her target sequence plan. Since the therapist knew that Grace loved the beach, she suggested that their next session occur early morning around the time of sunrise a local beach. Grace and her parents agreed.

Transitioning EMDR Therapy to a Beach Setting

The sessions on the beach were as confidential as possible, without any noticeable indication that Grace was engaging in a therapy session while her parents waited in the car. During one session, Grace and her therapist sat cross-legged in the sand for a brief assessment to identify key components of a painful memory of her biological father shaming her in the school carloop line several years prior. Grace began to lightly cry as the therapist asked her what the worst part was. She identified the worst part as the sound of laughter from her peers in the background. The therapist directed her to draw an image in the sand with her fingers to illustrate the worst part of her peers laughing. Grace drew five stick figures depicting the scene with her finger in the sand, then quickly erased it with her hand. The therapist then named potential associated emotions of embarrassment, humiliation, hurt, betrayal, anger, sadness, and overwhelm. Grace confirmed the accuracy of the named emotions and added that she felt really scared as well. The therapist then asked her to scan her body to find where she felt the emotions. Grace reported that she felt like crying in her eyes, a knot in her throat, and a heaviness in her chest. The client was then asked if the negative thought about herself was "I am shameful," which Grace then nodded her head with a "yes" motion as tears slowly rolled down her face. The therapist then asked her how activated the felt sense was on a scale of 0 (neutral) to 10 (the most intense) and Grace reported that it felt like an eight. The therapist then asked her what she would rather believe about herself instead of "I am shameful" and she said that she did not know. The therapist suggested the positive cognition, "I'm good enough" and Grace said that she would like to believe that, but it "did not feel true at all."

The therapist described to Grace that she would ask her to hold an image and a thought in her mind while walking on the edge of the water. She was directed to notice what came up in her mind and what she felt in her body. The therapist asked Grace not to talk while they were walking, but to merely just walk in silence until she was directed to stop. At that time Grace was directed to briefly describe what she was feeling or any thoughts in her mind. Then, they walked together to the water's edge to begin the reprocessing of her target memory. At that time, the therapist directed her to think of the stick figures that she drew in the sand and the "I am shameful" thought. Then, both Grace and her therapist began walking vigorously for about two minutes, and when the therapist stopped walking. During the pauses in their walk, the following conversation continued:

Therapist: "What are you noticing now?" [For about the first eight stops, Grace replied with a comment that suggested related distress.]

Grace: "That's how his dad talks to him. He hates his dad because he was so mean to him. I know he loves me though. He just doesn't know how to be a dad, that's all. I don't care if those kids were laughing. It's none of their business anyway."

Therapist: "Can you go back to the memory of the carloop incident and rate how distressing it felt in her body at that time."

Each time they paused, Grace's level of distress associated with the memory, also known as the subjective unit of distress, or SUD in EMDR language, lowered as the reprocessing continued until it was down to an identified "zero" with no associated disturbance. At that time, the therapist asked Grace if the thought "I'm good enough" still matched what she would like to believe about herself when she thought about that memory and Grace confirmed that it was an accurate positive cognition. Grace mentioned another positive cognition as well, "I'm a good kid." The therapist then asked her to write it in the packed sand near the shoreline with her finger (Figure 8.1).

Once Grace had done so, she was asked how true it felt on a scale from one (not true at all) to seven (the most true) when she thought about that memory in the carloop with her father. Grace said that it felt like a seven, the rating of most true. They both engaged in a butterfly hug, crossing their arms on their chest and tapping on either shoulder alternatively. With 15 minutes to spare in the session, the therapist and Grace built a rudimentary sandcastle in the sand, while they chatted about something unrelated to the target memory of her father yelling in the carpool line. At the end of the session, both were smiling and ready for the rest of the day (Figure 8.2).

In the following session, the therapist lightly described the same memory of the session to Grace and asked her to scan her body for any tightness, tension, or unusual sensations. Grace reported that she did not feel anything and asked if they could play outside again. Grace and her therapist continued to use EMDR and nature-based play and expressive therapies to reprocess her targets in sessions. Parents reported that the frequency and intensity of her tantrums had reduced, while they noticed an increase in flexibility in social interactions. For additional creative ideas for how to integrate nature play into the phases of EMDR therapy, refer to Appendixes A, B, and C ["I AM LIKE A ...", "NOTICING NATURE", "NATURAL ART EXPRESSIONS"].

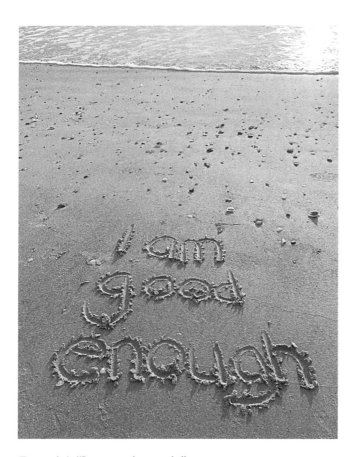

Figure 8.1 "I am good enough."

Source: Photo courtesy of author, Jackie Flynn.

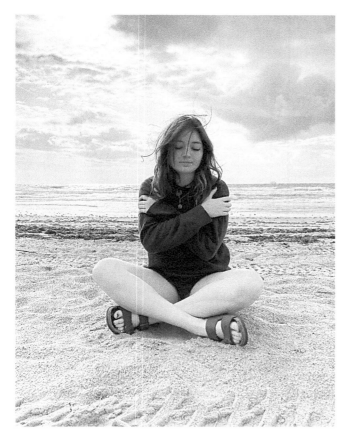

Figure 8.2 Butterfly hug.

Source: Photo courtesy of author, Jackie Flynn.

Summary

EMDR Therapy is enhanced with child and adolescent clients by incorporating nature-based play and expressive therapies. In regard to the topics covered in this chapter, clinicians need to keep in mind that working with traumatized children through the integration of EMDR and nature-based play and expressive therapies requires extensive training and consultation. As shown in Grace's case, this robust integration can offer a substantial amount of safety while reprocessing highly distressing trauma in children and adolescents. The grounding presence of nature is ideal for clients reprocessing early childhood trauma.

Reflective Questions and Suggestions

1 Think about a time you have played in nature, then scan your body to notice physical sensations associated with the experience.
2 What are your thoughts on integrating nature into trauma therapy sessions with children and adolescents?
3 Reflecting back on the case study in this chapter, and taking on the role of the therapist, consider three other nature options from the beach to utilize within sessions. What nature settings, other than the beach, would be appropriate for a scenario similar to the case study?
4 Visit EMDR International Association's website at www.emdria.org to explore the science of EMDR and training options.

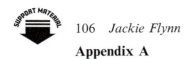

Appendix A

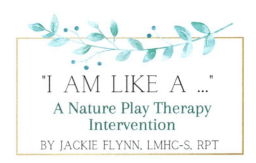

"I AM LIKE A ..."
A Nature Play Therapy Intervention
BY JACKIE FLYNN, LMHC-S, RPT

DESCRIPTION:

Nature is full of elements that represent personal resources such as determination, flexibility, helpfulness, perseverance, confident, compassion, love, empathy, confidence, emotional/ physical strength, and more.

This activity can bring children's awareness to, and support development of, their own inner resources through the power of metaphors in nature to make it more real and tangible.

SUPPLIES NEEDED:

Outdoor spaces with elements such as the beach, clouds, mountains, trees, water, valleys, streams, stones, twigs, leaves, sand, dirt, moss, and more. Imagery can be substituted if such spaces are not readily accessible.

GOAL:

To develop and strengthen a child's inner resources.

INSTRUCTIONS:

Provide examples of how elements of nature share some of the same personal strengths as humans—such as trees are resilient because they can weather big storms and still remain standing for years to come (to strengthen the "I can handle it" cognition). Another example is, ants can do difficult things when they work as part of a team because each one serves an important role (to strengthen the "I matter" cognition).

Ask the child, "What is a strength of something in nature that you also have?"

Then playfully take turns finishing the "I am like a ..." statement. It is important for clinicians to be mindful of the benefits of limiting personal disclosure which should only be used when therapeutically essential.

Suggestion for EMDR Therapists:
"I Am Like A..." intervention can be used to support Phase 1: History Taking.

EXTRA PROCESSING:
Invite the child to scan their body to notice where in their body they "feel" their identified strength(s) from this activity.

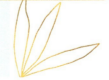

Appendix B

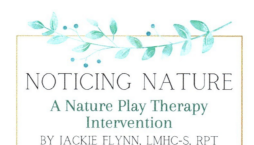

NOTICING NATURE
A Nature Play Therapy Intervention
BY JACKIE FLYNN, LMHC-S, RPT

DESCRIPTION:

Grounding through the senses can help children's ability to stabilize when experiencing dysregulation.

SUPPLIES NEEDED:

Outdoor spaces are rich with sensory input to facilitate the mindfulness of sight, sound, touch, smell, and taste (when appropriate).

GOAL:

Supports children's capacity to engage in self-soothing and affect regulation.

INSTRUCTIONS:

Go outside to a space abundant with sights, sounds, textures, smells, and tastes if possible. The therapist and the child take turns mindfully exploring the sensory characteristics of their surroundings while responding to the following questions:

- What are 5 things you can see?
- What are 4 things you can hear?
- What are 3 things you can touch?
- What are 2 things you like to smell?
- What are 1 thing you like to taste (or imagine tasting)?

Suggestion for EMDR Therapists:

"Noticing Nature" intervention can be used to support Phase 7: Closure.

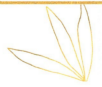
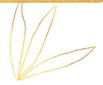

EXTRA FUN:

Bring a toy from the indoor play therapy space to hide in nature. Then, the therapist and child take turns hiding and finding it.

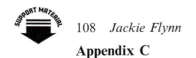

Appendix C

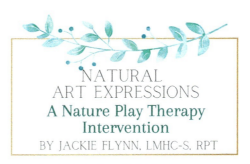

NATURAL
ART EXPRESSIONS
A Nature Play Therapy
Intervention
BY JACKIE FLYNN, LMHC-S, RPT

DESCRIPTION:

Much like Sandtray Therapy, this activity offers opportunity for creative expressions to process through experiences that are limited by words alone. In this intervention, children create scenes with recently gathered natural elements to portray their world in sand or dirt.

SUPPLIES NEEDED:

Open Area of Sand or Dirt Space

Container (Bucket, Bowl, or Basket)

Selection of Natural Elements

GOAL:

Creative Expression for Assessment, Processing, and Resourcing

INSTRUCTIONS:

The therapist and client go outside to collect a random selection of natural elements (sticks, leaves, pine cones, and other items found in outdoor settings). Once the container has enough natural elements to the satisfaction of the child, find a space outside for the child to create a scene for the "show me your world with all of these items from nature in the sand or the dirt." Then the therapist asks the client to describe their image as developmentally appropriate.

Suggestion for EMDR Therapists:

"Natural Art Expressions" intervention can be used to support Phase 3: Assessment.

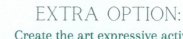

EXTRA OPTION:

Create the art expressive activity with the natural elements indoors in an office setting.

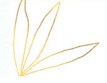

References

Beckley-Forest, A., & Monaco, A. (2020). *EMDR with Children in the Play Therapy Room: An Integrated Approach* (1st ed.). Springer Publishing Company.

Cornell, J. B. (2018). *Deep Nature Play: A Guide to Wholeness, Aliveness, Creativity, and Inspired* Learning (1st ed.). Crystal Clarity Publishers.

Courtney, J. A. (2020). *Healing Child and Family Trauma through Expressive and Play Therapies: Art, Nature, Storytelling, Body & Mindfulness* (Illustrated ed.). W. W. Norton & Company.

Dana, D. A., & Porges, S. W. (2018). *The Polyvagal Theory in Therapy: Engaging the Rhythm of Regulation* (Illustrated ed.). W. W. Norton & Company.

Dana, D. A., & Porges, S. W. (2018b). *The Polyvagal Theory in Therapy: Engaging the Rhythm of Regulation* (Illustrated ed.). W. W. Norton & Company.

Ewert, A., Klaunig, J., Wang, Z., & Chang, Y (2016). Reducing levels of stress through natural environments: Take a park; not a pill. *International Journal of Health, Wellness, and Society*, 6(1). https://doi.org/10.18848/2156-8960/CGP/vo6i01/35-43

Janov, A. (1984). *Imprints: The Lifelong Effects of the Birth Experience*. Perigee Books.

Levine, P. A. (1997). *Waking the Tiger: Healing Trauma*. Berkeley, CA: North Atlantic Books.

Norton, B., Ferriegel, M., & Norton, C. (2011). Somatic expressions of trauma in experiential play therapy. *International Journal of Play Therapy*, 20(3), 138–152. https://doi.org/10.1037/a0024

Parnell, L. (2007). *A Therapist's Guide to EMDR: Tools and Techniques for Successful Treatment*. W.W. Norton.

Schaefer, C. E., & Drewes, A. A. (2014). *The Therapeutic Powers of Play: 20 Core Agents of Change*. Wiley.

Shapiro, F. (2017). *Eye Movement Desensitization and Reprocessing (EMDR) Therapy: Basic Principles, Protocols, and Procedures* (3rd ed.). The Guilford Press.

Swank, J. M., & Shin, S. M. (2015). Nature-based child-centered play therapy: An innovative counseling approach. *International Journal of Play Therapy*, 24(3), 151–161. https://doi.org/10.1037/a0039127

PART IV

Nature Play Therapy Models and Other Individual Therapeutic Applications

9 Cultivating Mindfulness Through Use of Nature in Play Therapy

Lynn Louise Wonders

Introduction

This chapter presents a recipe for healing and growth that includes three key ingredients: *Mindfulness, Nature and Play*. There are bodies of research that support the healing and growth potency of all three of these ingredients. Combined, there can be a powerful effect in helping children and families experience interpersonal and intrapersonal transformation. When nature and play are combined, there is a natural vessel in which the therapist can introduce clients to the experience and practice of mindfulness. In this chapter, there will be an examination of how the research supports the concepts and practices of the three ingredients in the recipe for healing and growth beginning with a look at the concept of mindfulness. Next, there will be consideration of what the research tells us about the benefits of being in and with nature followed by a review of the established efficacy of the therapeutic powers of play. Finally, there will be a case study presented with specific expressive and play-based interventions utilizing elements from nature to foster the beneficial cultivation of mindfulness for clients.

Mindfulness

Mindfulness is largely defined as the ability to consciously attend to what one is experiencing in the present moment and to have awareness with full acceptance. It is a concept found in many practices including yoga, meditation, breathing practices, and stress reduction programs (Van Dam et al., 2018). Mindfulness is most often defined as the moment-to-moment awareness that is cultivated by paying careful attention to the present moment, without judgment. While the practice of mindfulness has its original roots in Buddhism, it has become widely revered and utilized in secular stress-reduction models particularly in the last three decades (Kabat-Zinn, 2011).

Research studies have shown that a particular form of mindfulness practice called Mindfulness Based Stress Reduction (MBSR), which includes a practice of focused, seated meditation, has resulted in positive changes to the brain including increased gray matter and improved learning, memory, and emotion regulation (Brown et al., 2015; Hölzel et al., 2011; Lazar et al., 2005). One study, for example, looked at a group of children who participated in a dynamic mindfulness practice in school. The results of this particular study showed that children who participated in the program demonstrated significant reductions in symptoms of anxiety and depression (Frank et al., 2016). Skinner and Beers (2016) discuss the ways in which elementary school teachers and their classes benefited when teachers practiced mindfulness skills. The teachers were better able to relate to the students and manage job stress and as a result saw improved learning and social connections for the children in the classroom. Bergen-Cico et al. (2015) found that a group of sixth-grade students who were introduced to a mindfulness program showed increased ability for global and long-term self-regulation. Other studies have demonstrated improved social cohesion within classroom dynamics after having children participate in mindfulness programs (Beauchemin et al., 2008; Meyer & Eklund, 2020). Flook et al. (2010) found that a group of second- and third-grade children who participated in a mindfulness awareness program showed significant improvement in executive functioning.

With ample research demonstrating mindfulness programs in school settings do provide benefits for children and teachers, it follows that psychotherapists working with children and families will also see the benefits of including mindfulness practices with clients within the process of play therapy services.

DOI: 10.4324/9781003152767-13

In the work psychotherapists engage in with children and families, there are numerous ways to introduce mindfulness through play-based therapeutic interventions.

Nature

As established in the first chapter of this book, the ingredient of nature in the recipe for growth and healing provided in this chapter is supported by the research literature. While more research is needed, Tillmann et al. (2018) found that interaction with nature had a positive effect on the mental health of children and adolescents. Alvarsson et al. (2010) discovered that nature sounds facilitate healing and recovery from psychological stressors while Wells and Evans (2003) found that children in rural settings who had regular contact and connection with natural plant-life were less impacted by life's stressors. Being in nature and connecting with nature provides children and adults opportunities to heal, grow and experience improved wellbeing (Barton et al., 2016). Sensory-rich exploratory play in biodiverse natural settings support children's healthy development (Beery & Jørgensen, 2016). Wilson (2009) wrote about an instinctual, intrinsic, natural drive all humans have to revere and be connected to all of life on Earth called *biophilia*. This innate love and respect for nature is something that is represented in a variety of indigenous cultures (Mills & Crowley, 2014) from which we can humbly learn.

The National Wildlife Federation (n.d.) has a project that encourages parents, caregivers, and educators to ensure children get a full hour of time in nature every day. The Center for Parent Education (2012) defines time in nature as any unstructured time spent in a natural setting and recommends parents and children schedule time to play together outdoors in order to increase and improve parent–child bonding. In an interview with Scholastic's Parent and Child (n.d), Richard Louv expresses the importance of parents and schools providing time and space for children to explore nature, emphasizing the research showing that nature contributes to the healthy development and well-being of children. Psychotherapists can provide opportunities for children and families to engage with elements of nature in the playroom and sometimes may have opportunity to take clients outside into nature for play therapy sessions. It also may be a very wise strategy to prescribe parents to play with their children in nature on a consistent basis to aid in achieving the benefits demonstrated by the research and recommendations of experts and related organizations as cited above.

The Power of Play

Play is an essential developmental activity as it provides children the opportunity to grow mentally, biologically, socially, and emotionally. Play also offers parents an ideal means for engaging fully and connecting meaningfully with their children (Ginsburg, 2007). Play is a healing agent for families in therapy as it helps lower defenses and contributes to stronger bonds (Gil, 2016). Play therapy is considered the most appropriate way of addressing children's behavioral, emotional, and developmental problems (Ray, 2011). Research reviews using meta-analysis of play therapy outcome studies have shown how play therapy is effective in treating children's mental, emotional, and behavioral needs across a span of ages and presenting issues (Bratton et al., 2005; Leblanc & Ritchie, 2001; Lin & Bratton, 2015). One meta-analytic study demonstrated that both nondirective play therapy and directive play therapy theoretical orientations are effective methods (Bratton et al., 2005). In the process of helping children and families cultivate mindfulness, it is advisable to use a combination of a humanistic, nondirective theoretical approach along with directive expressive and play-based interventions. Schaefer and Drewes (2014) established the four powers of play asserting that play itself (1) facilitates communication; (2) fosters emotional wellness; (3) enhances social relationships; and (4) increases personal strengths. The therapeutic powers of play enumerate a total of 20 core agents of change in play therapy, and these core agents of change are believed to be the "heart and soul" of the play therapy process (Schaefer & Drewes, 2014).

Under the arch of play therapy, there are often creative and expressive therapeutic experiences that facilitate growth and healing for clients. According to the *Recommended Toy List* at the Center for Play Therapy at University of North Texas (n.d.), a playroom should include creative and expressive supplies including art supplies. While creative arts therapies and expressive arts therapies are a distinct category of "action therapies" (Wiener, 2001), there is often complementary overlap between the two fields of expressive arts therapies and play therapy in helping children and families (Courtney, 2020; Malchiodi & Crenshaw, 2015). Lindsey et al. (2018) found that when adolescents were provided opportunity for participating in expressive art activities along with mindfulness training over a 12-week period, there was a significant reduction of anxiety and stress symptoms. Southwell (2016) found use of expressive therapies with preschool age children provided positive outcomes for those who suffered developmental trauma or attachment problems.

Utilizing the power of narrative in therapy is a way to help children and families creatively explore, express, connect, and develop skills (Cattanach, 2008; Cavett, 2018; Courtney, 2020; Mills, 2012). Storytelling is a natural complement to the work of play therapy that aids in facilitating experiences for children to identify and connect their own problems with that of the characters in stories (Carlson & Arthur, 1999). Story-telling and bibliotherapy are effective within family play therapy, helping parents to hear and accept ideas from the characters in a story and to provide the language of metaphor for children (Pernicano, 2015).

The use of play and expressive therapies itself provides an incubator for nurturing healing and growth for children and families. With the basis of play therapy as the context within which a therapist introduces elements of nature to have opportunity for the practice of mindfulness, the potential for healing and growth becomes all the more promising and potentially transformational.

Bringing Play, Mindfulness, and Nature Together in Play Therapy

Incorporating connections with nature into the play therapy process provides effective, natural, and often simple means for introducing the experiential practice of mindfulness. In a meta-analytic study, Schutte and Malouff (2018) found a significant reciprocal relationship between mindfulness and nature. It was discovered that mindfulness allows individuals to feel more connected to nature which in turn further fosters the experience of mindfulness. Noticing the interconnectedness humans have to nature is at the heart of mindfulness practice. For example, the air that a person breathes in is the air plants are breathing out and the air plants are taking in is the air humans are exhaling. The experience of touching or drinking water while noticing how water expresses as rain, lakes, rivers, clouds, or snow in nature can be an exercise in mindfulness practice (Van Gordon et al., 2018).

Both mindfulness and a connection with nature have been shown to be affiliated with lower anxiety, greater vitality, an experience of purpose and meaningfulness, joy, greater creativity, quality social relationships, and respect for the natural environment. The research shows that mindfulness actually mediates the relationship between nature, connectedness and wellbeing (Van Gordon et al., 2018). When clinicians seek ways to provide playful, nature-based therapy interventions with children and families within play therapy services, they invite nature to act as co-therapist in the process (Courtney, 2020). Courtney and Mills (2016) discuss the ways that elements of nature can provide both a sensory experience of connection with nature and provide metaphorical value contributing to a client's healing. Holding a heavy stone in the palm of the hand might represent the emotional heaviness of grief. Observing a single leaf being carried by a flowing stream and then becoming stuck, swirling in an eddy pool, could be a powerful metaphor for a client's experience of the flow of life. The experience of physically touching a stone, a leaf or a pinecone with the therapist's invitation to become absorbed in the tactile experience, noticing the physical properties of the item and any feelings that may be evoked is in itself a mindfulness practice through connection with nature (Courtney, 2020).

Through nature-based sensory play, games, stories, and expressive activities, therapists can bring together those three ingredients of nature, play, and mindfulness to facilitate an experiential and holistic healing experience for clients. There are many ways to incorporate nature-based play in the traditional playroom if therapists are unable to take clients outdoors into nature. The following case study demonstrates the nature-based play therapy journey of a child named Carla whose parents had been through divorce.

Case Study: Carla, Age Seven Years: Healing the Divide of a Family Through Nature-Based Mindfulness Play

This composite case is presented to demonstrate the common challenges children and families face when there is a divorce (Wonders, 2019). This case shows how the use of nature-based play therapy can foster mindfulness skills to support a child's adjustment to the new family structure and to help the child develop skills for healthy expression, coping and resilience.

Background

Juanita initiated therapy services reporting that her daughter, Carla, age seven, was having difficulty adjusting to her parents' recent divorce. After speaking with Juanita, I also spoke with Carla's father Jason and both agreed to meet with me together. Both parents verbally acknowledged the importance of setting aside their disagreements in order to meet on common ground to support Carla's healing and growth.

Initial Intake Session With Carla's Parents

Juanita and Jason arrived early for our first session and Juanita clutched a large notebook that was brimming with loose papers. Jason was scrolling on his phone when I entered the waiting room to greet them. They were clearly uncomfortable being in the therapy room together, so I made an effort to help them feel more at ease by reflecting on how it takes courage to come to therapy to help their child through a difficult time of transition. I affirmed this was likely a time of transition for all three of them and that being here together probably felt uncomfortable, which was completely normal. I invited them both to tell me about Carla.

Juanita explained that Carla had always been a happy and outgoing child until recently when she had become withdrawn with frequent crying. Juanita reported that Carla was struggling in school and didn't want to go on visits to see her dad. Hearing this, Jason took a deep breath and held up his finger signaling he would like to speak. Juanita ignored him and continued to share details of Carla's sadness about the divorce and resistance to seeing her father. I asked Juanita to pause and I turned to Jason. "Jason, I'm interested also in hearing what you are noticing about Carla. Would you please share your perspective with me?"

Jason looked over at Juanita hesitantly. Juanita gestured for him to go ahead, tightened her lips, and tucked her hands under the notebook in her lap. Jason told me that Carla's transitions from her mom to him did seem hard for Carla, but that once she rode in the car with him on the way to his apartment, she perked up, and by the time they arrived she was eager to go inside and see the little dog he had adopted after the divorce. Jason reported that he believed Juanita was making the transitions more difficult for Carla. Juanita appeared defensive, but refrained from objecting aloud. Noticing the tension between them, I gently reminded them both that it is normal to have different views and complex family dynamics when there is a divorce and that different styles of parenting were typical. I assured them that we will work together to help Carla. They both nodded in agreement.

I managed to help both parents feel they were heard and I gathered a great deal of information about Carla's early childhood, family history and culture. Juanita reported she was the middle child in a large family that immigrated from Mexico and she remembered her growing up with so many siblings with fondness. She expressed sadness that Carla was an only child, asserting that Carla suffered from loneliness as a result.

Jason shared that he was the only child of a Filipino mother and an African-American father. He waved off Juanita's concerns about Carla being an only child affirming that he had turned out "just fine" as an only child.

As I explored what Carla's home life was like at each of their homes, it became clear that both Juanita and Jason worked long hours from home and relied on electronic devices to entertain Carla in the afternoons and evenings. They both lived in an urban area where there was little access to outdoor time. Carla rode a bus to and from school and occasionally was invited to a birthday party. Otherwise, she had little opportunity to play with other children. When I asked if Jason and Juanita engaged Carla in play at home, they both indicated there was little time, but that Carla did love her dogs at both homes, and they both read books with her at bedtime.

After helping both Jason and Juanita to feel heard and supported in their parenting, I shared with them about my use of nature-based play therapy and the practice of mindfulness. I explained to them what we know from the research about the benefits of play, the benefits of connecting with nature and the practice of mindfulness. I expressed my understanding that it can be challenging for parents when they are busy working and when they live in an urban location but assured them that there are interventions we can use in therapy that can bridge that gap. Juanita and Jason both agreed that the divorce had been hard on Carla and that play therapy was a good idea.

We scheduled Carla's first play therapy session and agreed we would schedule future sessions on alternating weekends so that each would have opportunity to bring Carla and sometimes participate in the sessions. Jason and Juanita both seemed to feel a sense of relief and hope as we ended our initial intake session and said goodbye.

Carla's First Play Therapy Session

When Juanita brought Carla for her first session, Carla appeared quite shy at first, clinging to her mother, hiding behind Juanita in the waiting room. I greeted Carla with delight and invited them both into the playroom. I had a large basket of nature items and one of my sand trays on a low table with several large floor cushions around the table. Carla looked around the room with wide eyes, sucking on her fingers nervously. She seemed entranced by the shelves of toys and my windowsill full of potted plants.

I gestured for Juanita to find a floor seat, and I sat across from her as Carla explored the room and eventually joined us at the low table in the center of the room. She peered into the bowl of nature items and looked at me for permission to touch them. I told her she was welcome to touch and play with anything in the room. Sensing her anxiety, I knew it was important to not rush or direct Carla's activity at this point. Carla began arranging the sticks and pinecones in patterned rows in the sand tray. I gently reflected Carla's discoveries and arrangements in the sand. Carla smiled and eagerly began pulling more items from the bowl creating a nature world in the sand tray. I wondered aloud if Carla would feel comfortable allowing her mom to go have a cup of tea and come back later. Carla looked at her mom. Juanita nodded and Carla waved saying, "Bye Mom!"

As soon as Juanita had closed the door to the playroom behind her, Carla began talking to me excitedly. She told me how much she loved to make things, and she asked me where I found all the pinecones, sticks, and rocks. She asked if she could crumple the dried leaves and sprinkle the bits so that all the people in the world could have some of the leaves. Carla completed her nature world in the sand and then bounced around the room eager to explore and engage with me. In the last 10 minutes of our time together, I asked her if she'd like to plant a little rooted sprout from one of my plants in her very own pot. Together we scooped some fresh soil into a new, small, empty planter, and we carefully placed the rooted cutting into the soil. I invited her to give it a drink of water and set it in the sunny window. I told Carla that next time she came to my playroom, we would check to see if it had grown. Carla was delighted with her new little plant and excitedly ran to tell her mother about it. We scheduled her next sessions and said goodbye for the day (Figure 9.1).

Carla's Second Play Therapy Session

The next week, Jason and Carla arrived for Carla's second session. Jason sat down and opened his laptop in the waiting room and told Carla to go have fun. Carla gave him thumbs up and skipped toward my playroom. I asked Jason to please come in with Carla for the first part of the session. He appeared surprised but agreed. Carla immediately went to the window to see her little plant. She squealed with delight, "Look! It's gotten taller! Daddy, did you see this? I planted this and it's gotten taller!" Jason stood awkwardly near the door, nodding at Carla. I invited him to come sit on a floor cushion and motioned to the low table where I had set out several baskets with different sizes of stones, rocks, acorns, leaves, and twigs. For this session, I had provided a long tub of water on big tray on the floor. Carla joined us and looked curiously at the water and all the nature items. "Can I put some of these in the water?" she asked. I replied that she is welcome to play with the items and the water and anything in this room any way she would like. Carla pushed up her sleeves and dropped items into the water noticing aloud how some sank and some floated. Jason looked on quietly. I brought out a ladle, some large wooden spoons and a small container of sand and added them to the collection. Carla urged Jason to play with her. Jason moved closer and asked her what he should do. She directed him to sprinkle sand into the water and see what happens and then she handed him a spoon and invited him to stir the water.

After some time observing the dynamics of Carla and Jason interact with the nature items and the water, I directed Jason to go help himself to a cup of tea in the waiting room and told him Carla and I would meet

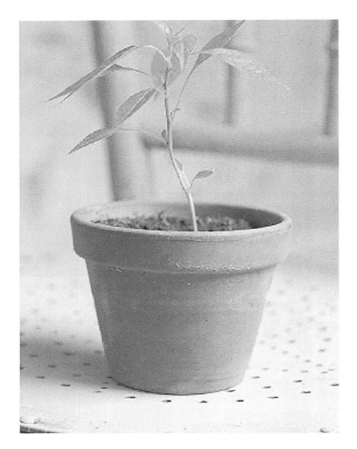

Figure 9.1 Planting a rooted cutting in soil with a child client can be a way to connect with nature in the playroom and serve as a metaphor for client growth.

Source: Lynn Louise Wonders.

him there when it was time to go. After Jason left the playroom, I told Carla that I had a special activity I would like to have her try when she felt ready. I reminded her of all the different kinds of rocks, stones, sticks, twigs, and other nature items I had in the playroom. I invited her to use these items from nature to tell me the story of her family choosing an item to represent herself, her parents, and anyone else she chose. I suggested she use the nature items to create a story of her own world. After thinking, Carla chose a large rock for her mother, a long twig for her father and a small pebble for herself. Incorporating mindfulness practice, I prompted her to notice the texture, the smell, and the weight of the items as she held them in her hands. Carla compared the outside of the two rocks and noted one was much heavier and larger than the other. She observed the long twig was rough and bumpy while the rocks felt smooth. Carla set up her world on the tabletop, placing the large rock on one end of the table and the small rock under the edge of the large rock. She then positioned the twig on the other end of the table. She took a strand of jute and stretched it between the pebble and the twig. She then shared the following:

Carla: *It's like this here in my life.* [She sat back and sighed].
Therapist: [Modeling mindful noticing, taking a slow, deep breath].
Carla: *I have to stay with my mama. She needs me. But I really miss my daddy. They don't like each other anymore, but I wish they would be friends again and that he would come back and live with my mama and me again. I hate divorce.*
Therapist: *It's hard for kids when their parents get divorced.* [Breathing deeply and slowly].
Carla: [Dipping hands in water and swirling them around].

Therapist: *I wonder how the water feels right there on your hands.*
Carla: *It feels cool and soft. When I move my hands, the water moves. I think it helps to wash the sad feelings.*

When Carla seemed finished with the water, I told Carla it was time to end our play session and gave her a small paper bag. I asked her to find five nature items she'd like to take home with her from the playroom. Carla chose three smooth river stones, and two pieces of mossy bark.

Therapist: *What do you notice about the way these items feel in your hands?*
Carla: [Caressing each items]. *The rocks feel so smooth and the wood with this green stuff feel bumpy.*
Therapist: *Ah! You notice the difference in how they feel in your hand…*

Carla remembered her little plant.

Carla: Oh! I need to give my plant a drink of water! [pouring water from the small pitcher into the potted plant.
Therapist: You remembered your plant! You want to be sure it's nourished so it will keep growing.

We went to the waiting room to find her dad and said goodbye for the day (Figure 9.2).

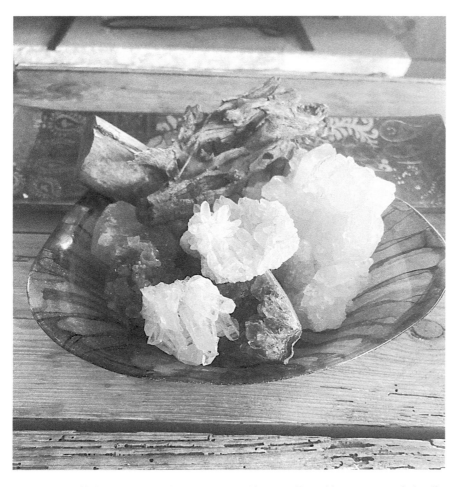

Figure 9.2 Offering stones, rocks, crystals, and items collected in nature can help clients creatively and mindfully feel connected to nature.

Source: Photo Courtesy of author, Lynn Louise Wonders.

Case Conceptualization and the Course of Treatment

My impression after meeting with Carla's parents and then with Carla twice was that her mother's sorrow about the divorce and added anxiety about Carla being lonely as an only child was causing Carla to feel it was her job to take care of her mother. What first may have appeared to be separation anxiety for Carla actually was a feeling of *loyalty conflict* (Wonders, 2019) as a result of her parents' conflict with one another. Carla felt torn between feeling a need to make sure her mother would be okay and a competing desire to also see and be with her dad. Her mother's anxiety made it impossible for Carla to tell her mother she wanted to be with her father fearing it would create more sadness for her mother.

Juanita needed her own counseling support along with some mindfulness skills training. The quality of connection with Carla would improve for both of them if they could learn to connect through dyadic nature-based play both in session and on some day trips to places in nature together. Jason's absorption in his work and his apparent discomfort with simply playing with Carla demonstrated a need for Jason to learn how to be in the moment with Carla. The quality of their connection also would be improved with dyadic nature-based play experiences both in sessions with me and on outings to places in nature I would help them find. I knew that I needed to help all three of them learn how to be more present through playful connections involving experiences with elements of nature.

We scheduled weekly sessions over six months with the first 15 minutes of each session including Carla and the parent who brought her to session. Juanita and Jason alternated weeks consistently. I utilized the mindfulness bell [see Appendix A] intervention at the first of every session to come into present time listening to the resonance of the bell until we could no longer hear it. We practiced playful breathing [see Appendix B] every session so Carla and her parents would be well rehearsed in how to access their breath to return to present moment. We used sensory exploration activities such as mud-painting and bean-sorting in session. I invited Carla to express her feelings through expressive and creative activities such as the All-of-Me Flower Petal Activity [see Appendix C] (Figure 9.3).

I met with the parents together and individually monthly. I referred both to their own counselors to support them in their own life transitional needs. I also referred them to a colleague who provides co-parenting counseling to learn how to communicate effectively for Carla's sake.

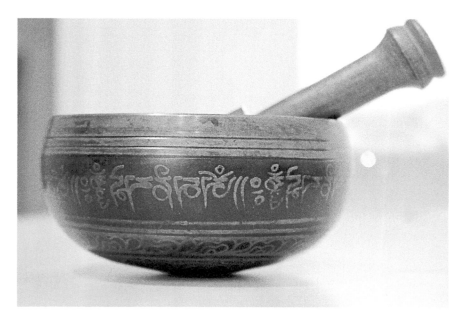

Figure 9.3 Use a Tibetan singing bowl for the mindfulness bell intervention to help clients come fully into the present moment.

Source: Lynn Louise Wonders.

The parents were both assigned with the task of taking Carla to a place in nature every weekend as weather permitted. I provided a list of parks and ideas for ways to engage with nature together. The results of this intervention were astounding. Jason found ways to incorporate his love of technology by allowing Carla to record nature sounds and take photos of things she saw in nature. He was able to print off the photos Carla took and affix them to her bedroom wall as reminders of their times together. Juanita found a play group with other nature-loving mothers and created a way for Carla to have interactive play time with other children at nearby parks. With Juanita's newfound peer friendships, she had her own need for social connection better filled and was happy to see Carla play with other children.

Termination

When the parents were working together more efficiently, Carla was transitioning between households with ease, her school performance improved, and Carla and her parents were consistently able to return to present moment when stressed, the goals of therapy had been reached. Through nature-based play therapy in session and at home, Carla and her parents had learned how to weather transitions, manage emotions, and communicate with one another effectively. We brought our counseling to a close over the course of the final six sessions, and on the final session, Carla took home the little potted plant she had nurtured from the very first session all the way until our final session together as a reminder of how we can heal and grow when we mindfully attend on a consistent basis.

Reflective Questions

1   How might a therapist consider embodying and modeling the practice of mindfulness as an important aspect of providing mindfulness-based interventions with children and their caregivers?
2   In what ways do elements of nature provide invitation for children and caregivers in therapy to engage with the here-and-now using mindfulness through sensory cues?
3   How does spontaneous explorative play that children naturally engage in promote the organic practice of mindfulness?
4   How might elements of nature contribute to the grounding practices that are often included in mindfulness-based activities?

Appendix A

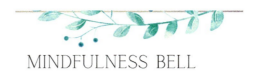

MINDFULNESS BELL

A Nature Play Therapy Intervention

Adapted from Thich Nhat Hahn (2011)
by Lynn Louise Wonders, LPC, CPCS, RPT-S

DESCRIPTION:

Utilizing our auditory senses, the lingering and enchanting chime that rings from the strike of a bell, a Tibetan singing bowl, or other bell-like instrument can help us to attune to the reverberation bringing us fully into the present moment. The mindfulness bell calls us to pay close attention.

SUPPLIES:

A Tibetan singing bowl, a meditation bell or any kind of instrument that when struck will create a lingering resonant chime.

GOAL:

Help us and our clients to tune into the present moment by anchoring our attention on the resonant sound of the chime from the bell.

INSTRUCTIONS:

Invite the child and caregiver(s) as follows:
As I ring this bell/bowl I would like for you to be very still and quiet while you listen very carefully and keep listening until you can no longer hear the chime. Let's see how long we can hear the ringing of this bell/bowl.

How to use:
Gently but firmly strike the singing bowl or the bell and join with your client in silent attuning to the resonant chime. Once you and your client have heard the last of the chime, with a whisper you can invite the child to notice how they are feeling in their body.

EXTRA FUN:

You will find that once you demonstrate use of the mindfulness bell, your child client will often want to be the one to strike the bell/bowl the next time and this can be a wonderful ritual for families.

Appendix B

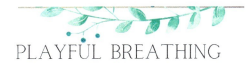

PLAYFUL BREATHING

A Nature Play Therapy Intervention
by Lynn Louise Wonders, LPC, CPCS, RPT-S

DESCRIPTION:

The breath is always with us and is a reminder of every present moment. This intervention provides a playful way for children and caregivers to practice engaging with their breath to elicit a connection to present moment and to invite a relaxation response in the body.

SUPPLIES:

All you need is your imagination and your breath!

GOAL:
Engage with the breath consciously for present moment connection and relaxation response.

INSTRUCTIONS:

After pretending to prepare a pizza (or a cake, or a giant cookie), we then bake the pizza, and when it comes out of the oven we smell the delicious aroma (inhaling deeply through the nose), and then we gently blow on the pizza to cool it off so we don't burn our mouths when we take a bite (exhaling long and slowly through the mouth). Practice belly breathing by selecting a stuffed animal or other light weight object from the playroom. We then lie on our backs, set the object on our bellies, and as we breathe in filling our lungs the item rises on our belly up into the air. As we slowly breathe out, we watch the item slowly lower back down.

EXTRA FUN:
Since our breath is always with us and our imagination is always available, playful breathing can be practiced anywhere, anytime!

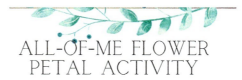

ALL-OF-ME FLOWER PETAL ACTIVITY

A Nature Play Therapy Intervention
by Lynn Louise Wonders, LPC, CPCS, RPT-S

DESCRIPTION:

Flowers are the perfect representation for the innate beauty within all of us. The parts of the flower also can symbolize the various aspects of who we are as people. Connecting with flowers in nature and bringing this metaphor into the playroom helps children to feel connected to who they are and their connections with others.

SUPPLIES:

- Precut flower petals
- Predrawn flower center
- Pens, pencils, crayons or markers
- Glue or tape

GOAL:

Create a physical visual of a flower that represents the various beautiful parts and connections of the child

INSTRUCTIONS:

With precut flower petals and a pre-drawn center of the flower, the child is invited to write or draw something on a petal that they know about themself, something they love about themself, something they don't like very much about themself, something their parents love about them, and something they wish would change or be better. The child then arranges the petals however they like around the center of the flower. Together we talk about that like a flower that has a stem, a center and many petals, we too have many parts that make up the whole of who we are.

EXTRA FUN:

Your client might create an entire garden of flowers representing all the people, places and beloved experiences they treasure in life.

References

Alvarsson, J. J., Wiens, S., & Nilsson, M. E. (2010). Stress recovery during exposure to nature sound and environmental noise. *International Journal of Environmental Research and Public Health, 7*(3), 1036–1046. https://doi.org/10.3390/ijerph7031036

Barton, J., Bragg, R., Wood, C., & Pretty, J. (2016). *Green exercise: Linking nature, health and well-being.* Routledge.

Beauchemin, J., Hutchins, T. L., & Patterson, F. (2008). Mindfulness meditation may lessen anxiety, promote social skills, and improve academic performance among adolescents with learning disabilities. *Complementary Health Practice Review, 13*(1), 34–45. https://doi.org/10.1177/1533210107311624

Beery, T., & Jørgensen, K. A. (2016). Children in nature: Sensory engagement and the experience of biodiversity. *Environmental Education Research, 24*(1), 13–25. https://doi.org/10.1080/13504622.2016.1250149

Bergen-Cico, D., Razza, R., & Timmins, A. (2015). Fostering self-regulation through curriculum infusion of mindful yoga: A pilot study of efficacy and feasibility. *Journal of Child and Family Studies, 24,* 3448–3461 (2015 https://doi.org/10.1007/s10826-015-0146-2

Bratton, S. C., Ray, D., Rhine, T., & Jones, L. (2005). The efficacy of play therapy with children: A meta-analytic review of treatment outcomes. *Professional Psychology: Research and Practice, 36*(4), 376.

Brown, K. W., Creswell, J. D., & Ryan, R. M. (2015). *Handbook of mindfulness: Theory, research, and practice.* Guilford Publications.

Carlson, R., & Arthur, N. (1999). *Play therapy and the therapeutic use of story. Canadian Journal of Counseling, 33*(3), 212.

Cattanach, A. (2008). *Narrative approaches in play with children.* Jessica Kingsley Publishers.

Cavett, A. (2018, May 3-4). *Play therapy with children impacted by trauma: Facilitating healing through narrative* [Paper presentation]. North Dakota Psychological Association Conference, West Fargo, North Dakota.

Courtney, J. A. (2020). *Healing child and family trauma through expressive and play therapies: Art, nature, storytelling, body & mindfulness.* W.W. Norton & Company.

Courtney, J. A., & Mills, J.C. (2016). Utilizing the metaphor of nature as co-therapist in StoryPlay. *Play Therapy, 11*(1), 18–21.

Flook, L., Smalley, S. L., Kitil, M. J., Galla, B. M., Kaiser-Greenland, S., Locke, J., Ishijima, E., & Kasari, C. (2010). Effects of mindful awareness practices on executive functions in elementary school children. *Journal of Applied School Psychology, 26*(1), 70–95. https://doi.org/10.1080/15377900903379125

Frank, J. L., Kohler, K., Peal, A., & Bose, B. (2016). Effectiveness of a school-based yoga program on adolescent mental health and school performance: Findings from a randomized controlled trial. *Mindfulness, 8*(3), 544–553. https://doi.org/10.1007/s12671-016-0628-3

Gil, E. (2016). *Play in family therapy.* The Guilford Press.

Ginsburg, K. R. (2007). The importance of play in promoting healthy child development and maintaining strong parent-child bonds. *Pediatrics, 119*(1), 182–191. https://doi.org/10.1542/peds.2006-2697

Hölzel, B. K., Carmody, J., Vangel, M., Congleton, C., Yerramsetti, S. M., Gard, T., & Lazar, S. W. (2011). Mindfulness practice leads to increases in regional brain gray matter density. *Psychiatry Research, 191*(1), 36–43. https://doi.org/10.1016/j.pscychresns.2010.08.006

Kabat-Zinn, J. (2011). Some reflections on the origins of MBSR, skillful means, and the trouble with maps. *Contemporary Buddhism, 12,* 281–306.

Lazar, S. W., Kerr, C. E., Wasserman, R. H., Gray, J. R., Greve, D. N., Treadway, M. T., McGarvey, M., Quinn, B. T., Dusek, J. A., Benson, H., Rauch, S. L., Moore, C. I., & Fischl, B. (2005). Meditation experience is associated with increased cortical thickness. *Neuroreport, 16*(17), 1893–1897. https://doi.org/10.1097/01.wnr.0000186598.66243.19

Leblanc, M., & Ritchie, M. (2001). A meta-analysis of play therapy outcomes. *Counselling Psychology Quarterly, 14*(2), 149–163. https://doi.org/10.1080/09515070110059142

Lin, Y., & Bratton, S. C. (2015). A meta-analytic review of child-centered play therapy approaches. *Journal of Counseling & Development, 93*(1), 45–58. https://doi.org/10.1002/j.1556-6676.2015.00180.x

Lindsey, L., Robertson, P., & Lindsey, B. (2018). Expressive arts and mindfulness: Aiding adolescents in understanding and managing their stress. *Journal of Creativity in Mental Health, 13*(3), 288–297. https://doi.org/10.1080/15401383.2018.1427167

Malchiodi, C. A., & Crenshaw, D. A. (2015). *Undefined.* Guilford Publications.

Meyer, L., & Eklund, K. (2020). The impact of a mindfulness intervention on elementary classroom climate and student and teacher mindfulness: A pilot study. *Mindfulness, 11*(4), 991–1005. https://doi.org/10.1007/s12671-020-01317-6

Mills, J. C., & Crowley, R. J. (2014). *Therapeutic metaphors for children and the child within.* Routledge.

National Wildlife Federation. (n.d.). Connecting Kids and Nature. https://www.nwf.org/Kids-and-Family/Connecting-Kids-and-Nature

Nha. (2011). *Planting seeds: Practicing mindfulness with children*. Berkeley, CA: Parallax Press.

Pernicano, P. (2015). Metaphors and stories in play therapy. In C. Schaefer & K. O'Connor , & L. Braverman (eds.), *Handbook of Play Therapy*, 259–275. https://doi.org/10.1002/9781119140467.ch12

Ray, D. (2011). *Advanced play therapy* (1st ed.). Routledge.

Schaefer, C. E., & Drewes, A. A. (2014). *The therapeutic powers of play: 20 core agents of change*. Wiley.

Schutte, N. S., & Malouff, J. M. (2018). Mindfulness and connectedness to nature: A meta-analytic investigation. *Personality and Individual Differences, 127*, 10–14. https://doi.org/10.1016/j.paid.2018.01.034

Skinner, E., & Beers, J. (2016). Mindfulness and teachers' coping in the classroom: A developmental model of teacher stress, coping, and everyday resilience. *Mindfulness in Behavioral Health*, 99–118. https://doi.org/10.1007/978-1-4939-3506-2_7

Southwell, J. (2016). Using 'Expressive therapies' to treat developmental trauma and attachment problems in preschool-aged children. *Children Australia, 41*(2), 114–125. https://doi.org/10.1017/cha.2016.7

The benefits of being out in nature for children- A natural fit. (2012, August 29). The Center for Parenting Education. https://centerforparentingeducation.org/library-of-articles/nutrition-and-healthy-lifestyle/nature-and-children-a-natural-fit/

The Center for Parenting Education. (n.d.). Retrieved November 3, 2021, from https://centerforparentingeducation.org/library-of-articles/nutrition-and-healthy-lifestyle/nature-and-children-a-natural-fit/.

Tillmann, S., Tobin, D., Avison, W., & Gilliland, J. (2018). Mental health benefits of interactions with nature in children and teenagers: A systematic review. *Journal of epidemiology and community health, 72*(10), 958–966. https://doi.org/10.1136/jech-2018-210436

Van Dam, N. T., van Vugt, M. K., Vago, D. R., Schmalzl, L., Saron, C. D., Olendzki, A., Meissner, T., Lazar, S. W., Kerr, C. E., Gorchov, J., Fox, K. C. R., Field, B. A., Britton, W. B., Brefczynski-Lewis, J. A., & Meyer, D. E. (2018). Mind the hype: A critical evaluation and prescriptive agenda for research on mindfulness and meditation. *Perspectives on Psychological Science, 13*(1), 36–61. https://doi.org/10.1177/1745691617709589

Van Gordon, W., Shonin, E., & Richardson, M. (2018). Mindfulness and nature. *Mindfulness, 9*(5), 1655–1658. https://doi.org/10.1007/s12671-018-0883-6

Webb, N. B. (2019). *Social work practice with children* (4th ed.). Guilford Publications.

Wells, N. M., & Evans, G. W. (2003). Nearby nature: A buffer of life stress among rural children. *Environment and Behavior, 35*(3), 311–330. https://doi.org/10.1177/0013916503035003001

Why kids need nature. (n.d.). Scholastic | Books for kids | Parent & teacher resources. https://www.scholastic.com/parents/family-life/parent-child/why-kids-need-nature.html

Wiener, D. J. (2001). *Beyond talk therapy: Using movement and expressive techniques in clinical practice*. American Psychological Association.

Wilson, E. O. (2009). *Biophilia*. Harvard University Press.

Wonders, L. (2019). *When parents are at war* (2nd ed.). Wonders Counseling Press. https://wonderscounseling.com/when-parents-are-at-war-divorce-book/

10 Nature-Based Child-Centered Play Therapy: Taking the Playroom Outside

Jacqueline M. Swank and Sang Min Shin

Introduction

In today's society, children are spending more time inside and less time in nature exploring the world around them. Louv (2005) noted concern about the decline in time children spend outside and the harmful health effects that may result, referring to this concern as nature-deficit disorder. It is crucial to provide opportunities for children to be in nature, as time spent in nature contributes to the development of children. McCurdy et al. (2010) reported being outside promotes physical activity that may help prevent various short- and long-term health problems (e.g., asthma and obesity). Additionally, in a review of 16 studies, Dankiw et al. (2020) found nature play among children positively influenced physical activity and cognitive play. Also, scholars suggested the connection between nature and social and emotional development (Swank & Huber, 2013; Swank & Swank, 2013), and Swank and Shin (2015a) found a therapeutic gardening intervention increased reported self-esteem, as well as children expressing they felt happy and calm and learned to work together. Moreover, in examining the benefits of immersive nature experiences for children and adolescents through a review of 84 publications, Mygind et al. (2019) found support for nature benefiting self-efficacy, self-esteem, resilience, cognitive performance, academic performance, and social skills. Furthermore, Weeland et al. (2019) reviewed 31 studies and found promising results for using nature with children to promote self-regulation and prevent mental health concerns. Thus, a wealth of research supports children spending time in the nature.

Nature-based therapies focus on the integration of nature within the therapeutic process, with nature becoming a cotherapist. This partnership may encompass a variety of approaches. Specifically, a nature-based counseling session may include similar activities to an indoor counseling session, except it occurs outside (e.g., sitting and talking, playing outside with therapeutic materials from the playroom). Additionally, sessions may involve interacting with nature (e.g., creating a collage using natural materials, gardening). Play therapists may also integrate the natural environment inside (e.g., window to allow a natural view, bringing natural materials inside) (Swank et al., 2020).

We believe the flexibility in ways to integrate nature within the therapeutic process provides opportunities for all clinicians to incorporate nature in their sessions with children, adolescents, and their families at a level that is comfortable for both the clinician and the client. In doing so, clinicians provide the opportunity for children to explore nature, which evokes multiple senses, promotes creative expression, and provides an opportunity to experience the therapeutic value of nature. We have integrated nature within counseling in a variety of ways; however, this chapter focuses on a model we created that embraces child-centered play therapy (CCPT) within the natural environment, known as nature-based child-centered play therapy (NBCCPT).

Nature-Based Child-Centered Play Therapy

Child-Centered Play Therapy

Nature-based child-centered play therapy (NBCCPT; Swank & Shin, 2015b) involves the integration of nature within a child-centered play therapy (CCPT) approach. CCPT began with Axline (1947) adapting Rogers' (1942) person-centered theory (Rogers, 1942) for counseling children. Within CCPT, the focus is on the relationship between the child and the play therapist. Sessions occur in a playroom containing a

DOI: 10.4324/9781003152767-14

variety of developmentally appropriate toys that provide an opportunity for children to express their thoughts, feelings, wants, and needs to the play therapist through play, the language of a child (Landreth, 2012). The play therapist is nondirective in the play session, providing an opportunity for the child to problem solve and take responsibility for their choices. In following the child's lead, the play therapist responds through tracking behaviors, reflecting feelings, encouraging, and facilitating the relationship. The play therapist sets limits only as needed to maintain safety.

In examining the effectiveness of CCPT, Bratton et al. (2005) found positive results, with nondirective play therapy (i.e., CCPT) yielding higher outcomes that directive, nonhumanistic approaches. Additionally, in a meta-analysis of 23 studies regarding play therapy in elementary schools, Ray et al. (2015) found improved behaviors among children participating in CCPT compared to children that received no intervention. Lin and Bratton (2015) also found support for the use of CCPT in a review of 52 studies. Furthermore, researchers reviewed studies that examined the effectiveness of CCPT specifically with marginalized children and found CCPT was an effective intervention for these children (Post et al., 2019). Thus, researchers support the effectiveness of CCPT as a treatment approach to working with children.

Components of NBCCPT

In the development of NBCCPT, Swank and Shin (2015b) applied the CCPT principles within the natural environment. This involves several considerations, including the play space, materials, limit setting, confidentiality, safety, and weather and other unpredictable conditions. In creating the outdoor playroom, the space will look differently depending on what the play therapist has access to for sessions and preference. This may involve a large grassy area, an area with dirt exposed, or a combination of the two areas. Safety, accessibility, and appeal are most important when selecting and designing the space (Swank & Shin, 2015b), and similarly to designing an indoor playroom, the play therapist may need to use their creativity to work with the space they have available when it is not an ideal space. Related to using NBCCPT with older children, Shin and Swank (2018) discussed allowing preadolescents the opportunity to name the space and not referring to NBCCPT as *play therapy* when describing it to older children, as they may consider this relating to younger children, and therefore be reluctant to participate. Other considerations for the nature play space include the availability of sun and shade, access to water and bathrooms, and man-made (e.g., fence) or natural (e.g., trees and shrubs) boundaries (Swank & Shin, 2015b). While we recommend minimizing man-made materials in the natural space, play therapists may integrate some nonnatural materials to make the space more comfortable (e.g., blanket, tarp, or chairs to sit on, something to provide a cover from the sun when natural shade is not available).

Play therapists should also consider confidentiality when selecting an outdoor space. While play therapists may not be able to guarantee confidentiality in an outdoor space, they should consider how they might minimize a breach. The play therapist should tailor the informed consent to NBCCPT, including the benefits of engaging in nature and NBCCPT, physical risks (e.g., injury during outside play), confidentiality concerns, allergies, weather conditions, and the presence of animals and insects. The play therapist discusses the consent form with the parents/caregivers and the child prior to beginning NBCCPT sessions (Swank & Shin, 2015b). This discussion may occur, when possible, in the outdoor, natural play space to introduce the family to the space that the therapist will use for NBCCPT sessions.

When possible, the play therapist may also consider having an outside, natural waiting area for parent/guardians and other family members to use when a child is having their NBCCPT sessions with the play therapist. This will depend on the amount of outdoor, natural space available and if the play therapist can separate this space from the natural play space used for the NBCCPT sessions, so that the play therapy sessions remain private. When this natural waiting space is available, it allows family members not involved in the NBCCPT sessions also to benefit from nature. Additionally, it may strengthen parents/guardians support of the NBCCPT approach, as well as encourage families to spend more time in and with nature. When a separate outdoor natural space is not available to use as a waiting area, the play therapist may consider integrating some natural materials within the indoor waiting area for families to engage with while they are waiting for the children participating in NBCCPT sessions (Figure 10.1).

Swank and Shin (2015b) discussed the integration of a variety of natural materials (e.g., sticks, tree cookies [cross-sectional pieces of trees], water, dirt, sand, leaves, and chalk) to replace the toys in the

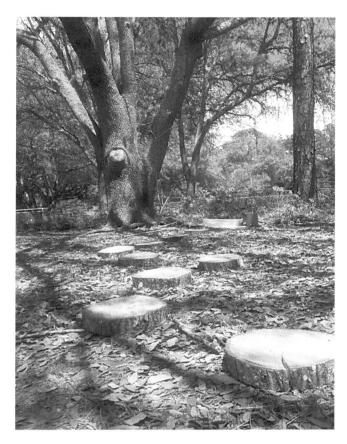

Figure 10.1 "Natural play space. A large tree with tree cookies as blocks or stepping stones."
Source: Sang Min.

playroom, while recognizing that some man-made materials may also be needed (e.g., gloves, shovels, buckets, or other containers to carry water). Some natural materials may already be present in the space, while the play therapist may also introduce other natural materials. When considering natural materials, it is important to think about what is developmentally appropriate for the age group the play therapist is working with, as materials available to older children and adolescents might be different from what is available for younger children (Shin & Swank, 2018). The play therapist may also consider the categories of therapeutic play materials discussed by Landreth (2012), when deciding on natural materials, to help with facilitating self-expression, as well as developing a sense of self and skill development. It may be challenging to think of how to represent every category, and we have found that children embrace creativity in using the natural materials available to express what they are thinking and feeling and work through the concerns they are experiencing in their lives. For example, children may use the tree cookies as blocks or stepping stones, play food, or use them as a canvas to draw on with chalk. Additionally, children may use sticks as building materials, weapons, or musical instruments. Thus, play therapists should provide children with the freedom and space to use the natural materials creatively in a way that meets their needs.

In facilitating sessions, play therapists use the CCPT principles similarly to how they would be used within an indoor playroom, including how they start and end sessions and the use of limit setting. However, it is important to be mindful that there can be heightened safety concerns in an outdoor setting. For example, due to less physical boundaries, a child may easily leave the natural play space and then be close to the street, instead of just leaving the playroom and running down the hallway.

Additionally, natural materials may become a safety concern, such as a broken stick with a sharp point or throwing rocks. Thus, it is important for the play therapist to anticipate potential safety concerns and to engage quickly in limit setting to maintain safety when needed (Swank & Shin, 2015b). Due to increased potential safety concerns and the play therapist having less control over the outdoor natural play space, we recommend that play therapists become skilled in using CCPT within an indoor playroom, including developing skill in limit setting, before engaging in NBCCPT sessions outside. We also recommend that play therapist receive training related to integrating nature in play therapy, such as NBCCPT. Play therapist may also explore integrating natural materials inside the playroom, as explained by Swank et al. (2020), before using NBCCPT in the outdoor play space. Other considerations discussed by Swank & Shin (2015b) include unpredictable conditions, such as weather, presence of critters, and change is space. Thus, there are multiple factors to consider when integrating NBCCPT into a play therapist's work with children.

In examining the effectiveness of NBCCPT, researchers have found promising results. Specifically, Swank et al. (2015) found NBCCPT was effective in reducing behavioral problems for two out of four participants and these participants maintained improvements in the post intervention phase. A third participant also showed improvements toward the end of the treatment phase that continued in the post intervention phase. Swank et al. (2017) also examined the effectiveness of NBCCPT with elementary school children ($N = 5$) using group instead of individual sessions (nature-based child-centered group play therapy, NBCCGPT) and found results ranging from debatable to effective among the treatment group for decreasing problem behavior and increasing on-task behavior. Additionally, children in the treatment group were more likely to demonstrate improvement in both areas during the treatment and follow-up phases compared to the control group ($N = 2$). Furthermore, Swank and Smith-Adcock (2018) compared the effectiveness of NBCCPT, CCPT, and no intervention for improving on-task behavior among children with attention-deficit/hyperactivity disorder (ADHD) ($N = 8$) and found children in both the CCPT and NBCCPT interventions were 4.59 times more likely to improve on-task behaviors compared to the control group. Thus, researchers have found some initial promising results for using NBCCPT to decrease problem behaviors and improve on-task behaviors.

School Adjustment Concerns

In the following case study, Peter experienced difficulty adjusting to school that was characterized by exhibiting internalizing behavioral concerns, lack of positive peer relationships, and academic difficulty. Some children have difficulty transitioning to elementary school and may exhibit externalizing (i.e., aggression toward others) or internalizing (i.e., withdrawn, anxious, lonely, and sad) behavioral concerns. A successful preschool experience can provide an opportunity for children to develop skills that promote success in elementary school. Specifically, the development of social-emotional competence in preschool can help children develop positive peer relationships and achieve academic success (Nakamichi et al., 2019). However, negative experiences in preschool may create anxiety and stress related to attending elementary school, creating difficulty for children to be successful in school.

A child's behavioral concerns may affect their academic performance as well as their interactions with others. Researchers found a negative relationship between internalizing problems and school adjustment and academic achievement (Pedersen et al., 2019). Researchers also found a correlation between lack of friends in kindergarten and internalizing problems in first grade, as well as a positive correlation between high-quality friendships in kindergarten and social skills in first and third grades, particularly for boys (Engle et al., 2011). Thus, it is crucial to address behavioral concerns and help children develop self-competency and social skills to promote academic success and positive peer relationships.

Case Study

Peter was a six-year-old boy who experienced adjustment issues at school, characterized by exhibiting internalizing behaviors (e.g., withdrawn, isolated, and anxious). His parents also reported that he was not doing well academically, lacked self-confidence, and had no close friends. They shared that Peter's difficulty began in preschool where his preschool teacher often scolded and punished him. They believed time in nature was good for children and that Peter could benefit from spending more time outside. They also reported that they thought Peter might enjoy NBCCPT.

Peter participated in 50-minute individual NBCCPT sessions once a week for three months (12 total sessions). There was also some brief time at the end of sessions for the play therapist, Sarah, to talk with Peter's mother. Sarah prepared the natural play area and natural materials following guidelines discussed by Swank and Shin (2015b). The area contained various trees, shrubs, and plants. There was a big sandbox under a large tree, a large plant bed, and access to water. Sarah also provided additional natural materials, including tree cookies, logs, sticks, straw, pinecones, seeds, dried moss, bark, and chalk. Additionally, man-made materials that encouraged Peter to explore nature were also provided including watering containers, a water hose, gardening tools (e.g., shovel and hoe), buckets, pots, a tarp, bubbles, and containers.

The informational session with Peter's parents occurred outside on the edge of the natural play space. Sarah discussed the informed consent form that included the benefits and risks of participating in NBCCPT, as well as the limits of confidentiality. She also asked Peter's parents about allergies and discussed appropriate attire for hot summer weather (e.g., hat and sunscreen). They also discussed a plan for bad weather. Sarah gave Peter and his parents a tour of the natural play space, as well as the natural waiting area for his parents to wait for Peter during sessions if they wanted to wait outside, instead of staying in the waiting room instead the office building.

Sessions 1–3

During the first session, Peter was initially hesitant and unsure of what to do in the space, asking Sarah what he was supposed to do. Sarah invited him to explore the space. He gradually began investigating the different natural and man-made materials in the play area. He was particularly interested in the gardening tools and various plant seed packets and asked if he could use them. He shared that he wanted to plant seeds in the pots. He asked Sarah to help him without attempting to open the seed packets by himself. Sarah encouraged him to select the seeds he wanted and to open the packets by himself. She consistently provided opportunities for Peter to engage in decision-making during this process. Peter finally decided on sunflower and pumpkin seeds and planted them in pots. Sarah provided continuous encouragement and reflected Peter's behaviors and feelings while he was planting the seeds. After planting the seeds, Peter noticed his knees and hands were dirty. He immediately asked permission to go to the bathroom and washed them. At the end of the first session, Peter asked if he could take the pots home. Sarah discussed with Peter how to take care of the seeds and he took them home.

Peter brought the pots back to the second session. It was obvious that he had not taken care of the seeds, as the soil in the pots was dry and hard. When he put his pots on the planting beds, he realized the soil in the other pots was not dry like his, and there were sprouts in the other pots. He complained about his pots and Sarah reflected his disappointment and frustration. Sarah also reminded him about the discussion from the previous session regarding how to care for the seeds, including placing them in a sunny area at his house and watering the seeds. Peter shared with Sarah that he had not watered the seeds at all during the week. Sarah used responses to return responsibility to Peter to facilitate decision-making. He asked if he could try again, and then he planted the seeds and took them home at the end of the session. He brought the pots back to the third session, this time he had took care of them, and he expressed feeling excited that the seeds had started to sprout. He expressed feeling proud of growing the plants and he continued to bring the pots to his NBCCPT sessions every week to show them to Sarah.

Sessions 4–10

In addition to caring for his potted plants, Peter watered the trees and other plants in the natural play space with the water hose, which demonstrated his desire to nurture and care for the garden. Sarah reflected his efforts to take care of his plants and used metaphors to relate his plant care skills to life situations (e.g., caring for his body so that he would grow and be healthy, trying his best at school and doing his homework so he would learn new things). Regarding his interactions with the insects/bugs, Peter initially was afraid and ran away from them. However, as therapy progressed, he gradually became more comfortable with them. Peter asked Sarah to approach the insects and directed her on what to do. Sarah encouraged him to approach the insects with her. Sarah's self-esteem-building responses led him to be able to look at the insects, observe them, and eventually touch them. He watched the ants and attempted to catch flying insects. In addition, Peter asked questions about Sarah's experiences and opinions on plants and insects: "Are these seeds for eating or planting?", "Do you think we can eat these seeds?" and "Have you killed flies?"

As NBCCPT progressed, Peter expanded his interests to sand and water play. He demonstrated two major play themes with the sand and water: (a) self-care/soothing, and (b) problem-solving and mastery. Regarding the self-care theme, he repeatedly dug in the sand with his hands, covering and uncovering his hands and watching the sand fall through his fingers. For the problem-solving and mastery theme, he tried new ideas with the sand and water. After repeated attempts with the dry sand, he discovered that he needed to get the sand wet to build sandcastles. He also wanted to make a rocket using the water hose and a small container. After several attempts and Sarah's help, at his request, he finally launched the rocket (container) into the sky with the water hose. He was thrilled to see his success after numerous attempts. He was persistent and patient throughout his failed attempts and kept trying. During this process, Sarah consistently used tracking, reflecting, and encouraging responses to facilitate his decision-making process and build his self-esteem. When he engaged in unsafe physical activities for his experiments, Sarah set limits to ensure safety, and he was able to comply with the limits. As therapy progressed, Peter also became more tolerant of being dirty and did not run to the bathroom to wash the dirt off during the middle of sessions. Along with his mastery play theme, he also played with bubbles. He challenged himself by blowing bubbles fast, making the bubbles unique shapes, and catching and popping them, and invited Sarah to participate with him in this activity. Thus, Peter engaged in multiple activities during sessions, and gradually demonstrated progress in problem solving, making decisions, taking responsibility for his behavior, and becoming more relaxed and comfortable in the natural play space.

Termination

At the end of the summer, Peter's mother shared with Sarah that Peter would need to stop attending NBCCPT sessions due to his conflicted schedule. Although termination was unplanned, Peter had two final sessions. He was quieter during his final two sessions. During the last session, his play was a combination of various activities that he had done across various sessions, including exploring insects, watering plants and trees, playing in the sandbox, blowing bubbles, and playing with the rocks. He asked if he could take a few rocks with him, along with his potted plants. Sarah said this was okay. He then gave one rock to Sarah and took the rest home along with the pots.

Post-Case Discussion

In his play, Peter displayed various themes, including relationship-building, nurturing, self-care, problem solving, mastering, and challenging. During the beginning stages of NBCCPT, he was reserved and only played with things that he was familiar with, such as gardening tools. Sarah used encouragement and responses that promoted decision-making and built self-esteem. Peter was also sensitive to getting dirty at the beginning of NBCCPT sessions. Furthermore, he initially did not take responsibility for caring for his plants. However, with time, taking care of his plants became a focus throughout his therapy and Sarah used the planting and growing process as a metaphor for situations in Peter's life outside of sessions. Through caring for the plants across his time in therapy, Peter demonstrated responsibility, improved self-esteem, and nurturing behavior.

The outdoor natural play space provided Peter with the opportunity to explore and experiment with problem solving and to take risks without concern of making a mess or fear of negative consequences. For example, Peter was able to play in the sand without worrying about getting in trouble if the sand went outside of the sandbox. He dug in the sand and allowed it to fall through his fingers, which was a relaxing, calming technique for him. Additionally, he was able to experiment with building sandcastles, testing his rocket, and watering the plants and trees without worrying about making a mess. Sarah gave Peter the freedom and space to be creative and take risks, without needing to set limits about the condition of the play space since they were outside. Thus, the natural, outside environment provided Peter with a safe space to focus on what he needed to work on without him or Sarah worrying about him making a mess or breaking something, which may have been concerns requiring limit setting in an indoor play space.

Peter's interactions with the natural environment changed as therapy progressed, with him becoming more comfortable with interacting with nature and less worried about getting dirty. He showed increased responsibility and ownership in caring for the plants and he became more comfortable being around insects and other creatures present in the outdoor play space. Peter appeared to begin considering his relationship and interactions with plants, trees, and animals in regard to coexisting or cohabitation rather than disengagement, detachment, or animosity toward them. Additionally, his attitude toward the weather changed with him being less anxious and nervous when the sky turned dark and there was a light rain. As therapy progressed, he showed an appreciation and enjoyment for playing outside during sessions when there was a light sprinkling rain. His adjustment to getting dirty, the weather, and insects and other animals reflected his gradual development of healthy coping skills and competence to adjust to various situations, even when they were not expected and unpredictable.

After termination, Peter's mom followed up with Sarah to let her know that Peter had made significant improvements in adjusting to school. Specifically, he had showed improvement in his academic performance, as well as his development of social skills. He exhibited increased positive interactions with peers, even initiating some interactions, instead of waiting for his peers to approach him. He was also able to adjust easier to change without becoming anxious. Peter's mother also reported that the time spent outside waiting for Peter during the NBCCPT sessions had also been beneficial for her and Peter's younger sister, providing them with an opportunity to engage in nature instead of sitting in an office waiting room while Peter had his therapy sessions. Thus, Peter's mother and sister were able to benefit indirectly from the NBCCPT approach.

Conclusion

NBCCPT is an innovative play therapy approach that combines nature with CCPT. Researchers support the effectiveness of CCPT as a therapeutic approach to working with children. Additionally, scholars emphasize the importance and physical and mental health benefits of spending time in nature. Researchers have also found promising results for the use of NBCCPT. Thus, with training and planning, play therapists may consider integrating NBCCPT within their work with children to promote holistic growth and development and healing for children.

Reflective Questions/Role Play/Experiential Learning Activities

1   What are your thoughts and feelings about being in nature? Do you like being outside in nature? What do you enjoy and dislike about being in nature (e.g., weather, animals/insects/critters, heat/cold, or getting dirty)? Reflect on your experiences being in nature and the influence they had on you.
2   What are your thoughts and feelings about facilitating NBCCPT sessions with children? What excites and worries you about using NBCCPT? What can you do to address your concerns to feel more comfortable and confident with using NBCCPT with children?
3   Consider the development of a natural play space to facilitate NBCCPT sessions with children. Where would you create this space? What would you want it to look like?
4   What natural materials would you want to be sure to include in your natural play space? Gather these materials to create a NBCCPT tote bag.

Appendix A

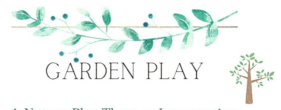

GARDEN PLAY

A Nature Play Therapy Intervention
Jacqueline M. Swank, Ph.D., LMHC, LCSW, RPT-S
and Sang Min Shin, Ph.D., LPC, RPT

DESCRIPTION:

Children engage in garden play through interacting with seeds and dirt.

GOAL:

Engage in self-expression and nurturing behaviors through interacting with nature.

SUPPLIES NEEDED:

Seeds of various sizes and species, pots/containers or designated outdoor space, soil/dirt, water, hand shovel, gloves, plants (optional)

INSTRUCTIONS:

This intervention can be nondirective or directive. If integrated with a nondirective approach, the play therapist has the materials available and the child decides what they want to do with them. This may include emptying all of the seeds on the ground or in the pot, planting only a few, or choosing to play in the dirt and/or water without using the seeds. The therapist may also be directive by working with the child on planting seeds and taking care of them each session or caring for them at home. The therapist can use this intervention in individual, group, and family sessions.

EXTRA FUN:

Have a variety of craft supplies available for the child to decorate the pot/container or make signs for the outdoor space.

References

Axline, V. M. (1947). *Play therapy*. Ballantine Books.

Bratton, S. C., Ray, D., Rhine, T., & Jones, L. (2005). The efficacy of play therapy with children: A meta-analytic review of treatment outcomes. *Professional Psychology: Research and Practice, 36*(4), 376–390. https://doi.org/10.1037/0735-7028.36.4.376

Dankiw, K. A., Tsiros, M. D., Baldock, K. L., & Kumar, S. (2020). The impacts of unstructured nature play on health in early childhood development: A systematic review. *PLoS ONE, 15*(2), e0229006. https://doi.org/10.1371/journal.pone.0229006

Engle, J. M., McElwain, N. L., & Lasky, N. (2011). Presence and quality of kindergarten children's friendships: Concurrent and longitudinal associations with child adjustment in the early school years. *Infant and Child Development, 20*, 365–386. https://doi.org/10.1002/icd.706

Landreth, G. L. (2012). *Play therapy: The art of the relationship* (3rd ed.). Routledge.

Lin, Y. W., & Bratton, S. C. (2015). A meta-analytic review of child-centered play therapy approaches. *Journal of Counseling & Development, 93*(1), 45–58. https://doi.org/10.1002/j.1556-6676.2015.00180.x

Louv, R. (2005). *Last child in the woods: Saving our children from nature-deficit disorder*. Algonquin Books.

McCurdy, L. E., Winterbottom, K. E., Mehta, S. S., & Roberts, J. R. (2010). Using nature and outdoor activity to improve children's health. *Current Problems in Pediatric and Adolescent Health Care, 40*, 102–117. https://doi.org/10.1016/j.cppeds.2010.02.003

Mygind, L., Kjeldsted, E., Hartmeyer, R., Mygind, E., & Bolling, M. (2019). Mental, physical, and social health benefits of immersive nature-experience for children and adolescents: A systematic review and quality assessment of the evidence. *Health and Place, 58*, 1–19. https://doi.org/10.1016/j.healthplace.2019.05.014

Nakamichi, K., Nakamichi, N., & Nakazawa, J. (2019). Preschool social-emotional competencies predict school adjustment in Grade 1. *Early Child Development and Care*. https://doi.org/10.1080/03004430.2019.1608978

Pedersen, M. L., Holen, S., Lydersen, S., Martinsen, K., Neumer, S. P., Adolfsen, F., & Sund, A. M. (2019). School functioning and internalizing problems in young schoolchildren. *BMC Psychology, 7*, 88. https://doi.org/10.1186/s40359-019-0365-1

Post, P. B., Phipps, C. B., Camp, A. C., & Grybush, A. L. (2019). Effectiveness of child-centered play therapy among marginalized children. *International Journal of Play Therapy, 28*(2), 88–97. https://doi.org/10.1037/pla0000096

Ray, D. C., Armstrong, S. A., Balkin, R. S., & Jayne, K. M. (2015). Child-centered play therapy in the schools: Review and meta-analysis. *Psychology in the Schools, 52*(2), 107–123. https://doi.org/10.1002/pits.21798

Rogers, C. R. (1942). *Counseling and psychotherapy: Newer concepts in practice*. Houghton Mifflin.

Shin, S., & Swank, J. M. (2018). Chapter 7: Nature-based play therapy with pre-adolescents. In E. Green, J. Baggerly & A. Myrick (Eds.), *Play therapy with pre-teens* (pp. 107–122). Rowman & Littlefield.

Swank, J. M., Cheung, C., Prikhidko, A., & Su, Y. (2017). Nature-based child-centered group play therapy and behavioral concerns: A single-case design. *International Journal of Play Therapy, 26*(1), 47–57. https://doi.org/10.1037/pla0000031

Swank, J. M., & Huber, P. (2013). Employment preparation and life skill development for high school students with emotional and behavioral disabilities. *The Professional Counselor, 3*, 73–81. https://doi.org/10.15241/jms.3.2.73

Swank, J. M., & Shin, S. (2015a). Garden counseling groups and self-esteem: A mixed methods study with children with emotional and behavioral problems. *The Journal for Specialists in Group Work, 40*, 315–331. https://doi.org/10.1080/01933922.2015.1056570

Swank, J. M., & Shin, S. (2015b). Nature-based child-centered play therapy: An innovative counseling approach. *International Journal of Play Therapy, 24*(3), 151–161. https://doi.org/10.1037/a0039127

Swank, J. M., Shin, S., Cabrita, C., Cheung, C., & Rivers, B. (2015). Initial investigation of nature-based child-centered play therapy: A single-case design. *Journal of Counseling & Development, 93*(4), 440–450. https://doi.org/10.1002/jcad.12042

Swank, J. M., & Smith-Adcock, S. (2018). On-task behavior for children with ADHD: Examining treatment effectiveness of play therapy interventions. *International Journal of Play Therapy, 27*(4), 187–197. https://doi.org/10.1037/pla0000084

Swank, J. M., & Swank, D. E. (2013). Student growth within the school garden: Addressing personal/social, academic, and career development. *Journal of School Counseling, 11*(21), 1–31.

Swank, J. M., Walker, K. L. A., & Shin, S. (2020). Indoor nature-based play therapy: Taking the natural world inside the playroom. *International Journal of Play Therapy, 29*(3), 155–162. https://doi.org/10.1037/pla0000123

Weeland, J., Moens, M. A., Beute, F., Assink, M., Staaks, J. P. C., & Overbeek, G. (2019). A dose of nature: Two three-level meta-analyses of the beneficial effects of exposure to nature on children's self-regulation. *Journal of Environmental Psychology, 65*. https://doi.org/10.1016/j.jenvp.2019.101326

11 Equine-Assisted Psychotherapy and Learning for Children: Why Horses?

Susan Jung

Introduction

It has been proven that contact with all aspects of nature can have a profound effect on people. A safe and structured nature-based environment enables children to discover their inner strengths in coping skills and social skills and improve their self-esteem. Offering play therapy in nature allows a more relaxed, client-centered approach. Children can focus and engage easier when the environment is more relaxed.

According to Swank et al. (2020):

> Nature-based child-centered play therapy (NBCCPT) is an innovative counseling approach that expands upon child-centered play therapy (CCPT) to emphasize the child's relationship with nature in addition to the relationship with the counselor. NBCCPT sessions occur within the natural environment with natural materials provided instead of man-made toys.

Integrating nature in the therapeutic process could involve having the child interact with nature or simply be present in the natural environment. Whatever the level of involvement, nature most likely will have a calming effect in the counseling process.

A Brief Introduction to Equine-Assisted Psychotherapy and Learning

Supporting Theoretical Literature

Animal-assisted therapy has been around for quite a while. There seems to be a natural tendency for humans and animals to form relationships with one another. Expanding nature therapy with animals seems to make it easier for children to talk in therapy and self-regulate. Having a nature-based setting with animals provides a child with additional conduits for developing social skills, problem-solving, and building resiliency.

More recently (the past 20 years), equine-assisted psychotherapy (EAP) and learning (EAL) have become recognized as a viable and effective treatment for mental health issues. The most extensively used model is the Eagala Model: (1) a team approach with a mental health professional and equine specialist, (2) 100% on the ground, (3) solution-focused, and (4) team members follow a strict code of ethics. It is a client-centered approach, and children usually respond well when placed in the arena with the horses.

Why Horses? (Eagala, 2009)

Horses have unique characteristics that impact positive results in EAP with children. Because horses do not judge or hold grudges, they provide emotional safety. Horses live in the here and now. They hold space and are accepting of people in the present moment. Children learn to change their behaviors based on their observations and relationships with their equine friends.

Horses are known in EAP to be honest and assertive messengers, which helps create lasting solutions to life's obstacles. Since horses are extremely sensitive and survive by paying close attention to their environment, children learn to be aware of what is going on around them. Horses seem to mirror what

DOI: 10.4324/9781003152767-15

children are feeling. Children feel empowered by experiencing immediate, honest, and observable feedback from horses.

Horses are also social animals. They have roles in their herds like humans do in their groups. Horses have distinct personalities, attitudes, and moods. While horses may seem stubborn and defiant at times, they also like to have fun. They are similar to humans in many ways.

Working with horses in a therapeutic setting can help children find solutions. The best solutions come from within and children grow from experiencing the horse–human relationship. Positive feelings, thoughts, and actions happen in EAP. Connecting with a horse can be a metaphor for developing a relationship in personal lives.

EAP allows children to discover, learn, and grow from the unique qualities of the horse–human relationship. Horses offer unique opportunities for children to discover inner strength beyond traditional play therapy. Horses also help children experience emotional safety, often helping children to overcome perceived obstacles in their lives and use problem-solving skills as they do in play therapy.

Review of Research

The first evidence-based study that specifically measured positive outcomes for children interacting with horses showed a reduction in stress hormones. This study describes how just 90 minutes weekly with horses reduced harmful stress and demonstrated that healthy stress hormone patterns may prevent physical and mental health problems later in life (Jurga, 2015).

Horses affect children therapeutically with their large, gentle presence. Quiroz et al. (2005) found that children who typically are averse to participating in or receiving affection are open to receiving it from a horse. In that same study, the authors went on to assert that children benefit socially and emotionally and that EAP most assuredly contributes to the improvement of mental health challenges with which children may struggle.

EAP is used to treat children who have experienced family violence. Researchers concluded that it was effective in improving the global assessment of functioning (GAF) scores of children diagnosed with adjustment disorder, mood disorders, post-traumatic stress disorder (PTSD), attention deficit hyperactivity disorder (ADHD), and disruptive disorders. The GAF scores were also significantly improved in the children who had experienced intra-family violence and substance abuse (Schultz et al., 2007). In a study of trauma, the researchers Buck et al. (2017) concluded:

> Equine-assisted psychotherapy (EAP) has emerged as a promising, evidence-based intervention for the treatment of trauma and stressor-related disorders. This experiential therapy offers an option for clients whose traumatic experiences render traditional talk therapies ineffective. Initial research on the most robust model of EAP, developed by the Equine Assisted Growth and Learning Association (EAGALA), indicates strong, positive effects for children, adolescents and adults who have experienced trauma. EAGALA was designed to allow for rigorous evaluation of efficacy, a clear theoretical base, standardized implementation, and ongoing training for practitioners. As the primary providers of mental and behavioral health services in the United States, social workers are keenly aware of the need for a portfolio of treatment methods to manage the increasing demand for services. EAP has emerged as an important addition to this portfolio, providing options for some of the most vulnerable client populations.

Another EAP study based on children's experience in an EAP therapy group yielded positive results. These were ground-based activities delivered in two-hour sessions for nine weeks. The group experience appeared to result in improved social relationships, improved behavior, and overcoming fears. The most important outcome was mastering challenges and translating that accomplishment into coping with future difficulties. (Dunlop & Tsantefski, 2018)

There is ample research that supports the position that horses provide a unique way to reach healing goals for children. Further, the literature shows that when horses are used as cofacilitators in play therapy, significant, positive changes in children's lives have been noted.

The Relevance of Play Therapy–Based Principles to Equine-Assisted Therapy

The Association for Play Therapy (2020) defines play therapy as, "The systematic use of a theoretical model to establish an interpersonal process wherein trained play therapists use the therapeutic powers of play to help clients prevent or resolve psychosocial difficulties and achieve optimal growth and development." In combining play therapy with EAP, we might consider that there is a use of a theoretical model to establish an interpersonal process within the presence of a trained equine-assisted mental health professional. Trained equine specialists use the horse's therapeutic powers to help clients prevent or resolve psychosocial difficulties and achieve optimal growth and development.

According to Schaefer and Peabody (2016), there are many approaches to providing play therapy services based on a variety of theoretical orientations. There is nondirective, child-centered play therapy, which emphasizes the therapeutic relationship above all else. There also are directive play therapy methods that offer facilitated experiences. Some approaches to play therapy are experiential such as sand tray therapy or sensory-motor play.

How do play therapy approaches relate to EAP/EAL? Nondirective play therapy is based on a client-centered approach. EAP is also client-centered and follows the client's lead, emphasizing creating a safe place for expression. Nondirective play therapy is akin to EAL in which situations are set up for the client, with specific learning objectives and outcomes. Child-centered, relationship, and experiential play therapies are very much like EAP. Just as children use toys to resolve issues, they may also use horses to help resolve issues. Elements of sand tray therapy has some presence within equine-assisted therapy as many children naturally like to draw in the sand at the arena and place objects in certain places that often symbolize the undercurrent of their struggles. Sensory-motor components often emerge in EAP as well.

Crawford et al. (2020) compared play therapy and EAP, noting the common factors. There were four areas of comparison: principles, the role of the therapists, the language of the therapists, and themes and patterns.

The principles of play therapy and EAP require a licensed mental health professional who follows a code of ethics. The therapist/facilitator serves both individuals and groups of children. The therapies are experiential and client-led, with a learning process involved. It is important that the therapist/facilitator trust the process. At the same time, the therapist observes patterns and focuses on the metaphors created by the child.

The role of the therapists in play therapy and EAP is to create a safe place where the child determines the direction of the therapy. The therapists provide toys and props (and horses) and allow the child to engage in a non-directive manner. It is up to the therapist to identify metaphors based on actions of the child. These metaphors may or may not be stated by the therapist, depending on the developmental stage of the child.

The language of the therapist is always respectful, using the child's words while avoiding judging or labeling language. It is important for the therapist to keep interpretations and assumptions out of the verbal reflections during the session, so that children develop their own metaphors. When the therapist uses the child's words the child is more likely to move forward with their own solutions.

The themes and patterns in play therapy correlate with SPUD'S (Eagala) model of observation in EAP/EAL:

> S – Shifts: The facilitators watch for any shifts in behaviors, such as "horses were running and now, they are standing, the horses were far apart, and now they are close, etc." Shifts indicate change. The change indicates movement. Movement often brings hope to children, especially when they have experienced trauma.
>
> P – Patterns: If a behavior occurs more than three times, it is a pattern. Sometimes a horse may go to some spot in the arena several times, or the horse may approach the child at least three times. When the facilitators voice those patterns, it may help children reveal patterns in their lives.
>
> U – Unique: The facilitators think, "Wow, I've never seen anything like that before!" A horse may act in an unusual way, such as putting his teeth on an item in the arena. Observing unique actions can have meaning for the child.
>
> D – Discrepancy: This is the only element of SPUD's that focuses on the human. For instance, the child says he/she is "having fun" but has not smiled at all during the session. A child may refuse to do something, then go and do it anyway.

'S – (apostrophe S) Self Awareness: What was on the minds of the therapist and equine specialist during the session? This element has more impact on sessions than any of the others. As with any therapeutic modality, therapists and facilitators must be keenly aware of their agendas, biases, reactions, and so on. With the team approach in the Eagala model, it is imperative to check in with each other so that they are completely present in the session. (Eagala, 2019)

Ethics and Liability Related to Working with Horses

There are several recognized models of EAP. Most are governed by ethical codes and require specialized training. Professionals can choose which model best aligns with their style of therapy. There are unique differences between office therapy and EAP. Regardless of the choice of models, it is essential to have specialized training, in order to meet the needs of professional competency and ensure we do no harm to clients. Training and certification programs offer authenticity, credibility, support, and resources. An example of a global organization is Eagala (Equine Assisted Growth and Learning Association). After a rigorous training process, the Eagala team is accountable to a code of ethics. In addition, the mental health professional must abide by their own profession's standards and equine specialist abides by the American Horse Council's Welfare Code of Practice. "The Eagala Code of Ethics serves as a standard by which to conduct business, and guide practice for all members. The Eagala Code of Ethics is based on providing for the fundamental overall safety and wellbeing of the client and horses" (Eagala, 2019).

Working with horses in a therapeutic session brings additional liability. Special insurance policies have been established to conduct equine-assisted sessions. Most require the professional team to be trained and certified by one of the recognized organizations.

Developmental and Theoretical Considerations Related to Case Study

In the following case, the main elements are trauma and resilience. The short-term treatment plan's objective is to address grief and anger resulting from the trauma and then subsequently build resilience. According to Cook et al. (2003), there are domains of impairment in children exposed to complex trauma. These domains include attachment, biology, affect regulation, dissociation, behavioral control, cognition, and self-concept. When a child presents with complex trauma, it is crucial to assess the areas affected most severely and design treatment goals accordingly.

Trauma affects a child's developmental stages. To determine reasonable treatment goals, the child's developmental age must be considered. Choosing a developmental theory to use as a framework is essential in working with children. Because EAP/EAL requires a certain degree of cognitive development, activities are more beneficial if the child's maturity level is considered in designing activities. Even when using a client-centered play therapy approach (modified with equine partners), it is essential to also have a further developed theoretical frame of reference in processing an EAP or an EAL activity with the client. Although minimal processing may take place with the client(s), as a mental health professional and equine specialist, applying a theory such as Piaget's cognitive development theory or Erickson's psychosocial stages of development will clarify the outcomes and benefits of the sessions.

One concept that is most frequently considered in EAP is that of resiliency. Resiliency is defined as, "a stable personality trait or ability which protects the individual from the negative effects of risk and adversity. Resiliency is a dynamic process that evolves as a normal part of healthy development" (Griffith, 2011). Resiliency can be diminished by abuse and neglect, separation or death of parents, complex trauma, and many other factors that children often face. By teaching and building resiliency within EAP, some children are enabled to succeed when faced with adversity and risk (Griffith, 2011).

Case Study of Sarina, Age Six

Background

Sarina had just come to her third foster home. She had been abandoned by her mother at age five, witnessed the arrest of her father at age six, and placed in foster care a week later. Sarina had been taken away from her home, her new puppy, and her school. Acting out her anger was such a problem, she was removed from the first home. The second home had an older sibling who physically abused her. When the case manager arrived to check in on Sarina, she found bruises on her arms and a cut lip. At first, Sarina would not tell her case manager what had happened. Finally, when Sarina shared what happened, the case manager decided that she would seek another placement. Now, Sarina was facing yet another transition and adjustment.

Her new foster parents were warm and accepting, but they were concerned about her withdrawing behavior and her refusal to talk. They wondered how they were going to help Sarina heal. When they heard about a therapy program using horses, they felt encouraged. When Sarina's foster parents called the farm, I explained to them how EAP works. I gave them details about using a team approach (a therapist, an equine specialist, and horses) and how sessions were structured. I also gave them information about why we use horses to help children heal. The foster parents agreed to come to the farm for an intake session. Sarina's case manager would also join the intake session to help provide information and start to develop a treatment plan.

Initial Intake

Sarina's case manager, Tonya, introduced herself. She shared background information about how Sarina came into foster care. Tonya explained to us that it was not likely she would ever be reunited with either of her parents. Sarina's mother had disappeared and was presumed to have been caught up in her substance abuse and addiction. Sarina's father was incarcerated and would not be released for many years. Tonya detailed the events that had taken place with Sarina's anger outbursts at the first home and the physical abuse by the hands of an older sibling at the second home.

I then asked the foster parents, Melinda and Bryan, to describe what they had seen since Sarina had arrived to their home. Sarina stayed to herself as much as she could and seemed reluctant to interact with their biological daughter Beth, same age as Sarina. They shared that in fact, Sarina had hardly communicated at all since she was placed with them. Teachers at Sarina's school reported that she appeared very withdrawn and refused to speak. At recess she sat on the wall with her head in her hands. Teachers and students who tried to help Sarina feel welcome gave up after Sarina did not respond.

Together Tonya, Melinda, Bryan, and I completed a pretest for assessment of trauma. We also completed a functional analysis of behavior that would help us develop treatment goals. We decided that addressing Sarina's grief and anger was the first step. After that, building her resiliency was critical due to the nature of foster care. So often when children are placed in the foster care system, they drift through several foster families before they age out of the system. We knew that changing Sarina's history was not possible but that perhaps helping her respond to her current environment in a healthier way would assist her in building the resiliency she needed.

We began developing our treatment plan. In EAP, the goal is to help in the healing of clients. Whereas, in EAL, the goal is to build resiliency, self-esteem and teach life skills (Jung & Cowles, 2009). With this case, both trauma and resilience needed to be addressed. The first sessions focused more on EAP, and the sessions toward the end focused more on EAL.

Before ending the intake session, I invited Melinda, Bryan, and Tonya to meet the horses. I took them out to the barn then showed them the arena where we would work with Sarina. I invited them to have a brief encounter with the horses to demonstrate how EAP works. They enthusiastically agreed so I asked the equine specialist to bring out two horses to the arena and join us. Horses are asked to be themselves in EAP and we remove any restraints, so they can roam at liberty. When everyone entered the arena, Pam, the equine specialist had a brief safety talk. Then, they were invited to meet and greet the horses in any way that they chose. After they finished, we talked about how that was for them and what they observed. All agreed that they thought this would be a positive experience for Sarina. The first session was scheduled, and Sarina began coming to the farm once a week to see her therapists (both human and equine).

Sarina's First EAP Session

Before Sarina arrived, Pam and I put out a variety of props in the arena, which included: poles, cones, buckets, ropes, jump standards, flags, ribbons, stuffed animals, dress-up clothes, hula hoops, scarves, masks, drawing utensils, foam squares, pool noodles, duct tape, and flags. These items are always in the arena when working with children, much like a playroom for play therapy. We decided to use just one horse in the first session, a small pony who was a proven expert with children.

Melinda and Sarina entered the barn. Sarina had her head down with her eyes on the ground. When Pam and I eagerly greeted her, there was no response. I stooped down and put my hand out to Sarina and said, "I have a special friend I would like for you to meet—will you come with me?" She gave no verbal response, but put her hand in mine and Pam, Sarina, and I walked out to the arena. Melinda stayed inside the barn in the waiting area. After we went through the gate we stood near the pile of props. The pony was on the other side of the arena grazing. Sarina began to look around but stayed frozen in one spot. In a couple of minutes, the pony began walking slowly toward Sarina. Soon he was face-to-face with her. They looked at each other and then he nuzzled one of her hands. She smiled and reached out to pat him on the neck.

The pony stood by Sarina for a few more minutes, letting her rub his neck. Then he went to the pile of props and put a stuffed animal in his mouth. He walked over to another spot and dropped the stuffed animal. Then he came back and picked up a pool noodle and moved it.

Pam said, "The horse is moving some things to a different place—I wonder what that's about?" Sarina looked at both of us as if to ask permission to move. She then went to the pile and took out a hula hoop and offered it to the pony. She put it on his neck, and he began to follow her on a walk.

When Sarina and the pony returned to us, she was smiling. I took a chance and asked her how that felt to have the pony walk with her. At first, she did not say anything. We showed a feelings chart and asked her to point to the face that showed how she was feeling. She pointed to the happy face. Then we asked her how she thought the pony felt, and she again pointed to the happy face. We told Sarina that our time was up for the day, but that she could say good-bye to the pony, however, she chose. She put her hand out to his nose, he nuzzled her again, and she said out loud, "Goodbye – see you next time." Melinda was waiting in the barn. Sarina was still smiling when we met back up with her. We scheduled the next session and they left.

Sarina's Second EAP Session

Bryan brought Sarina to the second session. She came into the barn and immediately started walking toward the arena. We had the pony and all the props already waiting for her. After a brief meet and greet for Sarina and the pony we introduced the feelings chart again. This time we added a feelings thermometer that measured feelings intensity on a scale from 1 to 10. Pam explained about horses living in the "here and now" and they are always watching around them to keep themselves safe. When they felt safe in the wild, they could lie down for short periods of time. We asked her how a horse might know it was safe and to point to where that might be on the feelings thermometer. She pointed to a "1," which indicated "chilling and peaceful."

We then invited Sarina to create a story using anything in the arena, including the pony. Sarina began looking through the pile of items. She chose four pool noodles and arranged them in a square. Inside the square she placed a towel and a stuffed dog. Then she took a rope and made it into a circle. Sarina stood inside the circle for a minute and ran to a mounting block (a two-step object for getting on a horse) and drug it to the center of the arena. She climbed onto the top step and again stood for a minute. Finally, she picked up six more pool noodles and made a shape. She put several stuffed animals inside and sat down on the ground in the middle of the animals.

It appeared Sarina was finished with her story. We asked her to tell us her story. She immediately went and put a hula hoop on the horse and encouraged him to come with her. She said that the first square was her home where she had to leave her puppy. The second circle with a rope was the first foster home where she was angry because she had to stay here away from her family. The mounting block represented a way to get away from that "bad boy who hurt me." The last shape she made was where she was now. The stuffed animals made her feel safe so she could sit down (just like a horse can lie down when they feel safe). Sarina took the pony with her to all the parts of her story. She stated that the pony made her "feel safe." At this point, our time was up. We invited Sarina to say goodbye to the pony in any way that she chose. She put her arms around his neck and said, "Thanks for keeping me safe. See you next week!"

In our debriefing session, Pam and I agreed that progress was being made. Sarina had talked quite a

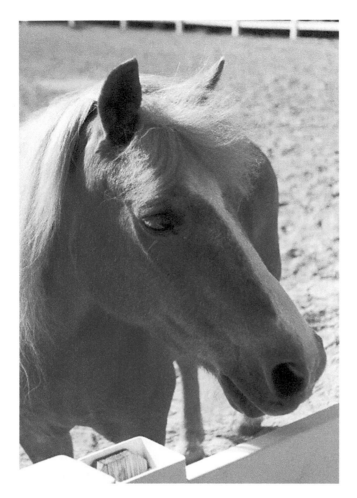

Figure 11.1 Chestnut colored horse with braided mane stands in horse ring.

Source: Susan Jung.

bit more this session and she seemed eager to express herself in her story. Bryan also told us that Sarina and Beth had played together several times during the week. Her teachers reported that Sarina still was not talking or interacting much at school (Figure 11.1).

Post-case Discussion and Summary of Treatment

We continued to see Sarina weekly for about six months. The treatment plan for Sarina called for trauma-focused activities early in the process. During and after each session, we constantly used the SPUD's observational model to evaluate what was happening in the sessions. There were many shifts and patterns during the sessions, which allowed us to determine when Sarina was ready to move forward into the next stage of treatment.

In the second phase of the treatment, we introduced concepts of understanding her feelings, providing some coping skills for everyday use in school and at home, and giving her some sense of empowerment. We wanted to provide Sarina with an experience of a nonjudgmental environment to explore changes in her behavior. In addition to working with Sarina in the arena, we spoke with Tonya, Melinda, and Bryan regularly to assess progress outside of therapy. There were certainly some ups and downs with Sarina's behavior throughout the process. Overall, Melinda said about halfway through treatment, "Sarina is at least smiling more, and we are beginning to feel more like she is part of our family. She's doing better in school, too!"

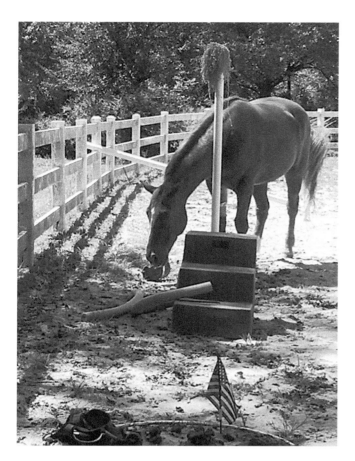

Figure 11.2 Dustin likes to play.

Source: Photo courtesy of Susan Jung.

About the last month of treatment, Sarina asked if Beth could join her sessions. We agreed and invited Beth to participate. The session went well and after two sessions, which included Beth, Sarina requested that Melinda and Bryan also join. The last three sessions of treatment were done with the family unit. At that point, we had added two other horses to the sessions. At the end, it was a celebration for them to all be together. The horses most definitely did their jobs. They were honest and provided important feedback. They showed attitudes and moods and they mirrored what Sarina was feeling. They liked to have fun. The nature-based play therapy with the horses proved to be a life-changing experience for Sarina. The following section is an example of session plans and procedures for EAP (Figure 11.2).

Session Plans and Procedures for the EAP Team

Session 1

For all sessions, have plenty of props in the arena, which may include poles, cones, buckets, ropes, jump standards, flags, ribbons, stuffed animals, dress-up clothes, hula hoops, scarves, masks, drawing utensils, balls, foam squares, pool noodles, duct tape, and flags.

Objective—Understanding and Communicating Feelings

Introduce a feeling chart and ask the child to name the feelings according to the pictures.

Discuss the role of body language in determining how humans or animals feel. Give a brief explanation of the word "empathy." Ask, "if you think you understand how someone feels, how important is it to respond? For example, if you see someone crying, what would you do?"

Have the child observe the horses in the arena. Discuss the following questions:

a   How are the horses feeling?
b   How do you know?
c   How do you know what people are feeling?
d   How can you tell by their actions?

**(These check-in questions can be used in all the sessions.)

Ask the child to lead a horse to different spots in the arena. Have the child "read" the horse's feelings at each location by paying attention to the horse's actions (body language). Ask them to determine what the feeling is and what action helped them come to this conclusion. Write their responses on separate index cards and place them in buckets labeled "feelings" and "actions."

After all the stations have been completed, review the cards in the buckets to reinforce the relationship between feelings and actions.

Debriefing:

1   Were the horse's feelings different at each spot?
2   How did you feel when the horse was feeling that feeling?
3   How did you respond to the horse's feeling?
4   How can you practice empathy during the coming week? (Jung, 2016)

Session 2

Objective: Becoming Aware of Personal Feelings

Introduce a feelings thermometer, a feelings wheel, or another instrument that helps the child identify and measure their feelings' intensity on a scale from 1 to 10. Ask the child to indicate the power of his or her emotion with certain activities like observing the horses, leading a horse, brushing a horse, etc. Explain that horses live in the here and now and that their goal is always to keep themselves safe. They are continually checking their surroundings and being present in the moment. Encourage the child to "check in" with their feelings throughout the day.

Ask the child to do some grooming of the horse. Use the check-in questions from Session 1 to help the child recognize feelings.

Session 3

Objective: Sharing My Story

Invite the child to create their story using anything in the arena. The horses can be characters in their story. The story may be in the form of a timeline, path, a circle, or any way they would like to express events and feelings. When the child has indicated they are finished, ask the child to share the story using curiosity questioning and the check-in questions about feelings. The SPUD's observational model will give important data for determining future directions in setting up the sessions.

Session 4

Objective: Defining Thoughts, Feelings, Actions

The difference between thoughts (using the mind), feelings (using the heart), and actions (things that are done) is discussed with the child. A large triangle is set up in the arena, with each point representing thoughts, feelings, and actions. Ask the child to choose some items that symbolize ideas and place them at the thoughts point. Then ask the child to place items that represent feelings on the feelings corner and items that illustrate actions on the action corner.

The child is asked to think of a real-life situation and take a horse to the Thoughts part of the triangle. Continue to move the horse to Feelings and then to Actions.

Debriefing:

1 What happened when the horse moved through the triangle?
2 What did the horse do with the Thoughts and Feelings?
3 How can you change negative thoughts, feelings, and actions into positive thoughts, feelings, and actions?
4 Who can help you do this at home, school, with friends?

Session 5

Objective: Rearranging Negative Thinking

Acknowledging that the child can stop negative thoughts (unhelpful thoughts, things untrue about themselves, the worst will happen, etc.) by Thought Stopping gives them a coping skill.

The child is asked to take a horse for a walk around the arena. Tell the horse to "go" and "whoa" in certain areas.

Debriefing:

1 What happened when you gave the horse the commands of "go" and "whoa"?
2 What were you thinking about during the activity?
3 If you use "whoa" to stop a thought in your brain, what might happen? If you have a terrible idea and tell it to "whoa," it helps you take charge of your thoughts and gives you power (EquiPower, 2015).

Session 6

Objective: Developing Self-Confidence and Empowerment

Ask the child to choose a horse and use anything in the arena to make the horse "the most powerful horse in the world" (see Appendix A).

Debriefing:

1 How did you decide what "powerful" means?
2 How does each of the items you used represent "power"?
3 Did the horse change any when he became "most powerful"?
4 When are times in your life that you feel "powerful"? (Jung, 2016).

Closing Comments/Chapter Summary

Believing the best solutions come from within, EAP/EAL allow children to discover, learn, and grow from the horse–human relationship's unique qualities. It creates a physically and emotionally safe environment as the horses and children are each free to interact. It requires nothing of the horse except to be a horse. Children can explore, problem-solve, and overcome challenges in their life. EAP helps children cultivate positive feelings, thoughts, and actions to enhance their well-being. EAP delivers life-changing outcomes.

EAP/EAL focuses on transformation, taking children at their current developmental level and moving them to their potential in that stage. "Helping them through the developmental stages of childhood, over the natural hurdles of life, prepares them for the next stage and builds their resiliency in handling those unforeseen events that create trauma and strife" (Jung & Cowles, 2009). Horses can transform lives.

Resources

Equine Assisted Growth and Learning Association. www.eagala.org
Natural Lifemanship. www.naturallifemanship.com
Path International. www.pathintl.org

Reflective Questions on Equine-Assisted Psychotherapy and Learning

1   In what ways are horses valuable in the therapeutic process?
2   How can the principles of play therapy be applied to equine- assisted psychotherapy?
3   What must be considered in designing a treatment plan using EAP?

Appendix A

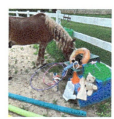

THE MOST POWERFUL HORSE

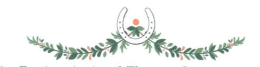

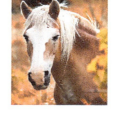

An Equine-Assisted Therapy Intervention
Susan Jung, EdS, LPC

DESCRIPTION:

This intervention utilizes the availability of an outdoor arena with a horse and equipment for a client to explore empowerment while assisted by a trained equine-assisted therapist.

RECOMMENDED SETTING:

An arena with a horse and several props, such as: cones, hula hoops, poles, flags, buckets, ropes, stuffed animals, dress-up clothes, masks, scarves, balls, duct tape, etc.

GOAL:

To develop self-confidence and empowerment.

INSTRUCTIONS:

Once in the arena, ask the client to choose a horse and use anything in the arena to make the horse "the most powerful horse in the world."

The client is then asked the following:
1. How did you decide what "powerful" means?
2. How does each of the items you used represent "power"?
3. Did the horse change any when he became "most powerful"?
4. When are times in your life that you feel "powerful"?

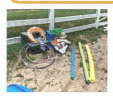

EXTRA FUN

The client can also be invited to choose items from the arena that would make them feel "most powerful." These activities could also be done in a sandtray or outdoor play using horse figures and other toys.

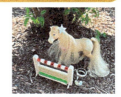

References

Association for Play Therapy. (2020). *What is play therapy?* Retrieved March 21, 2021 from https://a4pt.org

Buck, P., Bean, N., & de Marco, K. (2017). Equine-assisted psychotherapy: An emerging trauma-informed intervention. *Advances in Social Work*, 18, 387–402. https://doi.org/10.18060/21310

Cook, A., Blaustien, M., Spinazzola, J., & can der Kolk, B. (Eds.) (2003). *Complex trauma in children and adolescents*. National Child Traumatic Stress Network. http://www.NCTSNet.org

Crawford, T., Shaffer, A., Stuber, J., Waibel, P., & Walterreit, L. (2020). A match made in heaven: Equine assisted psychotherapy and play therapy—Hopewell Ranch Presentation at Eagala Conference, Lexington, KY.

Dunlop, K., & Tsantefski, M. (2018). A space of safety: Children's experience of equine-assisted group therapy. *Child & Family Social Work*, 23(1), 16–24. https://doi.org/10.1111/cfs.12378

Eagala (2009). *Fundamentals of Eagala model practice* (6th ed.). Santaquin, UT: Equine Assisted Growth and Learning Association.

Eagala (2019). *Fundamentals of the Eagala model* (9th ed.). Santaquin, UT: Equine Assisted Growth and Learning Association.

Griffith, K. (2011). *Building resiliency*. Warminster, PA: Mar-Co Products.

Jung, S. (2016). *Head 'em up! Move 'em out!: An equine assisted learning program for school counselors*. Conyers GA: Winning Strides LLC.

Jung, S., & Cowles, D. (2009). *Colts and fillies: EAL for children*. Conyers, GA: Winning Strides LLC.

Quiroz, R., Jimenez, B., Mazo, R., Campos, M., & Molina, M. (2005). From kids and horses: Equine facilitated psychotherapy for children. *International Journal of Clinical and Health Psychology*, 5(2). https://www.researchgate.net/publication/26420305_From_kids_and_horses_Equine_facilitated_psychotherapy_for_children

Schaefer, C. E., & Peabody, M. A. (2016). Glossary of play therapy terms. *Play Therapy*, 11(2), 20–24.

Schultz, P., Remick-Barlow, A., & Robbins, L. (2007). Equine-assisted psychotherapy: A mental health promotion/intervention modality for children who have experienced intra-family violence. *Health and Social Care in the Community (2007)*, 15(3), 265–271. https://www.kreac.nl/media/onderzoek10.pdf

Swank, J., Walker, K., & Sang, S. (2020). Indoor nature-based play therapy: Taking the natural world inside the playroom. *International Journal of Play Therapy*, 29, 155–162. https://doi.org/10.1037/pla0000123

The Jurga Report at EQUUS magazine.com. (2015). Horse in' around in childhood can really change your life. Retrieved January 7, 2015 from: http://equusmagazine.com/blog/horsing-childhood-wsu-evidence-cortisol-stress-hormone-16393#sthash.lMltemQj.dpuf

PART V
Nature-Based Family Interventions

12 Tiny Hearts and Hands: Nature Sensory Play Promotes Infant Mental Health

Janet A. Courtney and Ashley S. Lingerfelt

Introduction

The field of infant mental health is growing exponentially and many practitioners from a range of professional disciplines are desiring to grow their expertise to work with infants and young children (Courtney, 2020a). In that, practitioners are searching for new therapy strategies to intervene with parents and infants. As the growing interest in nature-based therapies increases, many practitioners are thinking about how to incorporate nature approaches for our youngest of clients (defined for purposes of this chapter as ages in utero to 36 months). While in attendance at the annual Zero to Three conference in October, 2020, this author (Courtney) learned that the association recently added a "green" initiative for infants with the original intention that infants and young children need access to unpolluted clean air. After the crisis of the COVID-19 pandemic and the healing benefits of nature came more to the forefront of awareness, the association began to widen their definition and recognized that infant mental health was supported by connection to nature overall—beyond just the physical health benefits (Figure 12.1). This is good news as Zero to Three is a highly influential infant mental health organization in the United States (refer to https://www.zerotothree.org/ to discover more about the organization).

Nature is Rich with Vital Sensory Experiences

At birth, infants have garnered millions of nerve connections that are chemically ready to encode sensory input (Schwartzenberger, 2020). Therefore, infants and young children need a wide range of sensory experiences to wire healthy brain development. Sensory input is directed through neuro pathways to the thalamus and across synapses to the amygdala limbic parts of the brain that are involved in emotion, motivation, and memory (Lillas & Turnbull, 2009). Nature experiences gives infants and their parents or caregivers the opportunity for direct contact with their sensory systems (Courtney 2020b).

It is important to recognize that children connect with nature differently than adults. For young children, nature is more than just a beautiful backdrop to admire—they want to engage whole-bodily with the environment. We are all familiar with our five basic sensory systems of sight (visual), hearing, olfactory (smell), gustatory (taste), and touch. Show a flower to a young child and they can delight in its beauty, they can smell for scent and feel the consistency of the varied textures of the leaves and petals. They will want to dig their hands into the dirt where the flower came from and may even place their ear near it to try and listen to its voice. Of course, infants may instinctively try to taste the flower too which calls attention to the need for safety measures and constant monitoring of young children in outdoor environments.

Spending extended time with infants in nature helps to invigorate all the vital sensory organs that assist us in navigating our interpersonal relationships as we grow. We know that the visual sense helps us to interpret nonverbal cues and discern eye contact and body language from others. Children that have a hard time processing visual stimuli may have problems within interpersonal relationships. The sense of smell is connected to our emotions and memories and is known as one of our oldest systems in our brain. Encouraging experiences in nature where young children can cultivate their sense of smell—such as breathing in the fresh air of an ocean or mountain breeze—may help to create a foundation of positive lifelong emotional regulation abilities stored within the implicit memory. The tactile and auditory systems are often cited with children who have been diagnosed with sensory processing disorder. Some children may have difficulty processing auditory input and might have problems with attention and directions and

DOI: 10.4324/9781003152767-17

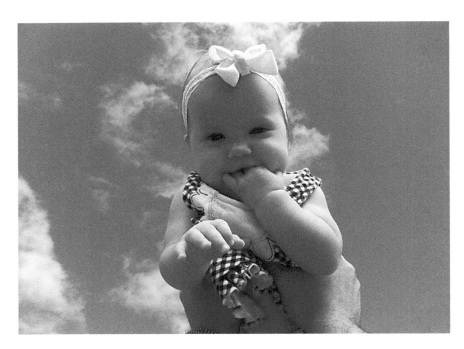

Figure 12.1 Sophia enjoys playing outdoors.
Source: Jesse Crowley used with permission.

become easily startled. The auditory sense helps to interpret sound frequencies and help us to understand and make sense of varied pitch sounds and speech. Thus, the natural world provides a wealth of auditory experiences from birds chirping to the sound of a splash from a stone thrown in a pond.

Touch is how children make sense of the world and is an important component of sensory integration (Courtney & Nolan, 2017). The development of touch is crucial to our ability to determine if something is safe to touch or dangerous—think hot stove—or a bush with pointed stickers. When a child touches something, the body sends that tactile information through the central nervous system up the spinal cord through the brain stem and to the somatosensory cortex that processes touch. Thus, providing opportunities for infants and young children to experience the natural world through direct kinesthetic contact such as pounding a mud pie, chucking rocks in a pond, pouring water in a bucket, gathering pinecones, or shaking a tree branch is vital to wiring synapses in the brain.

In addition to nature kindling the five senses, infants are developing their essential vestibular, proprioceptive, and interoceptive systems. The vestibular and proprioceptive senses are referred to as the sixth and seventh sense, respectively, and are much less recognized. The vestibular sense is all about balance, equilibrium, and coordination. It is the sense that helps children to put on their shoes, comb hair, walk across a narrow plank, or stack stones on top of each other. Inverting our head is one way to enliven our vestibular sense such as hanging upside down from a tree branch! Our proprioceptive sense helps us to make our way spatially in the world. It stimulates the receptors in our joints and muscles every time we move our body. Our proprioceptive awareness is focused in the right hemisphere of the brain, which is linked directly to the "physiological changes in the body when we experience emotion" (McGilchrist, 2009). McGilchrist elaborated, "The right hemisphere's superiority in the emotional realm is explicitly linked to this close physiological relationship with the body" (p. 69). Both senses work together wherein vestibular stimulation supports our bodily functions toward coordinated balance and self-independence and our proprioceptive sense assists to organize our body's spatial and emotional regulation. Time out in nature for children to run, jump, skip, roll, and somersault grows these two vital interrelated senses (Figure 12.2).

Interoception is one of our newer discovered senses. It relates to the physiological internal sensors that provide an awareness of what our internal organs are feeling. They play a crucial role in regulation and

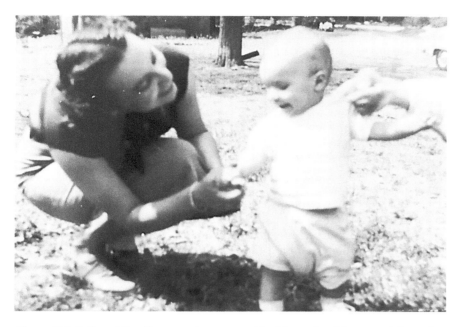

Figure 12.2 Infant Allen Courtney is supported by his mother Margaret Adams Courtney to learn how to walk and explore in nature growing his vestibular, proprioceptive, and interoceptive sensory systems.

Source: Janet A. Courtney.

assist to detect internal responses, including hunger, thirst, heart rate, respiration, and elimination. Interoception helps us to connect internally with our own bodies and works with the proprioceptive and vestibular systems. It is suggested that interoception is the key foundation of our ability to perceive our inner emotional feelings that supports self-awareness. Interoception works with the vestibular and proprioceptive senses to determine how a person understands their own bodily states. Taylor et al. (2009) postulated that the anterior insula-cingulate system may integrate Interoceptive information with emotional information to form a bodily sense of self. Young infants who are learning how to crawl, walk, and run are sprouting their developing vestibular, proprioceptive, and interoceptive systems. If adults can provide opportunities for infants and young children to practice these developmental milestones in a safe outdoor environment, then the opportunity for optimal wholistic growth to occur are bountiful.

The following case study examines how nature can provide a rich growing experience for a mother–infant relationship where they can develop and optimize their wide-range sensory systems and coregulate interrelational experiences while also exploring the boundaries of autonomy, attunement, risk taking, and safety within a series of therapist directed nature-based play therapy interventions.

Case Study of Elizabeth and Grace (18 Months)

This case study highlights the intersection of infant mental health and nature play therapy with a mother–daughter infant dyad, Elizabeth and Grace (18 months).

Background

Elizabeth is an attentive, responsive mother who suffers from perinatal anxiety. She first experienced symptoms of anxiety when pregnant with her daughter, Grace, age 18 months at time of intake. Her anxiety increased after she was advised by the medical doctor that she had an abnormal fetal ultrasound at 20 weeks. Fortunately, an additional scan a couple of weeks later revealed no abnormalities. However, despite this good news, Elizabeth continued to feel an overwhelming sense of fear and uncertainty regarding her daughter's ongoing health, even after birth. This anxiety has significantly affected her overprotective parenting style, which she feels may be adversely affecting Grace. Elizabeth brought up these concerns with her daughter's pediatrician, who then referred her to a counselor that specializes in infant mental health and infant play therapy modalities that included nature-based interventions. Concerned about the impact of her anxiety on her daughter's development, Elizabeth contacted the counselor and scheduled an intake appointment.

Session 1: Intake

During the initial intake appointment, the counselor gathered relevant history regarding Elizabeth's pregnancy and Grace's development. Elizabeth shared that she had noticed an increased sense of reserve and fear in Grace, and when compared to her peers, Grace seems more timid and not as "adventurous" or "independent." She shared, for example, that when playing with other toddlers at the local park, Grace often expresses interest in running and playing with her peers, but she quickly withdraws and clings to her mother. The counselor asked how Elizabeth has responded to Grace's attempts to explore in the past. Elizabeth shared that she does not like for Grace to pick up nature items from the ground at the park, and does not let her venture farther than an arm's reach at any given time due to wanting to keep Grace safe.

The counselor responded with empathy, understanding that Elizabeth's medical scare during pregnancy heightened her need to create safety for Grace. When the counselor asked about (or suggested) this connection, Elizabeth became tearful and said that ever since the misdiagnosed ultrasound, she has felt a deep need to keep Grace safe and healthy out of fear that something could hurt her at any moment. She explained that her entire world came crashing down when she was 20 weeks pregnant, and the only thing she could do was focus on keeping her child safe. Elizabeth could not shake the terrifying feeling of being out of control and having no control over her daughter's wellbeing.

In addition to the intake interview, the counselor offered the following assessments (Nowakowski-Sims & Powers, 2020):

a　*The Ages and Stages Questionnaire*, 3rd ed. (ASQ-3),
b　*Ages & Stages Questionnaires®: Social-Emotional*, 2nd ed. (ASQ®:SE-2), and
c　the Child Development Inventory as screeners for development.

In addition, the counselor screened Elizabeth for anxiety using:

d　the Perinatal Anxiety Screening Scale (PASS), and
e　the Generalized Anxiety Disorder-7 Scale (GAD-7).

Scores from the assessments and screeners revealed that Elizabeth does suffer from moderate to severe anxiety. Developmentally, Grace scored average or above average in the domains of cognitive, and emotional development, but her social and relational domains were slightly delayed, indicating a need for support in these areas.

Following the intake, the counselor created the following treatment plan.

Case Study Treatment Plan

Session Type	Objective	Nature Intervention
Session 1: Intake	Gather background history and formulate treatment plan	
Session 2	Increase co-regulation in the parent-infant dyad	"Earth Imprints"
Session 3	Increase parental reflective capacity and attunement	"Shadow Dances"
Session 4	Increase co-regulation and attunement	"Nature Touches"
Session 5	Increase opportunity to for natural risk-taking and sensory input	"Special Tracks"
Session 6: Termination	Support parental confidence and sustain progress at home	

Knowing it is not uncommon for young children of anxious parents to also demonstrate anxieties and insecurities of their own, the counselor explained to Elizabeth the potential impact of her anxiety on her relationship with Grace in a warm, nonjudgmental manner.

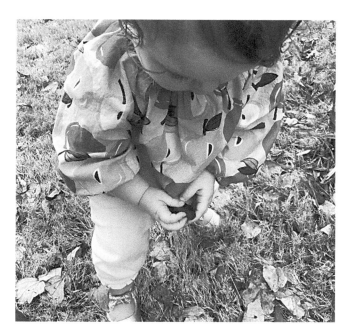

Figure 12.3 Tiny hands explore kinesthetic sensory play.

Source: Ashley Lingerfelt.

Counselor: "Thank you so much for sharing all of this with me today, Elizabeth. I know how difficult it can be to talk about our own worries and insecurities. Please know that you are not alone in this. One in seven women experience feelings of postpartum depression or anxiety. It's common, but not spoken about often. It's normal to need help with these thoughts. I'm so proud of you for seeking support! Together, we can help you overcome your anxiety and can support your relationship with your daughter to the fullest extent. How does that sound?"

Elizabeth: "Thank you. It is such a relief to know that I can repair my relationship with my daughter and set a healthy example for her going forward. I just feel so lost, though. I'm not even sure where to begin!"

Counselor: "That is understandable! That's what I'm here for. I have a few specific interventions in mind that will help foster a sense of exploration within Grace, while also supporting her connection with nature and most importantly, with you. Are you open to some suggestions?"

Elizabeth: "Yes, absolutely!"

Counselor: "Perfect! I am excited to work with you and Grace."

Session 2: "Earth Imprints"

The following week, Elizabeth met with the counselor to discuss the continuing plan of support. The counselor explained an intervention called "Earth Imprints" (see Appendix A) that helps to increase co-regulation within the parent-infant dyad as described in the following dialogue:

Counselor: "The first intervention I want you to practice is called 'Earth Imprints.' When shifting your parenting style, you're going to want to be consistent, but gradual with any proposed changes you make to your relationship with your child. While our goal is for Grace to have the trust and security to explore her natural world freely, we need to build up to that point with a few lower exposure interventions that focus on you and her being together, without high pressure or expectation. This intervention does just that. Not only will it help familiarize Grace with elements of the natural world and spark her sense of wonder and exploration, but it will also help you find peace and beauty in Grace's perfect little body, just as it is. I can't wait for you to try it!"

The counselor went over the instructions with Elizabeth, giving her an opportunity to ask questions and receive clarity before her appointment ended.

Elizabeth: "I'm nervous, but excited. I can't wait to see how Grace responds!"
Counselor: (In a reassuring manner) "It's okay to be nervous! This will be new for both of you.

Follow Grace's cues and go at a pace that is comfortable for both of you. I can't wait to hear how it goes!"

Session 3: "Shadow Dances"

During the next session, the goal was to monitor progress and introduce additional activities to support the parent–infant relationship. With that in mind, the counselor checked in with Elizabeth about last week's intervention, "Earth Imprints" (see Appendix A) and then introduced a new activity called, "Shadow Dances" (see Appendix B).

Counselor: "Hi, Elizabeth! So, tell me, how have things been since we saw each other last week?"
Elizabeth: "Well, things have been okay. I have been more aware of how I approach Grace and how much autonomy I give her when we are playing. It is hard to take a step back and trust in Grace's abilities. I find that to be rather difficult."
Counselor: "I completely understand. You're right, it is hard to make these changes. The good thing is that you've started to build awareness around your relationship with Grace and you are eager to support her. That's so good to hear. And did you have a chance to practice the Earth Imprints intervention with Grace?"
Elizabeth: "Thank you so much. I did! We practiced it one time. It was actually quite fun. We practiced it in our backyard. I followed the instructions and included Grace in gathering the nature objects. Grace found some sticks, stones and leaves and put them in the basket I had. When we got to the part of making her imprint, I was a little nervous because I was worried she would be uncomfortable and not enjoy lying on the grass."
Counselor: "And how did Grace respond?"
Elizabeth: "She was great! She laid there and I talked to her, just as the activity instructed. I labeled her arms, her head, and made a little story about the nature objects I was placing around her body. She looked at me and seemed very interested in what was going on. When she got up and saw the outline of her body, she smiled a huge smile. It was really nice to share this moment with her. I realized just how small, yet beautiful and strong she really is."
Counselor: "It sounds like this was a beautiful, positive moment you two shared."
Elizabeth: "It really was."
Counselor: "Did you find that it was difficult to continue the activity when you felt worried about Grace's reaction to lying in the grass?"
Elizabeth: "I honestly felt very worried about it, but instead of feeling overwhelmed and stopping the activity, I took a chance and followed through with it. I felt like our first session together gave me permission to share in this time with my daughter and that I should see it through."
Counselor: "I am so happy to hear that you persevered, even in the face of uncertainty. These small moments will go a long way in helping you feel secure in your relationship with Grace. It sounds like you gave Grace the opportunity to decide for herself what was too uncomfortable for her. From what you are sharing, it turns out, she greatly enjoyed lying in the grass and having you dote upon her! How wonderful that you both shared in this opportunity together. And, that was so creative that you added a story about the objects you were placing around her body."

Elizabeth:	"It was a little difficult at first, but yes, it was wonderful in the end."
Counselor:	"If it's okay with you, I would like to make another suggestion for this week's activity. Are you comfortable with trying something new?"
Elizabeth:	"Yes, of course."
Counselor:	"Great. The next intervention is called 'Shadow Dances.' This intervention will focus on helping you become more attuned with Grace, which will help you better discern her cues for support, independence, and more. How does that sound?"
Elizabeth:	"That sounds wonderful."
Counselor:	"Okay, let's go over it together before you leave today."

The counselor then explained the "Shadow Dances" activity (see Appendix B) and gave Elizabeth the opportunity to ask questions.

Session 4: "Nature Touches"

For their fourth session together, the counselor and Elizabeth discussed the previous week's progress and assessed Elizabeth's level of comfort with the current interventions. Elizabeth reported feeling confident about the "Shadow Dances" intervention and stated, "I enjoyed the opportunity to connect with Grace in such a fun, creative way." When the counselor asked about any difficulties Grace and Elizabeth experienced during this activity, Elizabeth admitted that it was hard for her to let go and be silly with Grace at first. She was unsure of how to move her body and dance. Elizabeth also admitted that she felt vulnerable moving so freely outside, but once Grace showed an interest in the shadows, a shift occurred and she was able to move freely to support the delight and amazement of her daughter commenting, "Nothing else mattered in that moment. Once I saw her eyes light up, I only wanted to enjoy this special time with her."

After processing the success and vulnerability of the "Shadow Dances" activity, the counselor asked Elizabeth if she felt comfortable being introduced to a new intervention. Elizabeth quickly agreed and the counselor explained an additional activity, "Nature Touches" (see Appendix C) that helps to heighten an infant and child's sensory awareness and preferences as well as increasing coregulation and parental attunement.

The counselor taught Elizabeth the new intervention and answered any questions she had. They agreed to meet the following week to monitor progress (Figure 12.4).

Session 5: "Special Tracks"

During the next session, the counselor and Elizabeth met to assess progress from the previous week. Elizabeth stated that she found the "Nature Touches" intervention "enlightening and informative." She said she had learned a lot about her daughter's sensory preferences through this activity and feels a heightened responsivity to her daughter's cues. For example, she shared that when brushing a feather across Grace's hand, she assumed Grace would enjoy it. However, Grace actually grimaced and quickly pulled her hand away and this reaction surprised Elizabeth. With the remaining nature objects, she paid careful attention to Grace's cues, such as her facial expressions, vocalizations, and body movements. Elizabeth realized that she had never paid such close attention to Grace in such an intentional way before. The counselor observed that this was the first time that Elizabeth had paid special attention to Grace's micro-expressions. Elizabeth felt as though she had gained a new understanding and appreciation for Grace's autonomy as a person.

The final intervention called, "Special Tracks" (see Appendix D), encourages parental support for natural risk taking. The counselor explained how each intervention has been building upon the skills of reflection, engagement, and attunement to strengthen Elizabeth's approach in each of these areas. She then explained that this fourth and final intervention is a culmination of these skills, with the addition of supporting appropriate risk-taking behavior by the child. The counselor shared the importance of risk taking and the role it plays in resilience and sensory development.

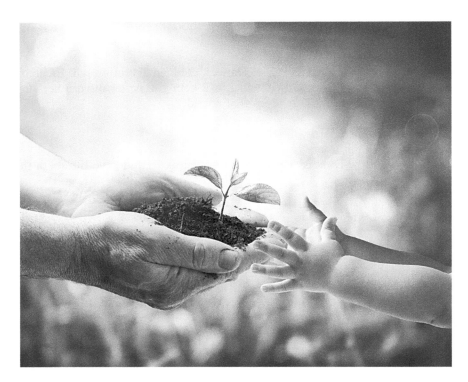

Figure 12.4 Sharing nature's treasures can begin at birth.

Source: RomoloTavani from iStock-641645848.

Session 6: Termination

The final session between Elizabeth and the counselor involved assessing how the previous week's intervention went. Elizabeth shared that "Special Tracks" was difficult for her to practice at first. She said that she took Grace to a local park to explore. This park had diverse terrain for Grace to explore, such as a small creek, a wooded area, a large grassy space, a paved walkway, and a bridge over a river. Elizabeth said that she let Grace lead the way, although it was difficult to remain a few steps behind Grace. Elizabeth shared that she "felt the urge to direct Grace's path," trying to keep her away from the rocks and divots in the natural landscape. However, Elizabeth said that as she observed Grace and allowed her the opportunity to explore the environment, she realized that Grace was actually quite capable of managing her safety naturally. Whereas before, Elizabeth did not allow Grace the opportunity for natural risk-taking during her play. Previously, risk-taking was difficult for Elizabeth to process. Elizabeth explained that there were a few occasions when Grace tripped as she toddled around, but to Elizabeth's surprise, she hopped right back up and kept going. When the counselor asked how Elizabeth would normally respond to Grace falling versus how she responded during this activity, Elizabeth said that she normally would not allow Grace the opportunity to fall, but if she did, she would respond immediately by picking Grace up and checking for injuries.

Elizabeth shared that this intervention felt foreign to her initially, but that thanks to the support during the therapy sessions and the previous interventions, she felt she could better identify Grace's needs via attunement. Using attunement, she was able to pick up on Grace's cues for independence and support. Additionally, if Grace did need a little bit of support, Elizabeth said she felt confident providing that support through coregulation. Overall, the counselor validated Elizabeth's perception of the intervention, agreeing that it must be difficult to allow Grace to explore freely when this is not something that is normally experienced within their parent–infant relationship. The counselor helped Elizabeth process this entire therapeutic experience, revisiting treatment goals and reiterating how much progress Elizabeth and Grace have shown. The counselor and Elizabeth agreed to meet on an as-needed basis going forward in an effort to support Elizabeth's growth.

Case Summary

Elizabeth, mother of 18-month-old Grace, sought counseling from an infant mental health specialist to increase her daughter's autonomy and independence in social settings. After undergoing assessments for both child and mother, it was determined that Elizabeth suffered from anxiety and that this was affecting her daughter's development. After completing a six-week treatment plan focusing on early developmental nature-based sensory interventions, Elizabeth experienced a reduction in anxiety symptoms and an increase in her ability to relationally engage with her daughter. Additionally, Grace participated in more independent play, risk-taking, and confidence when engaging in play with her mother and her peers.

Reflection Questions:

1   In thinking about working with young children ages birth to three years of age, what specific safety considerations might you take into account when suggesting nature-based outdoor play between a parent or caregiver and a young child.
2   Look over the four nature play activity appendixes in this chapter and with a partner discuss how you might use them in practice with a parent and young child.
3   Looking over the case study in this chapter, try to think of some other ways that you could support the mother Elizabeth with her young daughter. What other interventions might you suggest?

Appendix A

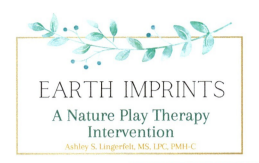

EARTH IMPRINTS

A Nature Play Therapy Intervention

Ashley S. Lingerfelt, MS, LPC, PMH-C

DESCRIPTION:

Let's focus on how special our bodies are!

In this activity, the caregiver traces the child's body with natural objects, leaving an imprint of their little body on the earth.

SUPPLIES NEEDED:

- Basket or small container

- Objects from natural environment, such as: leaves, flowers, pebbles, sticks, pinecones, acorns, and any other fun things!

GOAL:

To increase co-regulation in the caregiver/child dyad.

INSTRUCTIONS:

Child and caregiver gather objects from their natural environment, such as flowers, leaves, sticks, pebbles, acorns, pinecones, and more.

Caregiver asks child to lay down on the ground (preferably a soft, comfy spot). Caregiver then begins to outline the child's body with the objects, beginning with the child's head and coming down their arms, then their stomach, then their legs, ending with their feet.

Caregiver pays special attention to child's features, such as the length of their legs, the dimples in their elbows, the outline of their hair, etc., as they outline their body.

Once the caregiver is done, they help the child up and both take a few moments to marvel at the "earth imprint" the child left behind!

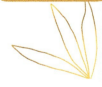 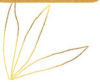

EXTRA FUN:

Encourage caregiver and child to place objects in the imprint signifying the child's heart, eyes, and any other special spots.

Appendix B

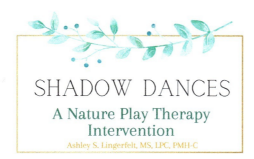

SHADOW DANCES
A Nature Play Therapy Intervention
Ashley S. Lingerfelt, MS, LPC, PMH-C

DESCRIPTION:

Let's dance!

Using your bodies, this nature-based intervention increases mind-body awareness and reflective functioning through organic movement.

SUPPLIES NEEDED:

- Comfortable clothes that do not restrict movement

- A safe, flat space outside

GOAL:

To increase reflective capacity and parent attunement.

INSTRUCTIONS:

Caregiver and child take turns watching their shadows dance.

Each person suggests a pose or movement and both try to achieve it!

Caregiver pays special attention to child's movements and reflects the speed, direction, intention, and emotion of the dancing.

Caregiver encourages child to notice the dances of other objects.

Do the trees and birds have shadow dances?
How about the weeds and bugs?

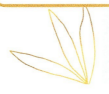
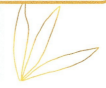

EXTRA FUN:
Introduce intentional tapping and stomping with hands and feet to create bilateral stimulation.

Appendix C

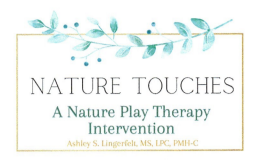

NATURE TOUCHES
A Nature Play Therapy Intervention
Ashley S. Lingerfelt, MS, LPC, PMH-C

DESCRIPTION:

Let's explore touch!

Using different natural materials, this activity focuses on sensory exploration with an emphasis on caregiver attunement.

SUPPLIES NEEDED:

- Basket or small container

- Objects from natural environment with varying textures, such as: leaves, flowers, feathers, twigs, grass, and more.

GOAL:
To increase co-regulation and caregiver attunement.

INSTRUCTIONS:

Child and caregiver gather objects from their natural environment, with an emphasis on collecting objects of varying textures and weights.

Caregiver asks child to hold out their arms and caregiver gently rubs the child's arm, wrist, and back of their hand with each item. Caregiver should apply an appropriate amount of pressure: not too hard, but not too light.

Caregiver pays special attention to child's response to each sensation. Some things to consider: Does the child seem upset? Do they seem to enjoy the touch? Are they smiling? Wrinkling their nose? Is the child pulling away?

As the caregiver goes through each item, give the child an opportunity to perform the same action on the caregiver.

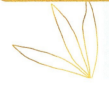

EXTRA FUN:
This activity can be repeated using the sense of smell. Can the child guess each item?

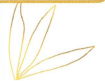

Appendix D

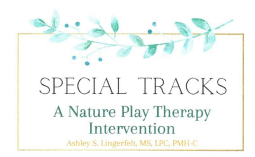

SPECIAL TRACKS
A Nature Play Therapy Intervention
Ashley S. Lingerfelt, MS, LPC, PMH-C

DESCRIPTION:

This activity encourages exploration via appropriate risk-taking behaviors. Caregivers will support movement, sensory exploration, and space as their child climbs, crawls, runs, sits, and more.

What kind of tracks does your child leave behind?

SUPPLIES NEEDED:

-A safe outdoor space with diverse terrain: hills, benches, streams, grass (boxes, chairs, pillows, and blankets can also be used for child to explore).
-Clothes that do not restrict movement

GOAL:

To increase opportunity for risk-taking and sensory input.

INSTRUCTIONS:

Caregiver tells child that they get to explore their world today. As they explore, caregiver narrates the child's journey and describe what kind of tracks the child leaves behind.

Caregiver follows child, narrating aloud as child plays. This may sound like: You are stepping over those rocks very carefully. You balanced on that log so well! What a fast animal you are! You are so brave.

Caregiver does not interfere with child's exploration unless child is in danger of being harmed.

While this activity is difficult for many caregivers, this intervention allows the child the opportunity to engage in appropriate risk-taking behaviors and enhances the development of their motor movements, sensory integration, and emotional resilience.

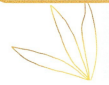

EXTRA FUN:

Encourage caregiver to ask child if they can imitate different animals. Can you run like a deer? Climb like a bear?

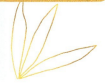

References

Courtney, J. A. (2020a). *Introduction infant play therapy: Foundations, programs, models and practice.* New York, NY: Routledge Publishing.

Courtney, J. A. (2020b). *Healing child and family trauma through expressive and play therapies: Art, nature, storytelling, body, mindfulness.* New York, NY: Norton & Co.

Courtney, J. A., & Nolan, R. D. (2017). *Touch in child counseling and play therapy: An ethical and clinical guide.* New York, NY: Routledge.

Lillas, C., & Turnbull, J. (2009). *Infant/child mental health, early intervention, and relationship-based therapies: A neurorelationship framework for interdisciplinary practice.* New York, NY: Norton.

McGilchrist, I. (2009). *The master and his emissary: The divided brain and the making of the Western world.* New Haven, CT: Yale University Press.

Nowakowski-Sims, E., & Powers, D. (2020). Trama-informed infant mental health assessment. In J. A. Courtney (Ed.), *Infant Play Therapy: Foundations, Models, Programs, and Practice* (pp. 67–79). New York, NY: Routledge.

Schwartzenberger, K. (2020). Neurosensory play in the infant-parent dyad: A developmental perspective. In J. A. Courtney (Ed.), *Infant Play Therapy: Foundations, Models, Programs, and Practice* (pp. 37–49). New York, NY: Routledge.

Taylor, K. S., Seminowicz, D. A., & Davis, K. D. (2009). Two systems of resting state connectivity between the insula and cingulate cortex. *Human Brain Mapping, 30*(9), 2731–2745. https://doi.org/10.1002/hbm.20705

13 Nature Play Therapy as a Healing Way for Children, Teens, and Families: Incorporating Nature with Play and Expressive Therapies

Jamie Lynn Langley

Introduction

Childhood and nature have often seemed such a natural pairing, until childhood literally stayed indoors with the influx of video games, television shows, and other media for entertainment. As clinicians, educators, and other professionals have become more concerned about children and youth and their loss of time in nature, a child and nature movement has taken root in recent years. This movement has especially flourished throughout the world since Richard Louv first pieced together research findings that the lack of time in nature was negatively impacting the physical and mental health of our children, declaring this as "Nature-Deficit Disorder" (Louv, 2005). Having grown up on a farm in early childhood and exposed to additional outdoor experiences via Girl Scouts and summer camp programs, nature was a large part of this author's early life experiences. It was concerning to realize the extent to which so many children have not had access to such experiences in nature, often due to the growing demands for their time for educational expectations, extracurricular activities, and the increasing screen time for entertainment. Already a champion for the importance of play for children, Louv's "call to action" provided the inspiration this author to understand the additional necessity of nature for childhood—and for play therapy itself.

History of Using Nature with Play Therapy

Traditionally play therapy has most often involved carefully selected toys within an indoor playroom, facilitated by a trained play therapist (Landreth, 2012). Incorporating nature with play and expressive therapies is different in that the therapist can go outside with clients and utilize nature's toys and playground for therapeutic play (Langley, 2019).This nature play can also include when items from nature are brought into the playroom or shared over a screen such as when part of telemental health (Langley, 2022). Although most play therapy practices and trainings have primarily emphasized the indoor playroom with toys as the primary setting, this has not been the only play therapy setting. It was recently learned from Dr. Linda Homeyer that one of the earliest play therapists, Dr. Margaret Lowenfeld, had a garden play area in the back of her building as early as the 1930s in which children could play outside as part of their therapy (Lowenfeld, 1991). This means that incorporating nature play as part of play therapy has been around almost as long as play therapy itself!

While not as well-known as a method of practice, nature materials and settings have been utilized by several play therapists in the nearly 90 years since Lowenfeld's practice. One of the longest known is registered art and play therapist Marie-Jose Dhaese of Canada, who has included nature-based practices as an integral part of her Holistic Expressive Therapy for over 40 years (Dhaese, 2011). She has a breathtaking natural outdoor play area and gardens, as well as many nature items indoors with which she conducts her therapy sessions and has provided inspiration for many child therapists (learn more here: https://centreforexpressivetherapy.com/).

There has been a resurgence of interest in the past few years for including nature as part of the play therapy experience. Even play therapists who had not previously considered nature-based practices have done more so since the COVID-19 pandemic, as they have wanted to continue providing therapy in a safer environment: the outdoors. This has included bringing normally indoor play materials outside to make a more formalized outdoor playroom (Walker, 2021). In addition, some play therapists have taken

DOI: 10.4324/9781003152767-18

clients outside with bubbles, pinwheels, and art materials to have a type of release and cathartic play after deeper or more intense play therapy sessions. In this way, clients can blow out or draw out those built-up feelings without concerns for walls, mess, or even volume for this play experience (see Appendix A). Nature Play Therapy can encompass various expressive arts as play often includes creative activities, movement, storytelling, and more. When utilizing specific activities and interventions within Nature Play Therapy, this author refers to these as NaturePlay.

Incorporating nature as part of play therapy has been an evolving practice for this author since that initial inspiration by Louv in 2005. As a practicing play therapist at that time for 15 years, nature had not previously been intentionally included in my play therapy provided. Once those seeds were planted, however, various ideas to include nature as part of play therapy began to sprout. This first began by taking games involving nature such as those played with my Cub Scout den and incorporating adaptions within play therapy. As these were successfully implemented, additional time was spent outside utilizing other nature-based therapeutic activities, games, and expressive arts as well as bringing aspects of nature to be incorporated in play therapy indoors and more recently over telemental health. In addition to offering these NaturePlay experiences during sessions, these are also prescribed to families as part of "nature missions" between sessions to continue and increase time spent in nature.

Making the Case for NaturePlay

Taking time for a "nature fix" was literally second nature for this author's family as an antidote to everyday stressors such as academic expectations and work pressures. Family activities including camping trips, day hikes, and even scout events that were often geared around nature. These nature experiences were later beneficial when working with children and their families who were not as accustomed to being outside. This has also helped when training therapists to incorporate nature in their play therapy practices. Some therapists and families have limited access to nature due to where they practice or live, especially in areas with little green space. Those who are not as comfortable with outdoor experiences are often concerned about the possible risks associated with being outside. Education and preparation are important keys to assisting both therapists and caregivers to be more comfortable with utilizing nature as part of play and expressive therapies.

The advantages of play for emotional health, brain development, and social interaction have become more recognized and understood in recent years (Wenner, 2009). Educating caregivers about the therapeutic powers of play (Schaefer & Drewes, 2014), as reviewed in Chapter 1, can be part of the intake interview to assist with their understanding of the need for play therapy. Helping them recognize that these mechanisms of change are also engaged via time in nature is instrumental (Ellard & Parson, 2021). To assist caregivers as well as therapists to better perceive the significance of these healing effects of nature, the following three research areas can be introduced to help "make the case" for NaturePlay: (1) emotional improvement, (2) positive results in short periods of nature exposure, and (3) long-term benefits into adulthood.

First: Time in nature improves emotional wellness, including increased attention, creativity, and problem-solving (Atchley et al., 2012), increased memory and decreased anxiety (Bratman et al., 2015), as well as improved mood (Berman et al., 2012), higher self-esteem (Barton & Pretty 2010), and enhanced creativity (Plambech & Konijnendijk van den Bosch, 2015). These are just a few of the many studies, but these findings appeal to most parents as they want their children to have improved emotional health.

Second: Being in nature can bring positive effects in a relatively short span of time. Research findings indicate the stress hormone of Cortisol can be reduced in as little as 20 minutes of daily nature exposure (Hunter et al., 2019). Prescribing nature with families between sessions for just 20-minutes in nature several times a week can be easily incorporated for families with busy schedules. This also makes integrating NaturePlay activities even more conducive to utilize in play therapy sessions. For therapists who find 20 minute increments difficult to incorporate within sessions, especially for clients (or therapists too) who may not be as comfortable with being outdoors, shorter periods of time can be implemented. As reported in the first chapter in this book, one study found that even five minutes outside in nature is beneficial to improve mood—even if it is simply sitting on a bench (Neill et al., 2019)! It makes sense that five minutes of play in nature would lead to even more improved mental health.

Third: These benefits of time in nature reach beyond the present into the future—for some children even into adulthood. Researchers are finding that more exposure to green and natural spaces in childhood leads to better emotional health as adults than those with less exposure (Preuß et al., 2019). We all want our children to grow up as emotionally and physically healthy as possible and time in nature can help achieve this!

These studies make a strong case for the inclusion of nature with play and expressive therapies. When these healing benefits of nature are combined with the therapeutic powers of play, Nature Play Therapy truly becomes a powerful dynamic duo. As such, it offers a double dose of healing for children, teens, and families.

Being Prepared and Safety Considerations for NaturePlay

There are some preparations needed for the therapist as well as the client and family prior to conducting Nature Play Therapy sessions. There are logistical issues such as consent forms, appropriate attire for various weather conditions, a medical history including conditions and any allergies, as well as a review of safety protocol such as the "buddy system." This latter involves not doing an activity outside without someone present to help with safety. In addition, it is helpful to review previous nature experiences for any participants, particularly if there have been any negative or traumatic situations in nature. If there has been a stressful association with nature, then some smaller steps to better acclimate would be encouraged before including activities outside. It is also advised to go over directions for outdoor NaturePlay activities before heading outside to review any guidelines, limits, and any safety precautions. Even non-structured NaturePlay activities will have some boundaries to review before beginning.

Scouting programs are known for their outdoor activities and adventures for youth and much can be learned from their experiences and resources. The motto for most scouting organizations all over the world is "Be Prepared." This motto originated from scouting founder Sir Robert Baden-Powell, who stated the following in his book *Scouting for Boys* back in 1908:

> The scouts' motto is founded on my initials, it is: BE PREPARED, which means you are always in a state of readiness in mind and body to do your DUTY;
>
> *Be Prepared in Mind* by having disciplined yourself to be obedient to every order, and also by having thought out beforehand any accident or situation that might occur, so that you *know* the right thing to do at the right moment and are willing to do it.
>
> *Be Prepared in Body* by making yourself strong and active and *able* to do the right thing at the right moment and do it. (Part I, p. 48)

Preparing a NaturePlay Kit: While most NaturePlay activities are not as extensive as scouting events and protocol, there are good considerations from the "Be Prepared" concept such as thinking ahead to prepare for situations. It is advantageous to put together a NaturePlay kit. In addition to what has already been recommended, other suggestions include having a water bottle for hydration, as well as sunglasses, hat and other weather-related gear when needed. Using a drawstring knapsack or similar container that can be carried, one can include such materials as binoculars, magnifying glass, whistle, compass, insect net, plastic tweezers, a small shovel, and a few baggies to hold found treasures. Insect repellant, suntan lotion, and hand sanitizer can also be added at the caregivers' discretion and application. Some youth might also want to include crayons, colored pencils or water paints, and a tablet or journal, as well as a camera or cell phone with a built-in camera. It is also recommended that the therapist have access to a portable first aid kit.

Taking the time to review the contents of the NaturePlay kit is helpful, especially for younger children as well as safety guidelines such as not exploring too far alone outside. The use of the whistle should be explained that it is for a signal for help or when assistance is needed, but otherwise not used as it can interrupt the natural environment. (Caregivers will appreciate this as well, otherwise the whistle may be blown above their comfort level.) A NaturePlay kit can also be assembled at home for use in conjunction with nature missions between sessions or for virtual sessions. For either of these situations, the therapist needs to emphasize with caregivers and clients that adult presence is needed nearby to assist for any safety issues if needed. This is especially critical for telemental health sessions due to the therapist presence being limited as it is over a screen and not there in an actual physical way to assist as it would occur with in-person sessions. (See also Chapter 1 to review the nature-based client consent form.)

Offering NaturePlay Activities Indoors

There are times when NaturePlay activities will occur indoors. This may be due to weather conditions, allergy seasons, or limited access to nature. There are also some situations in which a child is not yet ready or able to go outside. As an example, for areas that are not enclosed or fenced in, if a child presents as a "runner," this could be a safety (and thus liability) issue if they were to run away from the therapist. There may also be times when a client or family member has had a negative or traumatic nature experience, or has reported another discomfort to being outside, such as a fear of insects. To help acclimate a child, adolescent, or other family member with one or more of these considerations, introducing them to nature in small doses is advised. The therapist can begin by having some nature items in the playroom that the client can explore and play with indoors. Some suggestions for these nature materials include sticks, stones, shells, pebbles, pieces of bark, acorns, pinecones, leaves, blades of grass, dried flowers, flower petals, walnut hulls, "helicopter" seed pods, sea glass, and feathers.

There are several NaturePlay activities that can be utilized both indoors and outside with these nature materials. The first type of play is that of simply following the child with what they choose to do or make with the nature materials. This free play allows for creativity and curious exploration, including additional therapeutic powers of play such as creative problem-solving and self-regulation. This type of play with random materials is often referred to as "Loose Parts Play" (Nicholson, 1971) and can be with objects of all sizes and materials, but with NaturePlay activities, the materials are gathered from nature or are products made of natural materials. This latter may include items such as wooden blocks, chips, or even sliced tree cookies. Loose Parts Play is more popular in Europe, Australia, and Canada, and is a type of both constructive and creative play in which the child can build, construct, or deconstruct as they desire with the various objects on hand. There are no instructions or directives for this creative play. There is often a natural calming effect that happens when these nature materials are held, touched, and felt during play.

Another NaturePlay activity that can be utilized indoors with nature materials is the making of a Nature Buddy or Comfort Critter (refer to Figure 13.1). The addition of a neutral clay or dough is also useful as desired for the connection of these nature materials. A client may choose to create a Nature Buddy or Comfort Critter to go on some of the nature adventures with them, which can be especially helpful for those new to outdoor experiences (see Appendix B). This expressive play lends to the

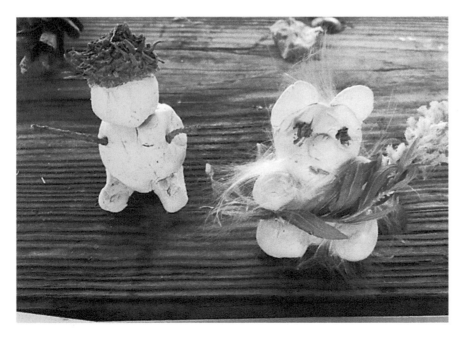

Figure 13.1 Nature buddies.
Source: Jamie Lynn Langley.

therapeutic powers of play such as creative-problem-solving and self-regulation as well as positive emotions, self-esteem, and self-expression.

Critter creations have also been used to assist with a fear of insects. Some clients have made representations of the insects that they are fearful of and can then hold them to become more comfortable prior to going outside. This graduated exposure play incorporates the additional therapeutic power of play of counterconditioning fears.

There are several other NaturePlay expressive art activities that can be utilized with these nature materials. Nature art can be made by a child or teen as part of their free play or there may be a directive or purposeful activity. Animals, people, and other figures can be made with leaves, sticks, or feathers and glued to construction paper, for example, to create a picture, or can be tied together with string to make doll or puppet representations for dramatic play scenarios. Nature feeling faces can also be made with these materials and a large tree cookie can be used to create various faces, which can then be used again for repeated therapeutic activities. These activities can be either nondirective or directive as needed by the child. In addition, for any clients who may have allergies, therapists can substitute some synthetic nature objects such as leaves, pinecones, shells, and more. This is also helpful when some items from nature are wanted for a particular art activity, but are not in season.

Creating nature mandalas is a favorite NaturePlay activity of many clients. Mandalas are often used for mindfulness, which can assist children and teens with self-regulation. In addition, creating mandalas often incorporates additional therapeutic powers of play such as positive emotions and creative problem-solving. A mandala is simply a circular shape with a center known as a bindu, which is often interpreted as referencing wholeness. The words "mandala" and "bindu" are from an ancient Sanskrit language. Mandalas have been used for many centuries by various cultures and religions and have been incorporated in both play and expressive therapies in a variety of ways (Bratman et al., 2015).

Children and teens can first be introduced to mandalas that are present in nature as well as artistically created by looking through pictures such as in *The Mandala Book: Patterns of the Universe* by Lori Cunningham (2020). The client is then invited to create their own mandala using whatever nature items they choose. The mandalas can be constructed on various surfaces such as the floor or a table. Various designs can be implemented around the bindu in the center inviting the opportunity for creativity without needing any artistic ability. Nature sounds with music are often played in the background as the mandala is being created, which can assist younger children to not go too quickly as they often like to "speed through" activities. This slower pace is often part of the regulating process, as well as to be more in touch with the soothing sounds of nature while creating. In addition, adding nature sounds brings in another healing element of the outdoors (Buxton et al. 2021).

This author also utilizes a round tray of sand with which to construct nature mandalas, which are called sandalas. This term came following a slip-of-the tongue when explaining a sand mandala to my son, and it came out as "sandala." Liking the sound of it, other therapists were consulted, and the response was incredibly positive. There is a nature creativity station in the play therapy office where the round tray is located and often clients choose to begin or end their sessions making a nature sandala at the station. A unique twist that they especially enjoy is that the sand is changed to reflect the seasons. In the winter, a sparkling white sand it used which the children refer to as the "snow sand." In the spring a light purple garnet sand is used, and in the summer, it is changed to a beach-colored sand. This is then replaced by a darker sable brown sand for the fall season. Another twist to the activity is with rocks, which have words on them, from which the bindu (center) can be chosen (see Figure 13.2). The client can indicate if this is something needed or appreciated, and then the design is constructed surrounding that center stone.

The nature creativity station (see Figure 13.3) is where nature mandalas and sandalas are often designed. Tree cookie art and loose parts play also occurs here.

Taking NaturePlay Outside

NaturePlay is admittedly at its best outdoors. When a child goes outside there is a natural release that accompanies this where play is often freer, more spontaneous, and more active. Our senses become more awakened once outside, and children by nature become louder when outdoors. Just go to a nearby playground and hear the children as they play! There are often many sounds that accompany this outdoor free play such as squeals of delight, screams of joy, and the like. This nondirective play provides

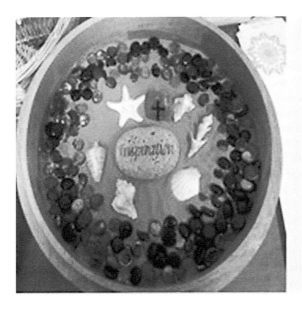
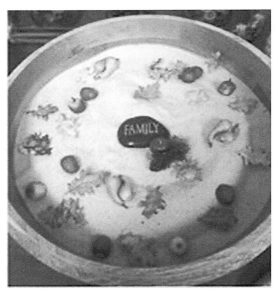

Figure 13.2 Nature Sandalas.
Source: Jamie Lynn Langley.

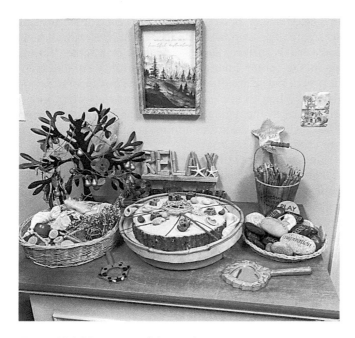

Figure 13.3 Nature creativity station.
Source: Jamie Lynn Langley.

for many opportunities of creativity and imagination as children explore their outside world. A therapist can follow this play, interacting as invited, for a child-centered approach. The therapeutic benefits are often cathartic, with higher positive emotions and limitless opportunities for creative problem solving. This type of NaturePlay can also be quite imaginative. Young clients may make stick figures to tell stories or look up at clouds to see all type of characters or animals to share about. Children can walk along a log pretending it is a pirate ship and having to "walk the plank," or sit on a stump to pretend to be flying a jet or driving a race car or pretend in any number of ways in the outdoor elements. Children can also experience some opportunities for risky play, such as if they walk and balance on a log or climb a tree. This assessment and mastery of risk adds to self-esteem and positive emotions as additional therapeutic powers of play.

Another element that adds to this outdoor play is that of discovery. The traditional playroom is primarily static in that the items are normally in specific places, often to provide a sense of comfort and stability. But when nature itself is the playroom, insects and worms and the like may appear, leaves can fall, birds can sing, and more. These additional elements add to the wonder for the child and oftentimes some moments of pure joy and awe. The NaturePlay kit is the perfect companion for this exploratory play, where items such as the magnifying glass and insect net can be used to view discoveries even closer. This investigation playfully encourages more executive function skills of focus and concentration.

The indoor NaturePlay activities previously described can also be conducted outside, but now the client has the added benefit of being able to participate in the actual gathering of the nature items. A basket or bag can be used to hold discovered treasures, where the client is encouraged to find things that have fallen on the ground, incorporating a nature-considerate approach to "pick up" rather than "pick" when possible, as was described in Chapter 1. However, there may also be times when selecting a few things to pick is warranted, such as a dandelion to blow and make a wish. Once items are found as desired, then the creative activities can be made on the ground, along a sidewalk, or at an outdoor table if available. A tablecloth can also be used, which is helpful if a client wants to paint their nature items or to use as the actual item with which to paint with. In addition, some children may choose to keep some of their found nature materials to include as part of a nature journal, or they may want to make a nature memory holder (see below.)

Another NaturePlay activity to use for kept nature treasures is making a nature calming jar or bottle. (See Figure 13.4) A client can select some different nature items and place in a container filled with water.

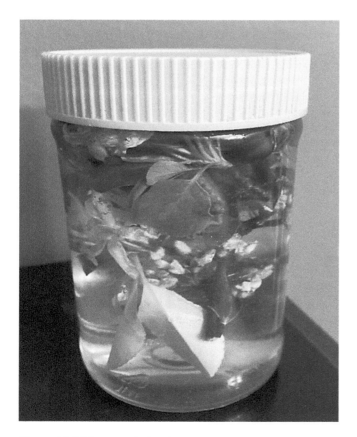

Figure 13.4 Nature calming jar.

Source: Jamie Lynn Langley.

Natures gifts of flower petals, clover, berries, leaves, and smaller wildflowers can be included, selecting varied colors when possible for visual impact. Also including a few heavier objects like small stones, acorns, shells, or walnut hulls add some sound effects. As the items are placed in the container, encourage the client to take a few moments to closely examine and feel their selected nature gifts, smelling them as well. This invites a more diverse sensory experience to the activity, which further assists with self-regulation. The client then secures the lid, and the jar can be turned upside down and then right side up again to enjoy the changing visuals and sounds (see Appendix C). The contents may need to be replaced every few days, depending upon the contents, which is a way to encourage ongoing nature outings with their family outside of sessions to gather new nature materials. A client may also want to make one as a memory holder for a favorite place such as a beach by using collected shells. Either way clients can use their nature calming jars to invoke positive memories and sensations from being out in nature.

There are also creative ways with which to use the contents of nature calming jars when they need to be changed. A client can pour out the jar contents as a way of returning back to nature, expressing gratitude to nature for the use of her gifts. Some children have also chosen to take the contents as the beginning of a nature soup or potion, adding in other nature materials. The stirring is quite regulating, and children benefit from the creative and calming experience. This nature soup can also be given back to nature once done.

Children and teens alike enjoy taking pictures and videos of these discoveries and their creations or they may choose to draw them as part of a nature journal. They can also make rubbings of the found nature items in their journals, which leaves the actual items to remain in nature. These nature rubbings provide additional opportunities for self-regulation and calming.

Nature mandalas are often constructed outside and are usually larger with the more open space, often resulting in the use of more abundant nature items like leaves and pinecones. Mandala creating can be utilized as sibling and family activities, exploring further connections as well as enhancing communication. Additionally, mandalas are found throughout nature, as with flowers such as daisies and sunflowers, as well as with snails, spider webs, and shells. Children enjoy looking for mandalas to discover once outside as part of a mandala nature walk or hunt. For those near beaches, mandalas can be made in the sand for outdoor sandalas. Tracing their fingers thorough the sand as part of the sandala design can add to the sensory experience. The following case vignette of Cassie illustrates the use of nature mandalas in practice.

The Case of Cassie, Age Nine Years

Cassie is a nine-year-old female who was referred due to excessive worrying and some perfectionistic tendencies. She tended not to try new things due to concerns of not being "good enough." When she began play therapy, Cassie quickly took to the nature station, often beginning her session with making a sandala. Music with nature sounds was played softly in the room, and there were times she would close her eyes in mindful silence, becoming enveloped in a peaceful state. Sometimes Cassie chose a word-stone bindu reflective of an event during her week and other times she chose an item related to how she was feeling in the moment. Sometimes she sat with a sand filled wooden bowl wherein she would sift her hands through the sand.

NaturePlay sessions outside were suggested, and Cassie and her mother agreed. Cassie admitted she did not spend much time outdoors, preferring to read a book or play a game on her computer. Sessions initially began with walking around outside, looking for certain colors and then shapes. In subsequent sessions, this deepened to listening for certain sounds. During one session, she decided to collect some treasures from nature to make a large mandala. She then cleared a space on the ground near the office where she intentionally placed each item in the mandala circle. Nearing completion, Cassie stated it was "not good enough" as her items did not all line up and match. It was suggested to her to consider that sometimes the beauty of the mandala is not with it being perfect, but more the uniqueness of it. She shrugged but continued until she had finished her mandala. Cassie then proceeded to create several nature mandalas in subsequent sessions. She was encouraged to look for positives about her creations, and during one session, she said: "That one's pretty good!" When asked how that felt, she laughed and said, "I feel pretty good too!" She got up and did a little celebratory dance and the therapist retrieved a stone for her to decorate. Cassie was asked to think about that feeling and write that on the stone with a marker. She wrote "Pretty Good!" on the stone and got up and placed it in the center of her created mandala, taking the flower she originally had as the bindu and placing it on top of her painted stone. She asked if a picture could be taken of her mandala which was then printed for her to take home. Cassie would subsequently use her "Pretty Good!" stone in other NaturePlay activities. By the time therapy was coming to a close, it was noted that her worries, and perfectionistic tendencies had decreased. As part of her "Wild Tea Party" celebration during the final session, the stone was given to Cassie as a transitional object and reminder of our NaturePlay sessions together. [See the Wild Tea Party activity (Closing Appendix B) at the end of this book.)

This case vignette illustrates that NaturePlay activities can follow the child in a nondirective approach, as well as include some directive activities. Such activities do not have to be complex for nature and play to provide healing. The therapist stayed with the client offering safety, guidance, and reflection as needed both indoors and outside. The client was able to both explore challenges and invoke creativity with gifts from nature as part of her healing process.

Games in NaturePlay

An additional category of outdoor NaturePlay activities involve playing various games. These games can involve many different therapeutic powers of play, from positive emotions and stress management to therapeutic relationship, attachment, and social competence, as well as creative problem solving, moral development, self-regulation, and self-esteem (Schaefer & Stone, 2020). Nature scavenger or treasure hunts of all types are popular, and can be changed for different seasons, to explore for various senses, or discover certain shapes or colors. A fun way to playfully incorporate scavenger hunts is to write the items to be discovered on small wooden discs that can be drawn per player. This makes the scavenger hunts easily adaptable for single client sessions, as well as siblings, families, or groups to do together. Items founds can then be used for other NaturePlay activities, or pictures of the items can be taken.

"Nature I Spy" is an easy game to play where participants try to see what the leader sees out in nature (see Appendix D). For example, the leader might say: "I spy with my little eye something in nature that is red" and then the partner tries to identify the source of red in nature that matches what the leader saw. This is also easily adapted to a game of "Do You Hear What I Hear?" to identify nature sounds that are heard by each player. These are easy to incorporate without much preparation as many are familiar with the basic concepts of these games.

Even a simple game such as "Follow the Leader" can be utilized outside for NaturePlay. It is particularly empowering for children to have adults such as the therapist or caregivers following their lead, especially when it is something the adult or therapist cannot do as well, such as with cartwheels.

The following game is one of the earliest this author utilized to incorporate nature with play therapy. It is called "Kim's Game" and was learned from time spent as a Cub Scout leader. It was created by scouting founder Robert Baden-Powell. Originally published in his booklet *Scouting Games* in 1921 (p. 16), this game involves collecting several articles that are then covered with a cloth, which is then lifted for one minute. The participant is to quickly scan the items before they are recovered with the cloth, and then identifies as many of the items that they can remember. As skills increase the number of materials can increase as well. A NaturePlay adaption this author calls "Nature See and Seek" is to have all these different items collected from nature. Once uncovered, revealed and then concealed, the client goes out in nature to retrieve the matching items. It is a fun activity incorporating movement outside while also improving executive function skills like focus and concentration. This game can also be used with siblings, families, and even groups by dividing up in teams.

NaturePlay over Telemental Health

When most therapists needed to move to telemental health services during the COVID-19 pandemic, many play and expressive therapy activities were adapted for use over a screen (Stone, in press). This successful implementation, along with a growing awareness of how much telemental health can be used for various reasons, has made it important to offer NaturePlay activities that can be utilized in a virtual manner. The main adaptions are exploring with the client and caregivers about safe ways to gather nature items that can then be utilized during the telemental health sessions. Most of the creative NaturePlay activities can still happen much as described previously, sharing the creations over a screen, as well as the therapist participating in some parallel play opportunities. For the game play activities, a client can take a tablet or phone outside with them to include the therapist for many of the activities. A caregiver would need to be nearby for such outdoor activities to help provide for physical safety (Langley, 2022).

Prescribing NaturePlay Between Sessions

An important part of this NaturePlay practice is to actually "prescribe nature" in-between sessions. As the research indicates, the more time spent in nature the better. Nature Play Therapy sessions usually occur on a weekly or ever-other-week basis. Therapists can make prescription pads in which "nature missions" or "nature adventures" can be prescribed for clients and their families to do together several times during the week. These adventures can then be explored for benefits and lessons learned when returning for the next session. For caregivers that struggle to find time for these nature missions, it is suggested to "exchange some screen time for green time," which can begin with half-hour increments.

There are also programs that include prescribing nature for treatment. Programs such as the Park Rx Program and Park Rx America (see www.parkrx.org and www.parkrxamerica.org) work with health care providers to offer nature prescriptions to clients. Park Rx America now has a web database that prescribers can log onto to assist clients in locating parks near them to help accessibility. The U.S. National Park Service partnered with these organizations in a program called Healthy Parks Healthy People. Similarly, some state park systems have also implemented programs that include nature prescriptions. In Tennessee, the home state of this author, there is the Health Parks Healthy Person TN program in which health providers are given prescription pads to prescribe nature. In turn, there is an app program in which participants can earn points by participating in these nature-based activities. These points can be redeemed for prizes such as overnight stays, ranger-led hikes, outdoor gear, and more. These rewards provide additional incentives for children and families to follow their nature prescriptions and have been utilized successfully by this author with many families worked with. (See www.healthyparkstn.com)

Conclusion

Nature Play Therapy provides a healing way for children, teens, and their families via both indoor and outdoor NaturePlay activities, which can also be done over telemental health. These NaturePlay activities are adaptable to follow the child for a more client-centered approach, or can incorporate more structured interventions depending upon the needs of the client. A NaturePlay kit can be constructed for use with in-person sessions, as well as for clients to have at home for telemental health or for prescribed nature missions between sessions. Additional benefits to this NaturePlay have been observed when families play outside together during these activities, as they are often more connected and involved with one another. Ultimately this connection with each other and with nature will have positive impacts for these children and adolescents.

As Penny Whitehouse of Mother Natured (mothernatured.com) has frequently shared: "Restore balance. Most kids have technology, school and extracurricular activities covered. It's time to add a pinch of adventure, a sprinkle of green time, and a big handful of play" (2021, May 12. www.facebook.com/mothernatured). As play and expressive therapists incorporating NaturePlay, we can help to restore this balance for nature and childhood for those we work with and hopefully encourage more to do so.

The following list summarizes the varied NaturePlay activities and games that were explored in this chapter:

*   Bringing Toys Outside (see Appendix A)
*   NaturePlay Kit
*   Nature Loose Parts Play
*   Nature Buddy/Comfort Creature (see Appendix B)

- Nature Art
- Nature Feeling Faces
- Nature Mandalas
- Sandalas
- Nature Journal
- Nature Calming Jar/Memory Holder (see Appendix C)
- Nature Soup
- Nature Photography
- Nature Rubbings
- Nature Mandala Walk/Hunt
- Nature Scavenger/Treasure Hunt
- Nature I Spy (see Appendix D)
- Do You Hear What I Hear? (see Appendix D)
- Follow the Leader
- Kim's Game / Nature See and Seek
- Nature Prescriptions / Nature and Adventure Missions

Reflective Questions

1   Refer to the case vignette of Cassie and her NaturePlay with creating nature mandalas. Discuss with a partner how she progressed in this process. Next gather some nature materials and create your own nature mandala. Think of a word to portray how you are feeling with this creative play, and paint or use a marker to draw this word on a stone. Then place this stone as your bindu (center). You and your partner can share your mandalas and this process. A picture can be taken of your nature mandala to reflect upon later.

2   In the "Making the Case for NaturePlay" section, three research areas are identified to support the use of nature with play as a healing practice. Do you agree or disagree that this research listed provided enough support to include nature as part of play and expressive therapies? Why or why not? Is there other research that needs to be included? Share your ideas with a partner.

3   This chapter explores beginning with indoor NaturePlay activities and then progresses to outdoor NaturePlay. Explore with your partner if this process assists conducting NaturePlay activities outdoors or does it prohibit in any way? Explain what you would need to feel comfortable to begin offering outdoor NaturePlay activities in your current practice.

Appendix A

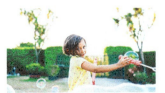

BRINGING TOYS OUTSIDE TO PLAY

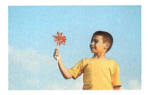

A Nature Play Therapy Experience
Jamie Lynn Langley, LCSW, RPT-S

DESCRIPTION:

There are times when children and/or the play therapist may bring toys from the playroom outside.

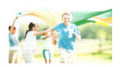

RECOMMENDED SETTING AND SUPPLIES:

A secure outdoor area.
The client and/or therapist can choose toys from the indoor playroom to bring outside.

GOAL:

Play therapy outdoors can provide a release for the client and offer opportunities for regulation, catharsis and creativity.

INSTRUCTIONS:

There are times a client may need a release following an intense play therapy session. Taking bubbles, pinwheels and even art supplies outside can provide a way for clients to release in a more open and powerful way once outdoors. This type of play can be particularly cathartic and regulating as well as a time for increased creativity. They can just blow or draw those contained feelings out!

Additionally, outdoor playrooms are being set up where practitioners bring traditionally indoor play materials outside. Clients experience additional sensory experiences with this outdoor element such as unexpected sights and sounds than when inside.

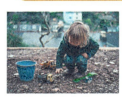 ## EXTRA FUN

Children may choose various toys for outdoor play such as cars, bubbles, pinwheels, buckets, shovels, animals, dolls and more. They can also utilize materials from nature to make structures, houses and roads as needed. Children may choose to make toys out of nature items, such as with sticks and rocks for dolls and puppets.

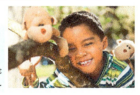

Appendix B

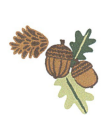

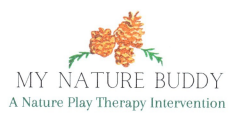

MY NATURE BUDDY
A Nature Play Therapy Intervention

Jamie Lynn Langley, LCSW, RPT-S

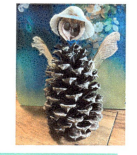

DESCRIPTION:

A child or adolescent can utilize materials from nature to assemble their own nature buddy.

SUPPLIES NEEDED:

Gather gifts from nature such as pinecones, twigs, shells, maple seedlings, acorns, walnut hulls. rocks, leaves and feathers.
Also have play dough or clay.

GOAL:

To become more comfortable with nature while also being creative.

INSTRUCTIONS:

Each client can make their own nature buddy. They can make any type of figure using chosen nature materials as well as a dough or clay. This dough can serve as a bonding agent or can be part of the actual buddy such as the body, head, etc.

The client can then have the nature buddy accompany them outside or when at home to go along on nature missions or for over telemental health. They can also be used in narrative play for storytelling as desired. Multiple buddies can be made.

EXTRA FUN:

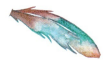

These materials can also be made into a comfort creature. In this case, they would make a creature they are afraid of or concerned about, such as a spider or insect, they they can then play with and become more comfortable about.

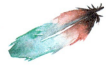

Appendix C

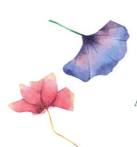

NATURE CALMING JAR

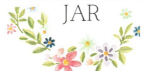

A Nature Play Therapy Intervention

Jamie Lynn Langley, LCSW, RPT-S

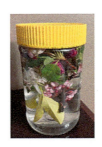

DESCRIPTION:

This intervention invites the child or adolescent to create a nature calming jar that can be taken home following a session. This jar can also be made during a telemental health session.

SUPPLIES NEEDED:

A container such as a plastic jar or bottle. Also gather found gifts from nature such as rocks, feathers, leaves, flower petals, pieces of bark, seeds, shells, acorns, sticks, and pinecones.

GOAL:

Utilizes a way to bring nature indoors for a client to access as needed for anxiety, stress, anger or worry.

INSTRUCTIONS:

This activity can be utilized with any age. Items from nature are gathered along a walk. These "treasures" are then placed inside a jar, bottle or other transparent container. Next add water to fill the remainder of the container and add the lid.

This jar can be placed upside down and then back right side up, as well as placed on its side and rolled around. The client views the items within the jar as they move around. This is calming and can be repeated as desired to assist regulation.

The contents can be replaced every few days, providing further time outside in nature as items are gathered. Seasonal changes will produce different elements to be included in each jar.

EXTRA FUN:

A client can use items from a memorable experience such as a beach vacation. Blue food coloring is added to the water first. Then shells from the vacation are placed in the jar. This is now a "Beach Memory Jar."

Appendix D

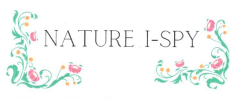

NATURE I-SPY

A Nature Play Therapy Intervention
Jamie Lynn Langley, LCSW,, RPT-S

DESCRIPTION:

For this activity we take the childhood game "I Spy" and bring in elements of nature or go outside to play.

SUPPLIES NEEDED:

For inside play: Gather nature items like shells, leaves, rocks, feathers, crystals, flowers, plants, bark, twigs, and more.

GOAL:

Builds connection, communication and executive function skills playfully.

INSTRUCTIONS:

This fun activity is a childhood favorite with a nature twist! Therapist and child can go outside in nature or items from nature can be brought into the playroom. When indoors, the therapist will explain we are looking for items from or about nature. Taking turns, each will take turns as "the spy" and state: "I spy with my little eye something _____" This could be something such as a color, a shape, something hidden, etc. Children especially love when this is done with a magnifying lens or a pair of binoculars. This activity can also be done with a group or family and can be playfully incorporated as part of a nature walk activity.

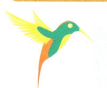

EXTRA FUN:

This activity can be changed slightly by listening for sounds of nature, becoming a game of "Do You Hear What I Hear?" Nature sounds are regulating and children often enjoy discovering new sounds.

References

Atchley, R. A., Strayer, D. L., & Atchley P. (2012). Creativity in the wild: Improving creative reasoning through immersion in natural settings. *PLoS ONE, 7*(12), e51474. https://doi.org/10.1371/journal.pone.0051474

Baden-Powell, R. (1908). Campfire yarn. no. 4. Scout law, part 1, p. 48. *Scouting for boys.* Dover Publications.

Baden-Powell, R. (1921). *Scouting games.* C. Arthur Pearson Ltd.

Barton, J., & Pretty, J. (2010). What is the best dose of nature and green exercise for improving mental health? A multi-study analysis. *Environmental Science & Technology.* https://doi.org/10.1021/es903183r

Berman, M. G., Kross, E., Krpan, K. M., Askre, N. M. K., Burson, A., Deldin, P. J., Kaplan, S., Sherdell, L., Gotlib, I. H., & Jonides, J. (2012). Interacting with nature improves cognition and affect for individuals with depression. *Journal of affective disorders, 140*(3), 300–305. https://doi.org/10.1016/j.jad.2012.03.012.

Bratman, G.N., Daily, G.C., Levy, B. J., & Gross, J. J. (2015). The benefits of nature experience: Improved affect and cognition. *Landscape and Urban Planning, 138,* 41–50. https://doi.org/10.1016/j.landurbplan.2015.02.005

Buxton, R.T., Pearson, A.L., Allou, C., Fristrup, L., & Wittemeyer, G. (2021). A synthesis of health benefits of natural sounds and their distribution in national parks. *Proceedings of the National Academy of Sciences, 118* (14), e2013097118. https://doi.org/10.1073/pnas.2013097118

Cunningham, L. B. (2020). *The mandala book: Patterns of the universe.* Sterling Publishing Co.

Dankiw, K. A., Tsiros, M. D., Baldock, K. L., & Kumar, S. (2020). The impacts of unstructured nature play on health in early childhood development: A systematic review. *PLoS ONE, 15*(2), e0229006. https://doi.org/10.1371/journal.pone.0229006

Dhaese, M. J. (2011). Holistic expressive play therapy: An integrative approach to helping maltreated children. In A. A. Drews, S. C. Bratton, & C. E. Schaefer (Eds.), *Integrative play therapy* (pp. 75–93). John Wiley & Sons.

Ellard, M., & Parson, J. A. (2021). Playing in the field: Scoping the therapeutic powers of play for nature play therapy. *British Journal of Play Therapy, 15*(Spring), 42–64.

Hunter M.R., Gillespie, B.W., & Chen S.Y.-P. (2019). Urban nature experiences reduce stress in the context of daily like based on salivary biomarkers. *Frontiers In Psychology,* 10, 722. https://doi.org/10.3389/fpsyg.2019.00722

Landreth, G. L. (2012). *Play therapy the art of the relationship* (3rd ed.) Routledge.

Langley, J. L. (In press). Nature play therapy and telehealth: How green time and screen time can play well together. In J. Stone (Ed.), *Play therapy and telemental health: Foundations, populations, and interventions.* Routledge.

Langley, J. L. (2019). Nature play therapy: When nature comes into play. *Playground,* (Spring/Summer), 20–24. https://cacpt.com/wp-content/uploads/2019/04/Playground-Spring-2019.pdf

Louv, R. (2005). Last child in the woods: Saving our children from nature-deficit disorder. Algonquin Books.

Louv, R. (Feb 28, 2012). http://richardlouv.com/

Lowenfeld, M. (1991). *Play in childhood.* Mac Keith Press

Neill, C., Gerard, J., & Arbuthnott, K. (2019) Nature contact and mood benefits: Contact duration and mood type. *The Journal of Positive Psychology, 14* (6), 756767. https://doi.org/10.1080/17439760.2018.1557242

Nicholson, S. (1971). How not to cheat children: The theory of loose parts. *Landscape architecture, 62*(1), 30–34.

Plambech, T., & Konijnendijk van den Bosch, C. C. (2015). The impact of nature on creativity – A study among danish creative professionals. *Urban Forestry & Urban Greening, 14*(2), 255–263. https://doi.org/10.1016/j.ufug.2015.02.006

Preuß, B. M., Nieuwenhuijsen, M., Marquez, S., Cirach, M., Dadyand, P., Triguero-Mas, M., Gidlow, C., Grazuleviciene, R., Kruize, H., & Zijlema W. (2019). Low childhood nature exposure is associated with worse mental health in adulthood. *International Journal of Environmental Research and Public Health, 16* (10), 1809. https://doi.org/10.3390/ijerph16101809

Schaefer C. E. , & Drewes, A. A. (2014). The therapeutic powers of play: 20 core agents of change. (2nd ed.). Wiley.

Schaefer, C. E., & Stone, J. (2020). *Game play: Therapeutic use of games with children and adolescents.* (3rd ed.). Wiley

Stone, J. (In press). *Play therapy and telemental health: Foundations, populations, and interventions.* Routledge.

Walker, K. L. A. (2021). Outdoor Child-Centered Play Therapy with Attention and Social-Emotional Competencies in Children, dissertation, May 2021; Denton, Texas. https://digital.library.unt.edu/ark:/67531/metadc1808455/m1/5/: University of North Texas Libraries, UNT Digital Library, https://digital.library.unt.edu

Wenner, M. (2009). The serious need for play. *Scientific American Mind, 20*(1), 22–29. https://doi.org/10.1038/scientificamericanmind0209-22

14 Using Nature-Based Interventions in Family Play Therapy

Jennifer Taylor and Bree Conklin

Some families love spending time in nature, but others feel much less comfortable spending time outside. Increasingly, therapists are taking clients outside for therapy sessions or including nature-based scenes, sounds, or elements within their offices and specifically as part of their treatment plans. Traditionally, therapists have also assigned homework for clients and families to complete outside of sessions to reinforce therapeutic goals. This homework has included "nature prescriptions" that are either structured (providing specific activities) or unstructured (simply education about outdoor resources) (Kondo et al., 2020). For children, however, an appropriate caregiver is often required in order to spend time in nature as prescribed. Sobel (2008) proposes that a sense of environmentalism comes from hours spent outdoors with an adult that shows and teaches respect for nature. Furthermore, it is through a caring and curious adult presence that children develop a "sense of wonder" about the natural world.

However, families often find that these open-ended prescriptions for nature-time can create anxiety. The caregivers of the child in play therapy sessions may not have grown up with this caring and curious adult presence in their own life. As noted in the Child Parent Relationship Training manual, "we cannot give what we don't possess" (Bratton et al., 2006). There are additional cultural considerations to explore for families whose connections to nature have negative associations or memories. Dungy (2009) noted in the poetry anthology, *Black Nature*, that Western, Anglo-Americans often express the "prevailing views of the natural world as a place of positive collaboration, refuge, idyllic rural life or wilderness," whereas in African American poetry nature is described through views of "moss, rivers, trees, dirt, caves, dogs, fields: elements of an environment steeped in a legacy of violence, forced labor, torture, and death" (p. xxi). Birch, Risbeth and Payne (2020, p. 8) reviewed both the benefits of nature and potential ways that "nature does not always help" by highlighting factors in urban environments where outdoor spaces are either not maintained well, less accessible, or potentially physically unsafe.

There is a need for additional resources for clinicians designing therapeutic interventions and between-session homework that will allow the client and their family the greatest opportunity for success in nature-based play and expressive therapies. In order to successfully create nature-based action plans for parents and children to use outside of therapy, a clinician must understand and address specific issues and offer step-by-step guidance along the way. In this chapter, clinicians will explore the potential challenges to using nature-based interventions with families outside of therapy sessions as well as find specific solutions that make action plans families will find enjoyable and easy to implement.

Introducing Nature-Based Play

The therapeutic powers of play factor into treatment planning and decisions about appropriate interventions. Therapeutic powers of play that are at work during nature play often include direct and indirect teaching, counterconditioning fears, stress inoculation, stress management, creative problem solving, self-regulation, self-esteem, and social competence (Schaefer & Drewes, 2011). For families where an open-ended prescription for nature-play is not working, but for whom the benefits of nature-play felt clinically relevant, a specific plan for introducing nature is required. Relying on an integrative approach using nature-based play and expressive arts therapies, as well as filial therapy, narrative therapy, and cognitive-behavioral therapy approaches, therapists can combine in-office interventions with between-session homework that both involves nature and feels realistic and achievable to caregivers. This approach gradually increases parental confidence and comfort in coleading nature-based play experiences with their children (Figure 14.1).

DOI: 10.4324/9781003152767-19

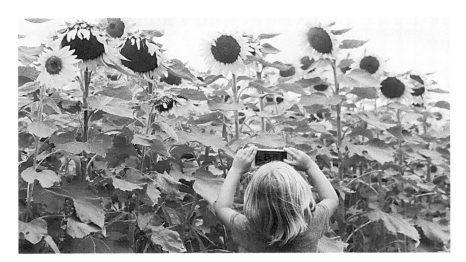

Figure 14.1 Grayson, age four, takes a "wonder wander" through the sunflower field.
Source: Jennifer Taylor.

Therapists can begin by introducing nature-based play through psychoeducation about the benefits children, teens, and their families may experience from time spent playing outdoors. For example, Boon (2020) asserts natural objects afford children the opportunity to transform in an infinite number of ways. Such items from nature offer substance, form, color, texture, and narrative while simultaneously allowing the freedom in which children may engage imaginatively and transform these objects into something entirely different. Parents living in homeless or domestic violence shelters in the Netherlands were observed to demonstrate increased need satisfaction and decreased need frustration after spending time in nature with their children (Peters et al., 2020). This effect was especially noted in parents with young children and positive psychological gains were noted with a single nature experience.

Even parents who cognitively understand the benefits of nature-based play or who have a desire for more outdoor nature experiences may still struggle with implementing interventions due to anxiety about being outdoors. Hyun (2000) noted that adults either teach children a "feeling of fear" or a "curiosity and inquiry to learn" depending on our own responses while in natural environments. Brussoni et al. (2018) noted that outside play often elicits anxieties in parents; they identified traffic safety, fear of strangers, serious injury, or disapproval from other parents as the most worrisome factors that prevented or reduced outdoor play. In 2018, those researchers began a study to measure the effect of a two-hour workshop aimed at reducing parental anxieties and strengthening parents' beliefs in the benefits of outdoor play. This workshop and the web-based version (www.outsideplay.ca) provide tools that guide caregivers through a reflective and educational journey on the perceived risks and the potential benefits of outdoor play.

For clinicians working with parents that have fears or insecurities about allowing their children to play outside, the online "Journey Map" provides a starting point for assessment of anxieties and teaching about the benefits of risky outdoor play. Using the website (www.outsideplay.ca), caregivers complete the Journey map which is a three-step process of: (1) reflection, (2) scenario-based psychoeducational (3) and an action plan. In the reflection stage, caregivers are prompted to think about and respond to a series of questions about their values and their own childhood activities and then consider those items in comparison to their own child's experiences. In the second section, caregivers are shown video clips of children climbing a tree, walking home alone from school and building a fort to help caregivers process their anxieties and see different ways of responding in each scenario. In the third step, an individualized action plan is created with specific goals about increasing outdoor play activities.

After this period of psychoeducation and assessment, the therapist can use in-office filial therapy sessions to teach parents how to act as the therapeutic agents of change for their children (Guerney, 2000). These filial play therapy sessions provide parents with specific language to use with their children including reflecting their thoughts and emotions, returning responsibility, encouragement, and limit-setting. The conjoint family sessions offer a place for parents to practice portions of between-session interventions with the supervision and guidance of the trained therapist. Once the caregiver has an understanding of the basic components of child-centered play therapy language, more directive interventions can be practiced and developed. These include narrative storytelling techniques, expressive arts techniques, and journaling exercises that can be used with nature items inside the office. Having completed this preparation process with the assistance of the therapist, the specific interventions can now be assigned as between-session homework with an increased likelihood of success.

The concept of between-session interventions (also known as homework) is a hallmark of cognitive behavior therapy (CBT) that extends the work being done in therapy to the time the client spends outside of therapy. Cronin et al. (2015) encourage therapists to provide "behavioral specificity" to their clients regarding between-session interventions, including discussions of when, where, and how often an intervention will take place. When prescribing these nature-based interventions to caregivers, the therapist should explore both the caregiver's perceived readiness and confidence in their ability to carry out the intervention. Upon return to the office, the therapist provides feedback, positive reinforcement, and also reviews any obstacles or challenges that occurred between sessions.

Literature Review

The biophilia hypothesis acknowledges our pervasive attraction to an emotional affiliation with nature (Courtney, 2020). Biophilia presumes the human relationship with natural objects extends beyond practical value. Nature is viewed as an active partner, or cotherapist, and serves as a container for the therapeutic work taking place, an observer of that work, and a provider of the natural materials that allow for a deeper connection between the inner processes of the human body and psyche and other processes found within the natural environment (Courtney, 2020; Nash, 2020).

As we observe and interact with the objects, materials, and processes found within nature, there is an evocation of thoughts, feelings, and memories tied to current events or significant memories within our biography (Kopytin & Rugh, 2017). We continually narrate our experiences through the creation of stories in autobiographical memory (Goodyear-Brown, 2021). These narratives shape the ways in which we understand ourselves in relation to the world around us. We continually narrate our experiences through the creation of stories in autobiographical memory (Goodyear-Brown, 2021). The theory of narrative identity suggests our personal narrative is an internalized and evolving story of self that is constructed throughout the course of life and establishes a framework within which experiences of the past are reconstructed, present is perceived, and future is anticipated (Adler, 2012). Narrative-based play and expressive therapies then focus on the process of making meaning through an individual's life story. Through the technique of externalization, the context is created in which one may examine, reflect upon, and deconstruct the problem(s) exerting influence over one's life. Problems are viewed as separate from the individual and it is assumed the individual possesses the skills, competencies, values, commitments, and abilities that will serve to guide change within the relationship between the individual and the problem (Beaudoin, 2005). The ultimate goal of narrative expression is to create space for the recognition of the problem-dominant narrative as a smaller part of a whole, multifaceted human shaped by the collective sum total of life's experiences (Malchiodi, 2020).

In order to create a reparative narrative, clients must engage in experiences that support safety, self-regulation, and inhabiting the body in both healthy and enjoyable ways. Creating a visual nature journal, for example, through taking pictures, or gathering items while interacting with nature is a mindfulness-based intervention that supports the goal of working toward the reconnection and return to experiencing oneself in the here and now. This process can begin with very young children. Johnson (2014) describes the use of nature journals with children from 18 months to 3 years. These nature journals are used to collect leaves, build letters out of sticks, draw pictures of things they have seen outside, and then become part of a discussion during circle time or other indoor activities. McMillan and Wilhelm (2007) found that middle school students who were given a 5-week assignment to observe nature by completing a moon-phase journal demonstrated increased feelings of gratitude and appreciation for the larger world while also increasing literacy skills and their understanding of nature-based figurative language. Johnson proposes that adults "let nature be the guide and the child's nature journal tell the story" (2014, p. 137). Kopytin (2017) states "this return to self by way of mindful attention to the relationship of self within

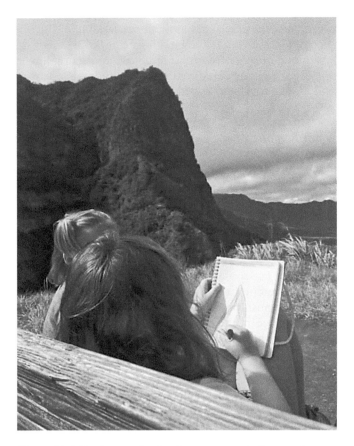

Figure 14.2 Sarah, age six, sketches a mountain for creating a story background while in Hawaii on the Kolekole trail.
Source: Jennifer Taylor.

nature helps to contain and organize, frame and reframe people's powerful and sometimes ambiguous reactions and experiences evoked by interactions with the environment" (Figure 14.2).

When introduced with the specific purpose of transforming problem-laden stories, expressive visual art is most helpful to clients when also introduced with metaphors that hold implications for imagining the future in some way that allows growth beyond the present circumstances (Malchiodi, 2020). Metaphors serve as bridges to intrapersonal connection that inspires solutions and strengthens one's inner resources and resiliency (Boon, 2020) The interaction of clients with nature often inspires reflection of the parallel between natural objects and one's biography thereby inspiring metaphors that express the inexpressible—to depict what words were unable to convey. Metaphoric story allows a more gentle and permissive way in which to consider solutions, comfort, change, and hope (Kopytin, 2017). For example, as noted by Malchiodi (2020), the metaphor of a tree stimulates thinking about the past (roots), present (trunk and branches), and future (what is growing or changing about the tree). With a coherent and organized story, the metaphor of the tree provides context of chronology for individuals and families with a beginning, current circumstance, and possibilities of a future.

Case Vignettes

Vignette #1 Mya, Age Nine Years

Presenting Background

Mya is a nine-year-old African-American child that is significantly overweight. She struggles with school and has difficulty paying attention in class. She refuses to complete assignments that are challenging and often hides under the desk when it is time to do her classwork independently. Her mother can respond harshly to Mya's behaviors and expects perfection and compliance, but also reported feeling anxious when they played outside because she could not predict what might happen. Her father is often overly lenient in regard to Mya's behaviors, and is also disengaged from the family life. He often ignores the child's requests for interactions and is inconsistently involved in his child's daily activities. The family spends very little time outside and often eats family meals in front of the television.

Family Play Therapy Nature Homework

Mya and her family participated in many family play therapy sessions in the office to work on parent–child relationship issues and regulating behaviors. The family identified a goal to increase their connections together by having family dinner once per week followed by an evening walk around their neighborhood. However, the family reported that the initial walk was awkward and unpleasant—the child complained about the weather the entire time, the father agreed to end the walk early to appease the child and the mother was disappointed that the plan was not "successful." The therapist introduced the mother to the Outdoor Play website assessment about safety outside and in nature and explored the mother's fears that the child would eat/touch something poisonous or dangerous.

The "I Wonder Wander" intervention was introduced by showing some items that the therapist had collected and brought into the office from her own walks in nature (sticks, rocks, etc.). The therapist and the family practiced the intervention by noticing something that they saw/heard standing outside of the office steps and did a very short three sentence story together (a beginning, a middle, and an end). The therapist then scheduled a specific date for the family to take an "I Wonder Wander" before their next session together.

At the next session, the mother reported that they completed the assignment but that the child still complained a lot, and the father only said a few words. However, the child did have a small rock to show the therapist. The family continued to add "I Wonder Wanders" to their life and over the next few months, the family was able to tell many stories about things that they noticed in nature, and also the silly stories that they told together.

Intervention: "I Wonder Wander" (see also Appendix A for a summary of this activity).

The purpose of an "I Wonder Wander" is to increase curiosity and connection to nature through joint attention between a caregiver and a child and a subsequent narrative story that solidifies the experience.

1   Start by inviting the child on a short walk with an open-ended question like, "Would you like to go wandering with me for a few minutes?"
2   Remind yourself that the destination is not important (especially on the first try). Take a deep breath as you walk outside and announce your curiosity. "Ok, I am really looking forward to our wandering today. I am so curious about what we might find."
3   Take note of the first thing that you notice with your senses (temperature, smells, sounds, sights). Make a neutral statement about something that you notice. "I see that the sky is really gray right now." Or "I just walked out the front door and I see the green grass."
4   Invite the child to participate by saying, "I wonder what you notice." If the child responds, make sure you provide joint attention to the thing brought up by the child. "I notice that too." If the child doesn't respond, that is okay. Allow the wonder statement to linger between you without demanding an answer.
5   Encourage the child to choose which way you should walk. A simple choice of "should we go to the left or the right?" is often good enough. Continue to pay attention to what you, as the adult, notice as you participate in your natural surroundings. You do not have to comment about everything you notice, but you do want to practice paying attention to the sights and sounds and smells that are coming up.
6   As you walk, you and the child can point out interesting or curious things. You might say things like, "I wonder what kind of tree that is." or "I wonder about the bird that I hear singing." It is not important to know the answers to any of the questions. "Hmm…that's a good question." Or "I'm curious about that too" is enough.

7   You can encourage your child to take pictures, or sketch, some of the things that they see. Look for a stick or a rock, or a flower (on the ground already) that you might carry or take home as a transitional object. These things can become part of the child's nature journal.

8   As you are walking, you can start to develop a story about the things that you have seen. (This is especially helpful if you are on your way home or when the child might be tired of being outside). You can invite the child to make up a story about something by saying something like, "You know, I'm really curious about that bird too. I wonder if we could make up a story about that bird." You can take turns adding one sentence to the story. "Once upon a time, there was a very loud bird in the tree. No one knew its name or why it was so loud, but…."

9   The next person adds a line to the story, "but, actually, he was really loud because he really wanted to have a cookie, but his mom said that birds don't eat cookies." Continue going back and forth adding any bit of information to the story. Do not worry if the story makes sense. Do not worry if the story takes a turn into something fantastical or ridiculous. When you are out of ideas or feel that the story is over, you can end by saying, "and that is the story of the very loud bird."

10   As you end your walk, be sure to thank the child for going with you.

11   Later, you can re-visit the experience by reviewing the photos, the sketches or the items you collected. You can also amplify the experience by finding some answers to the questions that came up during the walk.

Vignette #2, Leo Age 10 Years

Background or Presenting Problem

Leo is a 10-year-old Caucasian male whose mother died by suicide four months before he entered therapy. Six-weeks after her death, he and his father moved into the home of the paternal grandparents, whom Leo identifies as two of his closest relationships. Shortly after this move, his father was arrested and facing a minimum of 10 years in prison if convicted of the current charges. Leo is having difficulty sleeping at night and often has vivid dreams with intrusive and frightening images of his mother. His grades have recently dropped from mostly A's and B's to C's and D's. Leo says he no longer cares about school and dislikes his teachers and fellow students. He spends most of his time at home in his bedroom playing video games. His grandmother makes consistent efforts to be engaged with Leo but does not want to "upset him after all he has been through." When asked to participate in an outdoor activity, Leo refuses saying he would rather play games with his friends online. In response to his refusal, his grandmother leaves him alone in his room. His grandfather is preoccupied with running the family business and has little time in his day to engage in family activities. When he does interact with Leo, he is often distracted and distant. Each member of the family unit spends most of their time alone in separate rooms and on electronic devices.

Family Goals

The family identified the goal of increasing quality family time together free of electronics. In addition, both Leo and his grandparents identified the desire to increase family conversations around both the number of losses and transitions within their family. The therapist introduced the idea of building family rituals as the repetition of activity provides support of children and increases the confidence of caregivers in providing support to their child (Goodyear-Brown, 2021). Over the course of four weeks, the family worked to incorporate one extended walk into their weekly routine. In conjunction to the weekly family walk, the therapist introduced brief 5–10-minute mindful walks in nature during the therapy session. Upon returning to the therapy office after this brief walk, Leo and his grandparents learned how to reflect on what they saw and what feelings surfaced in response. The therapist then introduced the Vision Family Journal intervention and scheduled a time for the family to attempt the intervention prior to the next session.

During the next session, the grandmother reported the family completed the intervention and were "surprised" by the emotional content that came up when reviewing the pictures taken during the walk. His grandmother indicated all family members were engaged in noticing objects and taking pictures throughout the walk and observed more silence than conversation. Once home, the family organized their pictures on their computer in one collective album titled "Family Strolls" and then created a subfolder within that album for each family member. When reviewing photos from the family walk, Leo's grandparents noted he took quite a few pictures of roots. Leo shared that he felt particularly drawn to the roots of trees and was not certain why. His grandmother encouraged further reflection and asked what feelings he felt both while taking the pictures and in the present moment. Leo shared that he felt excited and curious when taking them but noticed a shift in that he felt sad "like I just want to cry" when reviewing the photos. When asked about parallels to current circumstances, Leo reported he felt sad and confused because his Mom died. The family then discussed and developed the metaphor: Roots give strength to reach even farther towards the sun.

Intervention # 2: "Visual Family Journal" (see Appendix B for a summary of this intervention).

The purpose of the "Visual Family Journal" is to allow the caregiver and child the opportunity to cocreate a visual journal by taking pictures of what captures the attention of each family member while taking a walk or hike. The family then reflects on the pictures taken and cocreates a narrative and explores any metaphors found in nature during their walk.

1   Decide as a family on a consistent day and time to enjoy a longer walk together. Creating a ritual around a weekly family walk. The walk can be a longer walk around the neighborhood or encourage family members to provide suggestions for a park or trail that is within reasonable driving distance.

2   Before starting the walk, make certain each family member has a way to capture pictures throughout the walk. Encourage each family member to take pictures of what captures their attention along the way.

3   Throughout the walk, mindfully reflect on what is capturing your attention. For example, "These flowers are such a unique color"; "The roots of this tree are so big and twisty!" Welcome silence for mindful reflection too!

4   Once home, organize the pictures taken by each family member into an album for easy access and review.

5   Have each family member review their pictures and briefly journal in response to the pictures. Encourage curiosity around feelings experienced both while actively taking the pictures and when reflecting back on the pictures.

6   Hold a family discussion of any themes present in the pictures. For example, "You took quite a few pictures of roots and the trunks of trees. What do you notice about how you felt while taking the pictures and now as we are talking?"

7   Based on the themes present in the pictures, encourage the development of a brief narrative that parallels in nature to what is currently happening in the life of the family. Notice if any metaphors can be created and how it may relate to the circumstances of the family.

Conclusion

Families that are "prescribed nature" may not immediately know what to do or how to implement those plans and the suggestion of spending more time outside with their children can trigger anxiety in parents and caregivers. These anxieties may arise from their general fears of injury, illness, or judgment from other parents, from unkempt or unsafe outdoor spaces or from a general feeling of incompetence about what to do in outdoor spaces. Clinicians that can introduce the benefits of nature-based play in a culturally sensitive manner will have a better understanding of any obstacles or challenges faced by their clients.

By utilizing online resources like the Journey Map, parents can overcome their initial worries about risky outdoor play and develop a plan of action to increase time spent in nature. Practice sessions utilizing nature-based play and expressive therapies with a trained therapist can further increase a parent's sense of competence in implementing nature-based interventions with narrative or metaphorical components between sessions. This comprehensive manner of helping families increase their time in nature provides a skill that will help develop a sense of wonder, awe and grounded mindfulness throughout their lives.

Reflective Questions

1   To what extent do you believe in the theory of biophilia? Do things like race, gender, socioeconomic status, attachment history, trauma history, or personality traits influence a person's "innate craving for nature"?
2   How is the use of metaphor in play therapy sessions similar or different from the use of metaphor in nature-based play and expressive therapies?
3   Spend a few minutes looking or wandering outside your current environment. What sparks your interest, wonder, or curiosity? A cloud, a flower, or even a sound. Name three characteristics of that item or think about the metaphor that the image represents.

Appendix A

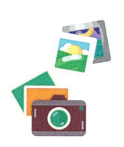

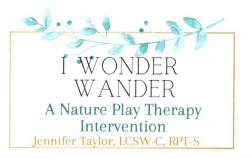

I WONDER WANDER
A Nature Play Therapy Intervention
Jennifer Taylor, LCSW-C, RPT-S

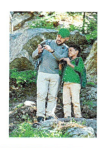

DESCRIPTION:

The purpose of an "I Wonder Wander" is to increase curiosity and connection to nature through joint attention between a child and a caregiver with a subsequent narrative story that solidifies the experience.

SUPPLIES NEEDED:

Two (or more) people out in nature

A sketch book and pencil and/or camera

An unhurried attitude

GOAL:

Create a nature-based experience that a parent and child can re-create together later.

INSTRUCTIONS:

1. Start by inviting the child on a short walk. Remind yourself that the destination is not important. Take a deep breath as you walk outside and announce your curiosity.
2. Take note of the first thing that you notice with your senses (temperature, smells, sounds, sights).
3. Invite the child to participate by saying, "I wonder what you notice."
4. As you walk, you and the child can point out interesting or curious things. that you have questions about.
5. You can encourage your child to take pictures, or sketch, some of the things that they see.
6. As you are walking, you can start to develop a story about the things that you have seen. You can take turns by each adding one sentence to the story.
7. Later, you can re-visit the experience by reviewing the photos, the sketches or the items you collected.

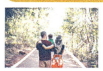

EXTRA PROCESSING:

You can also amplify the experience by finding some answers to the questions that came up during the walk.

Appendix B

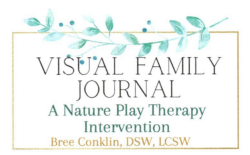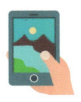

VISUAL FAMILY JOURNAL
A Nature Play Therapy Intervention
Bree Conklin, DSW, LCSW

DESCRIPTION:

A family nature walk that develops awareness and understanding of life experiences by journaling and co-creating metaphors about what is observed and experienced in nature during the walk.

SUPPLIES NEEDED:

Two (or more) people

A camera or cell phone with camera

Your sense of wonder!

GOAL:

Deepen awareness and understanding of life experiences within the family system in shared journal and co-creation of metaphors

INSTRUCTIONS:

Start by creating a ritual around a weekly family walk. Whether around the neighborhood or a decided upon by the family, let this walk be a longer walk to allow more time for curiosity and observing of nature. Before starting the walk, make certain each family member has a way to capture pictures or images throughout the walk. Encourage each person to take a picture of what captures their attention. During the walk, mindfully reflect on what is capturing your attention (i.e., "These roots are so big and twisty!"). Once home, organize the pictures taken for easy access and review. Have each family member review their pictures. Encourage curiosity around feelings experienced both while taking and in reviewing the pictures. Allow time for reflection through writing in a journal. Hold a family discussion around any themes noticed in the pictures. Based on the themes present in the pictures, encourage the development of a brief narrative that parallels in nature to what is currently happening in the life of the family. Notice if any metaphors can be created and how it may relate to the circumstances of the family.

EXTRA PROCESSING:

Encourage each family member to journal about what the co-created metaphor means and the ways in which that may allow a new and/or different perspective about a life experience

References

Adler, J. M. (2012). Living into the story: Agency and coherence in a longitudinal study of narrative identity development and mental health over the course of psychotherapy. *Journal of Personality and Social Psychology, 102*(2), 367–389. https://doi.org/10.1037/a0025289

Beaudoin, M. N. (2005). Agency and choice in the face of trauma: A narrative therapy map. *Journal of Systemic Therapies, 24*(4), 32–50.

Birch, J., Rishbeth, C., & Payne, S.R. (2020). Nature doesn't judge you – how urban nature supports young people's mental health and wellbeing in a diverse UK city. Health and Place, 62.

Boon, L. (2020). The wild inside: Offering children natural materials and an ecopsychological understanding of self within art therapy. In Heginworth, I. S. & Nash, G. (Eds.), *Environmental arts therapy: The wild frontiers of the heart.* Routledge.

Bratton, S., Landreth, G., Kellam, T., & Blackard, S. R. (2006). *Child parent relationship therapy (CPRT) treatment manual: A 10 session filial therapy model for training parents.* Routledge.

Brussoni, M., Ishikawa, T., Han, C., Pike, I., Bundy, A., Faulkner, G., & Mâsse, L. C. (2018). Go play outside! Effects of a risk-reframing tool on mothers' tolerance for, and parenting practices associated with, children's risky play: Study protocol for a randomized controlled trial. *Trials, 19*(1), 2. https://doi.org/10.1186/s13063-018-2552-4

Cacciatore, J. (2017). *Bearing the unbearable: love, loss, and the heartbreaking path of grief.* Wisdom Publications

Carson, R. (1965). *The sense of wonder.* Harper & Row.

Courtney, J. (2020). *Healing child and family trauma through expressive and play therapies.* Norton & Company, Inc.

Cronin, T.J., Lawrence, K.A., Taylor, K., Norton, P.J., & Kazantzis, N. (2015) Integrating between-session intervention (homework) in therapy: The importance of the therapeutic relationship and cognitive case Conceptualization. Journal of Clinical Psychology, 71(5), 439-450.

Dungy, C. T. (2009). *Black nature: four centuries of African American nature poetry.* University of Georgia Press.

Guerney, L. (2000). Filial therapy into the 21st century. *International Journal of Play Therapy, 9*(2), 1–17.

Goodyear-Brown, P. (2021). *Parents as partners in child therapy: A clinician's guide.* Guilford Press.

Heginworth, I. S., & Nash, G. (2020). *Environmental arts therapy: The wild frontiers of the heart.* Routledge.

Hyun, E. (2000, April). How is young children's intellectual culture of understanding nature different from adults? Presented at the Annual Conference of the American Educational Research Association, New Orleans, LA.

Johnson, K. (2014). Creative connecting: Early childhood nature journaling sparks wonder and develops ecological literacy. International Journal of Early Childhood Environmental Education, 2(1), 126-139.

Kopytin, A. & Rugh, M. (2020). Environmental expressive therapies. New York, NY: Routledge.

Kondo, M. C., Oyekanmi, K. O., Gibson, A., South, E. C., Bocarro, J., & Hipp, J. A. (2020). Nature prescriptions for health: A review of evidence and research opportunities. *International Journal of Environmental Research and Public Health, 17*(12). https://doi-org.ezproxy.memphis.edu/10.3390/ijerph17124213

Kopytin, A., & Rugh, M. (2017). *Environmental expressive therapies: Nature-assisted theory and practice.* Routledge.

Malchiodi, C. (2020). *Trauma and expressive arts therapy: Brain, body, and imagination in the healing process.* Guilford Press

McMillan, S., & Wilhelm, J. (2007). Student stories: Adolescents constructing multiple literacies through nature journaling. *Journal of Adolescent and Adult Literacy, 50*(5), 370–379.

Nash, G. (2020). Weaving the threads of theory and experience: a review of the literature. In Heginworth, I. S. & Nash, G. (Eds.), *Environmental arts therapy: The wild frontiers of the heart.* Routledge.

Outside Play. (2021). Outdoorplay.ca Collaborative. https://outsideplay.ca

Peters, E., Maas, J., Hovinga, D., Van den Bogerd, N., & Schuengel, C. (2020). Experiencing nature to satisfy basic psychological needs in parenting: A quasi-experiment in family shelters. *International Journal of Environmental Research and Public Health, 17*, 8657. https://doi.org/10.3390/ijerphy17228657

Park, B.J., Tsunetsugu, Y. Kagawa, T., & Miyazaki, Y. (2010). The physiological effects of shinrin-yoku (taking in the forest atmosphere or forest bathing): Evidence from field experiments in 24 forests across Japan. *Environmental Health and Preventative Medicine, 15*(1), 18–26.

Ramshini, M., Hasanzadeh, S., Afroz, G., & Hashemi, H. (2018). The effect of family-centered nature therapy on children with autism spectrum disorder. *Archives of Rehabilitation, 19*, 2.

Schaefer, C.E., & Drewes, A. A. (2011). The therapeutic powers of play and play therapy. In C. E. Schaefer (Ed.), Foundations of play therapy (pp. 15–25). John Wiley & Sons Inc.

Sobel (2008). *Childhood and nature: Design principles for educators.* Stenhouse Publishers.

PART VI

Nature-Based Storytelling Interventions

15 Into the Great Forest: Fairy-Tale Themes of the Wild Take Shape in Sandplay

Rosalind Heiko

They won't tell you fairytales
of how girls can be dangerous and still win.
They will only tell you stories
where girls are sweet and kind
and reject all sin.
I guess to them
it's a terrifying thought,
a red riding hood
who knew exactly
what she was doing
when she invited the wild in.

—Nikita Gill, "Girls of the Wild"

Introduction

Every successful girl heroine's journey story incorporates travel into the heart of the Great Forest, that representation of the archetypal source of both the challenges and resources in the outside world and the client's psyche. Becoming attuned to the outer world of nature, as well as the inner world of the self, allows our clients to mindfully gather these macro- and microcosms together into a sense of experienced harmony. The essential core of both fairy tales and the practice of Sandplay is rooted in acceptance of our own wild nature, in what we have tamed within ourselves, and how we learn our place within the greater whole. This acceptance can be integrated in our personal lives, our homes and communities, and the larger world. Respect for our spiritual nature, for the environment we share with our brothers and sisters, and for our world is vital to this therapeutic individuation process and manifests in the stories children and teens share in the sand.

Clarissa Pinkola Estes (2003) points out that the word "wild" when applied to a fully realized life, means: "to live a natural life, one in which the criatura, creature, has innate integrity and healthy boundaries" (p. 8). She speaks of stories as "soul vitamins," and states:

> Fairy Tales, myths, and stories provide understandings which sharpen our sight so that we can pick out and pick up the path left by the wildish nature. The instruction found in story reassures us that the path has not run out, but still leads women deeper, and more deeply still, into their own knowing. The tracks we all are following are those of the wild and innate instinctual Self. (p. 4)

Poet and storyteller Terri Windling speaks of Tolkien's "great soup of Story," and the great power, danger, and transformative aspects of the old stories.

DOI: 10.4324/9781003152767-21

Over the centuries the symbols and metaphors that give marchen [tales] their power have been worked and reworked by storytellers of each generation and each culture around the globe. Tolkien envisioned this as a great soup of Story, always simmering, full of bits and pieces of myth, epic, and history, from which the storyteller as Cook serves up his or her particular broth…The fairy tale journey may look like an outward trek across plains and mountains, through castles and forests, but the actual movement is inward, into the lands of the soul. The dark path of the fairy tale forest lies in the shadows of our imagination, the depths of our unconscious…this ability to travel inward, to face fear and transform it, is a skill they will use all their lives. (Datlow & Windling, 2019, p. 10)

The Multisensory Role of Sandplay

Sandplay therapy is a nonverbal, nondirective therapeutic method, built on the therapeutic alliance between clinician and client, which fosters the use of symbolic language and representations in the service of psychological growth and healing. This method is used worldwide and "is especially applicable in working with children, and with adults with trauma, distress, disabilities, and migration issues", demonstrating "significant improvements with moderate effect sizes for a variety of child and adult mental health problems". (Roesler, 2019, p. 84)

In Sandplay practice, clients are presented with trays filled with sand and with water available, in a room filled with shelves of images and figures, which reflect the clinician's worldview and world cultures as well as personal mythology. Clients engage with sand forms and choose figures and images to symbolically represent their struggles. They create places and worlds, which manifest their hero or heroine's journeys in the sand and water. Clients are offered this "safe and protected space" (Kalff, 2020, p. 7). The clinician holds and contains the client's emotional states and conflicts. The Sandplay therapist continually engages in a process of "coming to understand," maintaining an open and observing attitude, witnessing the Sandplay journey unfolding, along with the client. The process of creating sandtrays over time enables the client to nonverbally express both conscious and unconscious material. This awareness of powerful emotional material can bring a deep, meaningful, spiritual self-understanding that includes their unique challenges, capacities, and connection to the larger world.

Sandplay is a multisensory experience that engages smell, sight, touch, and movement of sand, water, and fire, which can strengthen neural integration and self-regulation as the clients manipulate actual elements or symbolic figures. Badenoch (2008) theorized that "the whole experience encourages vertical brain integration, linking body, limbic region and cortex in the right hemisphere" (p. 221). Within the Sandplay process, and accompanied by a trusted therapist, both left and right hemispheres are engaged. A recent study has shown Sandplay to be effective in reducing anxiety symptoms, and possibly promoting subcortical brain function and health (Foo et al., 2020).

"In Sandplay a self-directed, natural process of meaning making occurs. The Sandplay therapist does not direct or interpret the creative process, but rather supports through attuned presence, curiosity and awaiting receptivity" (Freedle, 2019, p. 97). The client decides whether to touch the sand or employ the figures and symbols on the shelves. The tray itself can be viewed as an extension of the client's embodied feelings and thoughts. Pattis Zoja (2004) stated that Sandplay

deals with preverbal and pre symbolic areas of experience by way of the shaping and manipulation of concrete objects. The hands assume the leading role, the body assumes the leading role. Not narrative not language. Sandplay follows the patient into his or her particular phase of development, and its flexibility is sufficiently great as to allow it completely to adapt itself to whatever the patient's current needs. (p. 19)

Engaging Therapeutic Powers of Play in Sandplay and Storytelling

The Therapeutic Powers of Play can bring about desired emotional and behavioral changes and well-being in clients (Schaefer & Peabody, 2016). The multisensory experience inherent in Sandplay provides an invitation to the client's unconscious through indirect guidance, as well as fostering emotional identification and expression. The Sandplay therapist's unconditional acceptance of client creations can strengthen attachment and coregulation in the therapeutic relationship. Sandplay therapists work to provide a nonjudgmental atmosphere of security and containment, which may also increase client mastery and self-reflection activities. Client engagement in storytelling fosters connection and attachment to the therapist-storyteller, and demonstrates a way to increase personal strengths in creative problem-solving and resilience.

Deep into the Forest: How Fairy Tales Illuminate the Sand Journeys of Children and Teens

Fairy tales engage us at a very basic level. There is a rich perspective that these stories grant us: the ability to listen to clues about our own instinctual nature (Heiko, 2018). Andrews writes eloquently about the aspects of the Forest that engage our senses and heighten our awareness as shown in the following:

> When you enter the woods of a fairy tale and it is night, the trees tower on either side of the path. They loom large because everything in the world of fairy tales is blown out of proportion. If the owl shouts, the otherwise deathly silence magnifies its call. The tasks you are given to do (by the witch, by the stepmother, by the wise old woman) are insurmountable - pull a single hair from the crescent moon bear's throat; separate a bowl's worth of poppy seeds from a pile of dirt. The forest seems endless. But when you do reach the daylight, triumphantly carrying the particular hair or having outwitted the wolf; when the owl is once again a shy bird and the trees only a lush canopy filtering the sun, the world is forever changed for your having seen it otherwise. From now on, when you come upon darkness, you'll know it has dimension. You'll know how closely poppy seeds and dirt resemble each other. The forest will be just another story that has absorbed you, taken you through its paces, and cast you out again to your home with its rattling windows and empty refrigerator - to your meager livelihood, which demands, inevitably, that you write about it.
>
> (Andrews, 2005, p. 84)

Warner (2014) speaks of the magic currents inherent in nature. When we go to the heart of a forest, we come up against "the indifferent and immense power of the archetype of Mother Nature's energy itself" (Heiko, 2018, p. 50). In these fairy tales, talking horses and birds share wisdom and resources with the hero and heroine. These characters must rely on their intuition and problem-solving abilities—as well as draw from the power of their connection to nature if they are to succeed. However, Mother Nature does not concern herself with individual lives, needs, and challenges. It is up to the hero and heroine to address these challenges with assistance.

Utilizing the Sandplay Journey Map in Sandplay

The journey to the wild heart of our metaphorical internal forest consists of a number of tasks that encourage completion if clients are to survive trauma and mature in whatever developmental stage they find themselves. In Sandplay, the children, teens, and adults must undergo similar steps as they:

- Prepare for a quest: figuring out what is best to take with us, actually and metaphorically.
- Manage internal conflicts and tensions: figuring out if we can trust ourselves and our tentative forays into the new.
- Find their way forward by discovering pathways to explore the new.
- Uncover the ability to identify helpers who guide and challenge us when they show up (animals, people).
- Forge a way to acknowledge and integrate parts of the shadow inside of us: that internal material that we either don't want to face, aren't ready to know about ourselves, or aren't yet capable of understanding and integrating.
- Celebrate the treasures of the heart's wisdom: connecting with that simple and authentic understanding and perspective which comes with the experience of journeying.

- Find a way to repair the broken inside of us: how do we find the will and capacity to mend what has been torn away, damaged, betrayed in our psyche.
- Return homeward with the treasure of connection to our essential nature.
- Begin to integrate our newfound wisdom and heart-opening with a return to life respecting ourselves and the environment in which we live.

Guide to the Gateways

The Sandplay Journey Map in Sandplay (Heiko, 2018) generally delineates this process in mandala form through four Gateways around a central core. This journey is called a "process," whereby clients choose figures and images to symbolically represent their world in sandtrays. The core, called the "Center," represents the inner beauty and wisdom found in illustrating images of the self. The beginning phase of treatment, represented by Gateway 1, is named "Pathways." Here is where the client chooses to begin the journey in their sandwork. Gateway 2 is "Discernment," in which clients courageously create trays that delineate the fears, tensions, and challenges they face. This second Gateway represents the middle phase of treatment. In Gateway 3, "Harmony," the client begins to reconcile those tensions and trauma. They begin to forge new connections in healing. This third Gateway represents the beginning of the final phase of treatment. Gateway 4, named "Re-turn," brings the journey full circle, and concludes the final phase of treatment. Here clients manifest images of abundance, and an appreciation for the treasure of connection to their inner nature and the outer world around them.

Introduction to Case Vignettes

In Sandplay, we venture into the heart of forested glades, with shadowed pathways and secret caves as well as the majestic glories of wind, earth, and water forms, which represent the storms and sheltered spaces within the psyche. Many of the themes in fairy tales echo and illustrate the fears, loneliness, betrayal, and sadness inherent when a child comes up against the cold unresponsiveness in the landscape of indifference that exists with inept and neglectful parenting.

The following section will present three different case vignettes. Each vignette begins with a brief case background description, followed by a series of Tray Detail examples that will contain which figures and images were used, or how the terrain of the tray was created. Each vignette will also include a section for Therapist Reflections and Concluding Reflections. The first vignette of Lainey will demonstrate how this girl explored pathways in nature in her quest for healing and courage.

Vignette #1: Lainey: Demonstrating That Nature and Forest Are Places of Healing

Lainey was a girl of six and a half when she began her Sandplay process, and nine when she finished. She was slight and quick in motion and in thought. She appeared shy at first; and soon demonstrated her capacity for and joy in connection by relating detailed and absorbing stories of her everyday life. She had to overcome overwhelming early neglect and trauma. Her casework is fully conceptualized and presented in this text (Heiko, 2018, pp. 69–91). For our purposes, we will focus on the way Forest and Nature itself become places where she can draw healing energy. Here are 9 of her trays, out of a total of 27.

Lainey Tray 1 (See Figure 15.1): Beginning Phase/Gateway 1

Lainey Tray Detail

This scene is a First Nations village on one side of a water path that appears to be blocked as it moves downward. A girl sets out on the river without a paddle. There is a bear family eating and playing on one side of the water; as well as a squirrel on the top of one of the trees, and beaver and rabbit families. The fenced in village is surrounded by a forest with four evergreens among the trees, and one downed tree. A contained and well-tended cooking pot over flames was placed in the center of the village; as well as uncontained flames nearby.

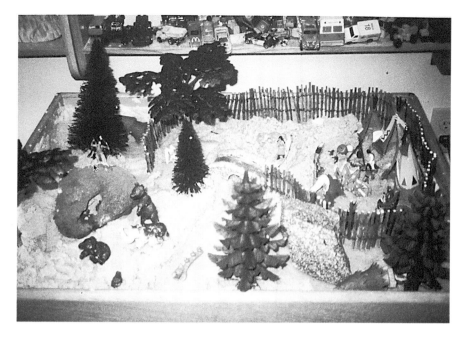

Figure 15.1 Tray 1: Setting out.

Source: Rosalind Heiko.

Therapist Reflections

In Sandplay, setting out on a path can represent a journey toward individuation, toward an under-standing and perspective on the self as developmentally appropriate. Most interpretations of Sandplay journeys consist of questions about the meaning of and patterns in the chosen symbols over the course of the process. Here, there is a wilderness, which surrounds the village, crossed by a bridge, which connects the two. This might point to the possibilities of integrating the disparate energies of family and com-munity to her instinctual nature. The squirrel has climbed high up in the tree, gaining a bit of perspective on the scene. There are dangers lurking in this tray: There is a warrior sighting the river path close to where the girl will pass; the bears are fearsome creatures when they protect themselves and their young; and there is the matter of the uncontained fire in the middle of the village. Fire can represent activation energy of a strong sort in sandtrays; and possibly strong emotional reactions. Can Lainey reconcile her fiery impulses and her need for continuity and connection within her psyche?

Lainey Tray 2: Beginning Phase/Gateway 1

Lainey Tray Detail

Lainey spent most of her time wetting the sand and digging down to into the blue bottom of the trays. Here, are found five evergreens inside a gated area, surrounding a lookout tower in the center. The ladder to the tower is blown down and one of the large evergreens is blown over, just like the small evergreen we saw in her first tray.

Therapist Reflections

In creating this tray, Lainey moved deeper into exploring watery paths. Water engulfs the tray, possibly representing the unconscious. Perhaps she has created the feeling of emotional upheaval through the scene of storms that blew through the landscape of the evergreen forest. Do the evergreens represent herself and the other four members of her family? Although there is a tower, no one is there to gain perspective on the scene, nor is there a way to get the ladder back up to the tower. A feeling of abandonment and loneliness permeated the creation of this flooded tray.

Lainey Tray 3: Beginning Phase/Gateway 1

Lainey Tray Detail

Here in Tray 3, is found a pond with a frog and goldfish in a very wet tray.

Therapist Reflections

Lovely flowering lotus plants abound in a quiet nature scene, which celebrates rest and a peacefulness. This illustrates how clients create trays that bring a sense of calm to their disordered and dysregulated experience of life throughout their sand process.

Lainey Tray 4: Beginning Phase/Gateway 1

Lainey Tray Detail

In this tray, domesticated animals are appropriately fenced off in different areas of the tray: pig families and horses.

Therapist Reflections

Horse energy can highlight the emotional connection between horse and rider, as well as the freedom of motion inherent in their nature. Does Lainey need the connection to her animal nature in the form of horses and farm animals to represent the familiarity, order, and domesticity of her life in the family?

Lainey Tray 5: Middle Phase/Gateway 2

Lainey Tray Detail

Tray 5 depicts large animals: lions, an elephant, and families of orangutans and giraffes within a savannah landscape, gathering around a water pond made of felt in a wet tray. A tiger is placed on top of a large cave.

Therapist Reflections

Large wild animal energies come to the fore in this tray around the water symbol. Is the tiger, possibly a symbol of solar energies, getting perspective on the scene? Is this Lainey's way of facing her fears and engaging with primal energy of these Big Game animals?

Lainey Tray 6: Middle phase/Gateway 2

Lainey Tray Detail

This flooded tray contains the flowering lotus plants used in Tray 3, and the lookout tower and ladder she used in Tray 2. A small green plant is placed at the entrance to the top of the tower.

Therapist Reflections

Buddhists say that the lotus stalk grows through the mud to bloom, just as our spiritual selves reach through troubled times to flourish. In this scene, the small green growth is placed in front of the tower in the center of the tray—and this time the ladder is placed strategically, in contrast to Tray 2. Does the flooding of this tray point to the emotional overwhelm Lainey has experienced? Will this threaten her well-being?

Lainey Tray 7: Middle Phase/Gateway 2

Lainey Tray Detail

Tray 7 was created with wet, packed sand. Again, five evergreens are present. The King's castle dominates the scene surrounded by the evergreens. A big snake lolls in one of the turrets, facing the water and overlooking the scene. Four sparklers and the water pond made of felt used in Tray 5 complete the tray.

Therapist Reflections

The feeling of watchful protectiveness in the forest is inherent in this scene. The King in his kingdom can't be seen; but the landscape is orderly and organized. The snake may represent the possibilities inherent in transformation and initiation from girlhood in the young feminine to young womanhood.

Lainey Tray 8 (See Figure 15.2): Beginning Final Phase/Gateway 3

Lainey Tray Detail

Lainey painstakingly dripped sand to create this tray to build up the mountain surrounded by water. Three battery-operated lit candles were placed on islands in three corners of the tray, with boats set around the mountain.

Therapist Reflections

The glorious drip mountain provides a centered, balanced feeling of the landscape, with the flow of ocean and water to and from the islands. Lainey has already begun to make substantial changes in her behavior, school performance, and social connections. She is well on her way to healing, demonstrating this through her strong connection to the earth and water energies of mountain and sea.

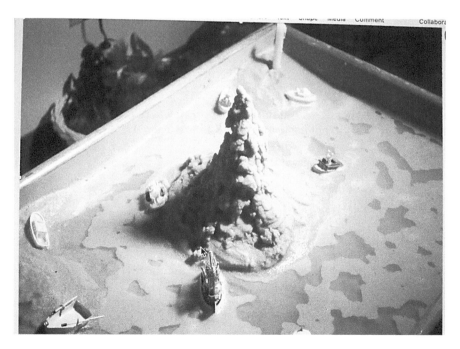

Figure 15.2 Tray 8: Drip mountain.

Source: Rosalind Heiko.

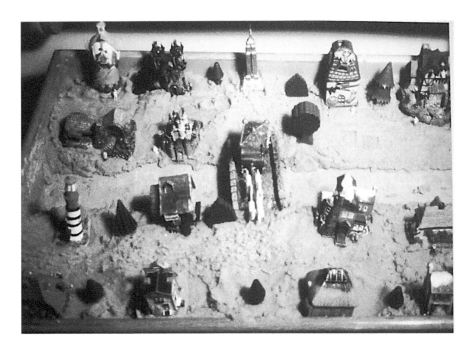

Figure 15.3 Tray 9: Coming home.

Source: Rosalind Heiko.

Lainey Tray 9 (See Figure 15.3): Final Phase/Gateway 4

Lainey Tray Detail

There is a town here, which includes a lighthouse, church, a fairy-tale carriage going over a bridge spanning both sides of a river, smaller evergreens scattered throughout the tray, a palace, fairy-tale tower, scary Halloween house, and a mill with both adults and children set around the scene.

Therapist Reflections

Here we come full circle from the First Nations village found in Lainey's first Tray (refer back to Figure 15.1), all the way to a scene of city life. This is a harmonious tray where both fearsome places (the Halloween House) and the fantastic (a palace and a fairy tale tower) are integrated within Lainey's unconscious with the solidity of the everyday town life. Now the water path flows consistently from east to west without blockage, again in contrast to her first Tray (refer back to Figure 15.1).

Lainey Vignette Concluding Reflections

Nature was a huge factor in Lainey's progress and healing in therapy through her sandplay process. She worked with big and small animal energies in her trays, and created forested areas. She engaged with different states of water, flooding many of her trays. Lainey symbolically represented water, through the use of ceramic streams, and made pathways through the sand to the blue "water" of the painted bottom of her trays. This brought her great satisfaction in connecting to the harmony of the natural world.

The next section will introduce a case vignette with Shaina. She was able to connect with the healing elements of water, fire and earth in her sandtrays to repair painful disconnection and trauma in her life.

Vignette #2: Shaina: Demonstrating Courage in Representing the Elements to Heal

Shaina was a preteen when she created these seven trays as part of a larger Sandplay process. She was introverted and gentle, focused on learning to handle a blended family, with high parental expectations for performance and behavior. Her difficulties manifested in extreme anxiety and fear of inadequacy.

Shaina Tray 1: Beginning Phase/Gateway 1

Shaina Tray Detail

In Tray 1, there is a very wet tray with a bit of the blue bottom of the tray showing around the middle portion of the mounded and worked sand.

Therapist Reflections

Shaina shared that this scene was a picture of the Universe forming. She spent the entire session working the wet sand to her satisfaction. A huge sigh marked the end of her creation. Was this a representation of the huge possibilities and vast energies, which confronted and surrounded her?

Shaina Tray 2: Beginning Phase/Gateway 1

Shaina Tray Detail

Tray 2 details a forest with caves hidden within the foliage. Large rocks, small plants, and animals are set around the forest. A gold chain necklace set on top of the trees decorates this forest scene.

Therapist Reflections

Shaina's connection to the landscape of forest is evident here. We can wonder if the hidden entrances to the caves represent the need for private space within her psyche. She appears to luxuriate in the beauty of the forest glen. These private spaces can bring energy and power to the psyche.

Shaina Tray 3 (See Figure 15.4): Middle Phase/Gateway 2

Shaina Tray Detail

Here there is a forested area set with palm trees, hedges, a waterfall, and splashes of water set around its base. Figures from the Star Wars universe have paddled into the scene. They have beached their canoes and are walking towards an area replete with colored glass stones.

Therapist Reflections

Every rebel warrior knows that they must find a place of repose where they can rest and recharge. Here the characters from Star Wars search for treasure amidst the trees on the beach. This is a place of tentative centering and connection to inner resources.

Shaina Tray 4: Center/Illustrating the Beauty of the Self

Shaina Tray Detail

An island formed of plants and trees flourishes in the sea. Rocks are scattered in the water.

Therapist Reflections

This is a scene replete with the bounty to be found in and on the earth. It is a glorious, colorful representation of wealth and beauty, a place where Shaina can draw emotional sustenance and connect to her inner core of strength.

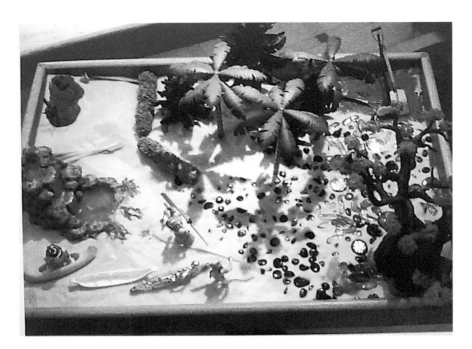

Figure 15.4 Tray 3: Rest and recharge.

Source: Rosalind Heiko.

Shaina Tray 5 (See Figure 15.5): Center/Illustrating the Beauty of the Self

Shaina Tray Detail

This tray contains rocks, glass and plastic treasure stones, large and small colored marbles, small gold colored bricks, tiles and glass shells.

Therapist Reflections

Throughout her Sandplay process, Shaina seems to reach for a peaceful haven. Can she revitalize her psyche through her connection to both man-made treasures and those beautiful gems found within the earth?

Shaina Tray 6 (See Figure 15.6): Beginning Final Phase: Gateway 3

Shaina Tray Detail

Shaina created a stream or river meandering through the landscape of colored glass and plastic stones, and marbles and large rocks.

Therapist Reflections

The center limestone rock comes from the Carpathian Mountains in Romania, formed primarily from shells or coral. Those mountain ranges were created with tremendous volcanic force. Here the persistence of water wearing away a path in the rocks seems formidable. Does Shaina relate to this quality in her own psyche as a way to manage the turbulence of her own life? Is she beginning to synthesize this understanding and inner wisdom through the representations of earth and treasure?

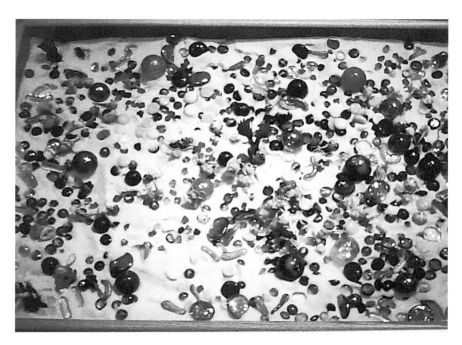

Figure 15.5 Tray 5: Treasures.
Source: Rosalind Heiko.

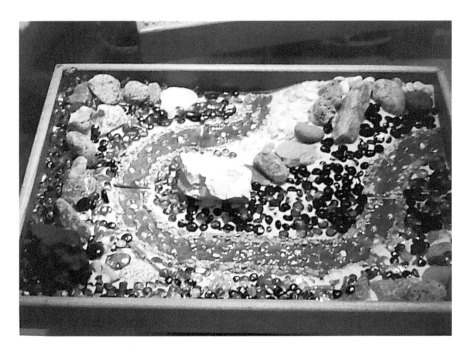

Figure 15.6 Tray 6: The strength of stream and stone.
Source: Rosalind Heiko.

Shaina Tray 7: Final Phase/Re-Turn

Shaina Tray Detail

Minerals, precious and semiprecious stones, shells, trees, and flowering plants are placed within this tray.

Therapist Reflections

In this landscape of forest and gems, Shaina brings forth all natural resources and treasures to again showcase the abundance and colorful variety of nature in all its beauty. Does she represent the treasures of the Self as well? As she created this scene, Shaina again sighed deeply, a smile gracing her face. This was a deeply satisfying tray to Shaina; a culmination of her work in connecting the inherent harmony and grace found in Nature within her psyche.

Shaina Vignette Concluding Reflections

The nature scenes in Shaina's trays were often abstract and gorgeously arrayed, and form a stabilizing and grounding process in Shaina's psyche, allowing her to access healing energy for her emotional development and sustenance. In all of these cases, bringing the concept of working with archetypal energies found in the therapist's play therapy collection to the outdoors, could also enliven and enrich the therapeutic engagement and experience (find the Nature Tray intervention in Appendix B).

The last vignette introduces Andi and examines how the lure of the wild can excite and overwhelm our psyche.

Vignette #3: Andi and the Tale of Little Red Cap (Riding Hood)

Andi was a teen who flirted with addiction to nonprescription substances, and with potentially dangerous sexually intimate relationships. As a budding writer, she was drawn to fantasy in reading and movies. She created several trays using the which focused on the tale of Little Red Cap. As a reminder to the reader, the story of Little Red Cap will be briefly reviewed here: The tale of Little Red Cap is a

> tale of initiation, an allegory of canal knowledge and social prohibitions, about innocent girlhood on the threshold of maturity, with the trackless forest standing in for the dangerous world, the predator for the seducer, the abuser of innocence. This view has since taken on a deep psychological meaning. (Warner, 2014, p. 115)

In this story, Little Red Cap must choose between doing what she knows she should and what she really, unconsciously wants to do. Bettleheim relates that in this story, the color red

> is the color symbolizing violent emotions, very much including sexual ones. The red velvet cap given by Grandmother to Little Red Cap thus can be viewed as a symbol of a premature transfer of sexual attractiveness, which is further accentuated by the grandmother's being old and sick, too weak even to open a door...Little Red Cap's danger is her budding sexuality, for which she is not yet emotionally mature enough. (1976, p. 176)

Andi Tray 1 (See Figure 15.7): Middle Phase/Gateway 2

Andi Tray Detail

Little Red Cap, Grandmother (in purple), a woman holding a rose, and the Wolf dressed in Grandmother's clothes, lurking off near the dead tree to the right can be found here in a forest scene.

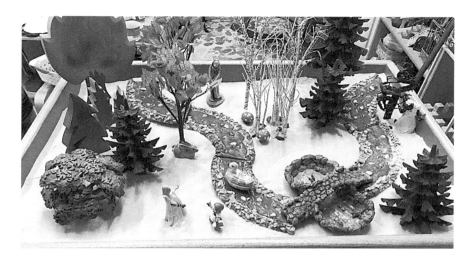

Figure 15.7 Tray 1: Choices.
Source: Rosalind Heiko.

Therapist Reflections

Andi created a scene in the Great Forest and its pathways. Warner speaks of forbidden desire and traumatic experience in fairy tales as: "something which ought to have remained hidden but has come to light. The forest, so bright with dancing sunbeams and fresh flowers, seems homely, but is uncanny ominousness grows as it tempts the little girl off the path" (2014, p. 120). The girl seems to be having a conversation with the woman. Does this woman represent her Mother? Or perhaps herself when older? The Grandmother figure waits farther along the forest path. The Wolf lurks off to the right, dressed in Grandmother's clothes. Will Little Red Cap follow the path her Mother wishes her to follow to her Grandmother? Does Andi unconsciously yearn to connect with the Wolf lurking nearby?

Andi Tray 2 (See Figure 15.8): Middle Phase/Gateway 2

Andi Tray Detail

Here is a wishing well off to the back right of the tray; a golden pathway to and from the pond and wishing well; a small spring of water next to a bench; two autumn trees near the pond; and a nest of two birds in the back of the tray.

Therapist Reflections

Does Andi need a place of reflection—somewhere she can take a break from her impulses and desires? The water in both the wishing well and pond allow a mirroring of that unconscious energy so that she can gather her thoughts while sitting on the bench and contemplate the path before her. Will she listen to the quiet whispering of her inner wisdom? Will she silence it?

Andi Tray 3 (See Figure 15.9): Middle Phase/Gateway 2

Andi Tray Detail

Woman and Wolf in the Great Forest, path detail of golden circles and gems, and Grandmother in front of her house and front gate looking toward them.

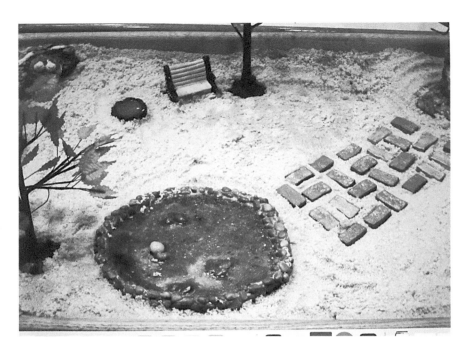

Figure 15.8 Tray 2: A place to contemplate.
Source: Rosalind Heiko.

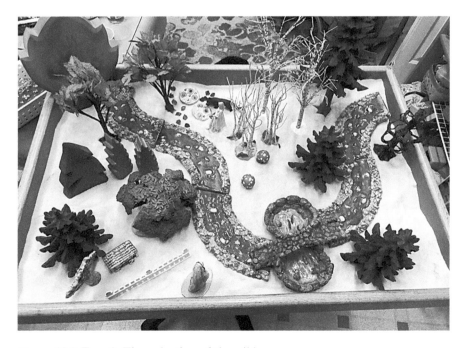

Figure 15.9 Tray 3: The seduction of the wild.
Source: Rosalind Heiko.

Therapist Reflections

In this scene, the figure of the woman seems to replace the figure of Little Red Cap. She appears to choose a path that leads to danger, walking with the wolf further into the Forest. Warner warns that

> fairy tales speak through beasts to explore common experiences - fear of sexual intimacy, assault, cruelty, and injustice and, in general, the struggle for survival…Monster bridegrooms can also take the form of animals that used to pose a very real threat - wolves and bears and pigs and warthogs… Often hybrid, huge, scaly, tusked, and bristling, such beasts endanger and even rape the heroine, in far-flung exotic settings or close to home. (2014, pp. 27–29)

The Grandmother, the strong wise woman who often warns of listening to one's intuition, waits closest to the place where Andi created this tray. Will the woman leave the Wolf and race back to her Grandmother? Will she disappear with the Wolf into the Wild?

Andi Concluding Reflections

Andi teetered on a destructive personal path while in treatment, choosing to make unwise connections in relationships in particular. At this point in therapy with teens and adults, I usually share the vicious and gorgeously descriptive poem "Silver and Gold"; and I did so with Andi. The poem clearly elucidates the menace and the power of seduction represented by the Wolf. The phrases from this poem found in Appendix 15.B are worthy of emphasis: "Sometime, I explain, it's hard to tell the difference between the ones who love you and the ones who will eat you alive" and "from what nearly destroys you, love may emerge". The chilling ending of the poem concludes:

> I will again leave the path and wander into that fragrant green wood and when I see coat of silver, eyes of gold I will follow.

(To read the full poem, see Appendix A. "Silver and Gold" by Ellen Steiber from *Snow White, Blood Red*, edited by Ellen Datlow & Terri Windling, an AvoNova Book, William Morrow & Company, Inc., 1993. Copyright ©1993 by Ellen Steiber. Reprinted by permission of Ellen Steiber.)

Themes of self-harm and self-destructiveness in the young feminine resonate and play out in Andi's sand creations. The vital questions therapy needed to address were to explore who and what Andi was running from; as well as what she was moving toward, trying to grasp. Had she lost sight of something essential? Was she herself "lost"? Within the crucible of the story and themes of Little Red Cap, we began to untangle these challenges for Andi in her treatment.

Closing Comments/Chapter Summary

Nurturing confidence and well-being and resilience in our children is essential to their journeys of in-dividuation. Maitland (2012) states that resilience is

> the simple honest awareness that horrible and dangerous things do happen, but that you can cope; with a modest application of good sense you can not only survive, you can gain from the experience…you can hide in a wood within earshot of your grown-ups, in a way you cannot usually on a mountainside or beach…The fairy stories themselves are also training grounds for resilience. Terrible, terrible dangers threaten the children in fairy stories—from cruel and abusive parents to giants, wolves and witches. But in every single case, not through special skills or miraculous interventions but through the application of good sense (and interestingly, good manners), the children do not merely survive, they return home wiser, richer, and happier. (pp. 100–101)

Our wild, instinctual nature must be respected and integrated into our psyche. Otherwise, we run the risk of one-sided perspectives and behavior. When we bring the natural world into our therapy process in our

Sandplay rooms, we open up vistas from archetypal stories that enliven and enrich our psychological growth and healing.

Permissions

I want to thank the following publishers and authors for permission to quote and reprint material for this book:

1   Nonexclusive permission was granted to reprint the nine figures cited from: A therapist's guide to mapping the girl heroine's journey in Sandplay (2018), Heiko, R. L., Rowman & Littlefield Publishers in this text. All rights reserved.
    Figure 8.1, p. 72; Figure 8.2, p. 73; Figure 8.5, p. 76; Figure 8.7, p. 78; Figure 8.12, p. 83; Figure 8.15, p. 86; Figure 8.16, p. 86; Figure 8.17, p. 87; Figure 8.20, p. 90.
2   Nonexclusive rights to include the following material: "Silver and Gold" by Ellen Steiber from *Snow White, Blood Red*, edited by Ellen Datlow & Terri Windling, an AvoNova Book, William Morrow & Company, Inc., 1993. Copyright ©1993 by Ellen Steiber. Reprinted by permission of Ellen Steiber.

Chapter Reflection Questions

1   In what ways do sand creations of clients reflect the natural world?
2   What natural materials can be gathered and used comfortably indoors in the sand room?
3   What elements are present in Sandplay scenes (i.e., common examples are: states of water, fire, earth, and wind or air)?
4   How do Sandplay creations reflect the landscape of the Great Forest?
5   How does an understanding fairy-tale themes enrich the experience of Sandplay therapy?
6   Utilizing the Nature Tray Activity, in what ways, does this enrich the experience of bringing Sandplay out of the office into the larger expanse of the outdoors for our clients?

Appendix A

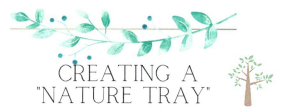

CREATING A "NATURE TRAY"
A Nature Play Therapy Intervention
Rosalind L. Heiko, PhD, RPT-S

DESCRIPTION:

This intervention asks the child, teen or parent to gather natural materials in nature and create a "nature tray" outside with the instruction: "make your own nature scene."

SUPPLIES NEEDED:
Found objects like feathers, stones, rocks, crystals, leaves, plants, bark, petals, sticks, pinecones, seeds.

GOAL:
Celebrating connection to self and the natural world, facilitating self-expression.

INSTRUCTIONS:

This activity encourages and allows clients to express their symbolic connection to the natural world and their place in it. The client is given about 45 minutes from start to finish for the activity. They are asked to gather materials outdoors to create the "Nature Tray" [about 10-15 minutes]. They bring items over to a chosen spot, bounding off the area for their "Nature Tray" in a roughly rectangular/circular shape, using the materials they've gathered. They arrange the material in any way they'd like, with the instruction: "See what your hands want to do to make your own nature scene" [about 20 minutes, with a 5-minute reminder]. Upon completion, they are asked if they have a title or story about their scene. The adult can record the activity if the child wishes.

EXTRA FUN:

A small group of children can work in different areas close by each other and then walk to each other's "Nature Tray" and tell a story of its creation, contents, and a title, if they wish to share.

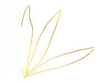

Appendix B. Poem Silver and Gold

"...Walk nice and quietly,
and do not run off the path,
and when you go into your grandmother's house
do not forget to say, 'Good-morning,'
and don't peep into every corner before you do it."
Mother's instructions.
The thick-knit cloak without which
I never dared venture into the world.
Is it any wonder that when the wolf appeared,
coat of silver, eyes of gold,
when the wolf sauntered toward me, kindly as you please,
and showed me fields of lavender and jessamine,
hawkweed and flax —
purple and yellow and flame run wild,
blue stolen from the skies;
when he bade me shed the heavy woolen cloak
and hear the birds calling their young,
spinning the moon light on their song;
when he taught me to follow the sunbeams
dancing through the trees,
warming the pine needles till their scent filled the air
and led me far from the path;
when he told me there was no reason to be so grave
when the wood was merry;
is it any wonder I went deeper and deeper into the green trees?
Now the doctor asks me
how it was I could not tell my own grandmother from a wolf.
The huntsman had no such problem, you see.
He strode right into the cottage, called out,
"Do I find you here, you old sinner? I have long sought you!"
He even guessed my grandmother was inside,
and was wise enough not to fire
but to take scissors
and cut open the stomach of the sleeping wolf.
A man who knows his enemies, hunts them down cleanly,
and disposes of them efficiently,
taking care not to harm
what good they may contain.

I was not nearly so clear.
The doctor asks me
whether I was not living among wolves from the start.
How could one confuse a grandmother with a wolf
unless the grandmother and wolf were kin all along?
It's complicated, I tell him,
thinking that in sunlight
my grandmother's hair is as silver as the wolf's pelt,
that at dusk her eyes have always glittered gold,
that always in the corners of her cottage
there have been small treasures waiting —

toys made from thimbles, ribbons for my hair.
Sometimes, I explain,
it's hard to tell the difference
between the ones who love you
and the ones who will eat you alive.
The explanation doesn't wash.
Open your eyes, child, he tells me.
Appearances may deceive.
Dangers seduce.
You must give thanks to the huntsman.
You needed an avenging angel,
a savior strong and unafraid,
a man to tear open the wolf's belly
and help you out.

I tell him I am grateful
that my grandmother still lives in her cottage
with gifts tucked in every corner;
grateful that I am alive,
that a stranger held out the hope
that from what nearly destroys you
love may emerge.
What I do not tell him is that
I will again leave the path
and wander into that fragrant green wood
and when I see
coat of silver, eyes of gold,
I will follow.

"Silver and Gold" by Ellen Steiber from *Snow White, Blood Red*, edited by Ellen Datlow & Terri Windling, an AvoNova Book, William Morrow & Company, Inc., 1993. Copyright ©1993 by Ellen Steiber. Reprinted by permission of Ellen Steiber.

References

Andrew, E. J. (2005). Through the dark night *from On the threshold: Home, hardwood, and holiness*. NY: Basic Books.

Badenoch, B. (2008). *Being a brain-wise therapist: A practical guide to interpersonal neurobiology*. NY: W. W. Norton & Company.

Bettleheim, B. (1976). *The uses of enchantment: The meaning and importance of fairy tales*. London: Thames & Hudson.

Datlow, E. & Windling, T. (Eds). (1993). *Snow white, blood red*. NY: William Morrow & Company, Inc.

Datlow, E., & Windling, T. (2019). *Snow white, blood red (Fairy Tale Anthologies)* (Kindle ed.). NY: Open Road Media Sci-Fi & Fantasy.

Estes, C. P. (2003). *Women who run with the wolves*. NY: Ballantine Books.

Foo, M., Freedle, L.R., Sani, R., & Fonda, G. (2020). The effect of Sandplay therapy on the thalamus in the treatment of generalized anxiety disorder: A case report. *International Journal of Play Therapy*, *29*(4), 191–200. https://doi.org/10.1037/pla0000137

Freedle, L.R. (2019). Making connections: Sandplay therapy and the neurosequential model of therapeutics®. *Journal of Sandplay Therapy*, *28*(1), 91–109.

Heiko, R. L. (2018). *A therapist's guide to mapping the girl heroine's journey in Sandplay*. Lanham, MD: Rowman & Littlefield Publishers.

Kalff, D. M. (2020). *Sandplay: A psychotherapeutic approach to the psyche*. Oberlin, OH: Analytical Psychology Press Sandplay Editions.

Maitland, S. (2012). *Gossip from the forest: The tangled roots of our forests and fairytales*. London: Granta Books.

Pattis Zoja, E. (2004). *Sandplay therapy: Treatment of psychopathologies: Understanding with the hands* (Kindle DX version.) Retrieved from amazon.com.

Roesler, C. (2019). Sandplay therapy: An overview of theory, applications and evidence base. *The Arts in Psychotherapy*, *64*, 84–94.

Schaefer, C. E., & Peabody, M.A. (2016). Glossary of play therapy terms. *Play Therapy*, *11*(2), 20–24.

Steiber, E. (1994). Silver and gold. In E. Datlow & T. Windling (eds.), *Black thorn, white rose* (pp. 306–309). NY: William Morrow & Company, Inc.

Warner, M. (2014). *Once upon a time: A short history of fairy tale*. Oxford, UK: Oxford University Press.

16 The Wisdom of Nature: StoryPlay®, Connecting Nature's Gifts of Thriving and Resiliency to Play

Danielle Woods and Joyce C. Mills

Introduction

The world of nature and the weaving of story through craft and play helps begin a story of safety, resiliency, and a message to thrive. The stories and metaphors from nature allow clients to find what is just right for them. As a caterpillar needs a safe leaf on which to settle to begin her journey to becoming a butterfly, our clients need a safe place to find who they can become. Within that safe space must be just the right nourishment. As recent neurological research suggests, allowing children to play in nature increases feelings of happiness, encourages their development, and their sense of well-being (Berrera-Hernández et al., 2020; Dankiw et al., 2020).

This chapter focuses on the beneficence of nature using resiliency focused StoryPlay®, developed by Joyce C. Mills, PhD. StoryPlay® integrates components of metaphor, story, and creativity with transcultural healing philosophies and natural resources (Courtney & Mills, 2016; Mills, 2011). Mills depicts StoryPlay® as the trunk of a tree with the work of Milton H. Erickson as the taproot, fed by creativity, transcultural wisdom and healing, creativity, stories and metaphor, play therapy, and the natural world.

The Role of Nature

Terms like Nature-Deficit Disorder (Louv, 2008) and "biophilia" signal the importance, and, indeed, the necessity, of experiencing nature. "Nature Therapy" with its basis in ecopsycology reminds us that nature is a partner in the therapeutic process (Berger, 2017). "This extraordinary formative influence of nature in children's health and development underscores this connection is not just a matter of physical fitness and intellectual capacity, but as well emotional capacity, identity, basic values, and even our moral and spiritual condition" (Killert, 2009).

The research-based program, Play and Grow, in Hong Kong, found that parents who saw their young children have a closer connection with nature reported less distress, less hyperactivity, and fewer emotional problems among their children (Sobko et al., 2018). A study by Tasia Oswald (2020), of the University of Adelaide, and colleagues finds that "more green time and less screen time" increases more positive psychological outcomes in children and adolescents.

Such research indicates that creative interventions involving nature become an essential part of a therapist's toolbox. Nature becomes the cotherapist through metaphorical storytelling, ritual, and multisensory experiencing (Mills & Crowley, 2014). Reconnecting with nature allows people to reconnect with their strengths and become a source for healing (Berger, 2017). Nature play improves motor skills, levels of attention and concentration, imagination, and resilience (Dankiw et al., 2020).

Metaphor, Story, and Nature as Healing Partners in StoryPlay®

The Natural World – Beyond the internet, books, and even toys lies our *Natural World Library,* which provides another valuable source of information for learning life lessons and achieving comfort for healing. StoryPlay uses the seasons, the weather, leaves, feathers, shells, butterflies,

DOI: 10.4324/9781003152767-22

animals, flowers, and even such annoying insects as flies as educational and healing instruments to facilitate transformational change.

(Mills, 2011, p. 12; Mills, 1999)

StoryPlay® partners with nature and the natural world through metaphor and discovery. Utilizing what the client brings to the session along with the neural importance of metaphor and creativity is a key component of StoryPlay® (Figure 16.1). Utilization, as defined by Lankton (2004), is "making use of common understandings and behaviors that the clients bring to the office so that these may be part of the motivation or reinforcements of therapy" (p. 107). Utilization also allows the therapist to adapt what is available in the client's natural world. For example, the natural world of inner city living offers different opportunities from living in the suburbs or on the farm. Sometimes the therapeutic moment can be as simple as: find a rock that you notice, hold the rock, and let the rock teach you something (Mills, 2011, p. 105).

"With treatments focused on the alleviation of suffering and symptoms, the exploration of patients' strengths, accomplishments, and joys have received short shrift" (p. 167, Russell, E., & Fosha, D., 2008). A cornerstone of StoryPlay® is resilience. Using the stories of the clients, understanding what they have done well, listening for the key supports they have used are all part of resiliency based StoryPlay®. It is what Brooks and Goldstein (2001) call having a "resiliency mindset." Recent research on brain activity and metaphor indicates that sensory motor regions of the brain activate when metaphor is used (Lai et al., 2019). "Whether problems are about courage to speak up for oneself, or issues around loss, abuse, or trauma, stories provide a medicine" (Mills, 1999, p. 3). This is a pathway for clients to discover the magic of their own healing.

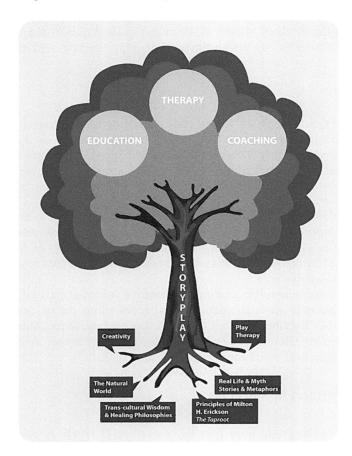

Figure 16.1 The roots of StoryPlay®.

Source: Mills & Crowley, 2014, p. 107.

The Medicine Within

Using metaphor, story and nature, the way is opened for reconnecting to cultural values (Mills, 2020). A Lakota elder states: "When we hear the drum, we feel like dancing" (White Bison, 2002, p. 4). He goes on to tell the story of those raised away from the traditions coming back and fitting in, because they have found who they are. The nature of the drum is the heartbeat.

Vignette A: Clayton, Adolescent *(Mills)*

Clayton (pseudonym), a male adolescent, lived in a residential treatment center due to extremely aggressive and self-harming behavior. His mother was deceased, and his father told him only that she was from the Lakota Nation and that she was an alcoholic. He knew nothing of her history nor the culture of the Lakota.

Since he knew nothing of his mother's history, his culture, or the Lakota stories, Clayton was disconnected from an essential part of himself. His mother was not just an alcoholic, she was born a Native American woman who endured cultural trauma and historical oppression. Siegel (2012) stated, "We are storytelling creatures, and stories are the social glue that binds us to one another…the mind, as a fundamental part of our humanity, is shaped by story" (pp. 31–32, italics in original). Without the story, there can be no attachment. Stories take many forms—art, oral, movement, dance, and more. Clayton, like his mother before him, experienced what Duran (2006) called "soul wounding."

Over the years, working with many people from different Native American nations, I had many items given to me as gifts for our work together. Clayton showed great interest in these and I shared the stories I had learned about these sacred objects and healing ceremonies. The spirit of the stories began ignited in Clayton a sense of determination to know more, an awakening of what I call "sleeping story memories," or memories resting in the unconscious. With the belief that we all have invisible umbilical cords, I hypothesized that Clayton was experiencing a reconnection to his mother's soul.

Clayton was especially drawn to several drums. The drum is not just an instrument, but the heartbeat of Native American culture. At times we drummed together and at other times, we took turns creating drumbeat sounds in nature, such as thunder, rain, and wind. My client made a special connection to the drum. Rather than buying one, a drum-maker from a nearby Nation made a large drum with my client. In a sense, his "heart-drum" was beating in rhythm with his new discoveries of life.

Finding Connection

E.J. White's 2015 study, "Insights from young children in nature," found that children connect with nature in creative and unique ways. In her two books for ill children, *Gentle Willow* and *Little Tree*, Mills uses trees as a metaphor for healing, changing, and for dying. In her book, *Reconnecting to the Magic of Life*, she writes,

A couple I worked with decided to renew their relationship after separating and bought a fruit tree for their yard. They planted it just as the sun was coming up, a time of day that symbolized new beginnings. They agreed to water it together to make sure it grew healthy and strong. (p. 185)

And, in her work in creating StoryPlay®, Mills uses the tree as the metaphor for creating a healing system. In his research about the sacred trees of Norway and Sweden, Douglas Hulmes (2009) describes the planting and caring for "a sacred tree in the center of the yard of the farm…is a moral reminder of caring for the farm or the place where one lives." It becomes the guardian tree. Hulmes (2009) captures the deep awe of connection in viewing an ancient living tree:

I could see snow spiraling and swirling down from clouds that shrouded the top of the tree. I stood agape, and I felt my entire body tingle, while the words came to my mind: the cells of my body are in absolute awe with the cells of the being that stands before me, for within this tree, that has stood for more than three thousand years, is a Will that began as a tiny seed, and has lived through the millennia transforming light from the sun into oxygen as its byproduct of photosynthesis and in the process, sustains life on the earth.

The following case vignette by author, Woods, gives an example of how a sacred tree metaphor was utilized with a child client.

Vignette B: Liam, Age Nine Years *(Woods)*

LIAM: *(pseudonym) is a nine-year-old boy whose history includes several foster placements and finally, adoption. His adoptive parents initiated counseling due to "rages and tantrums." He described his favorite things to do as "making up really long stories" and "running fast." When asked to draw what "running really fast" was like, Liam included his house with a tall saguaro cactus in the front. Noticing the saguaro, the therapist asked him if he knew the story of "sacred trees."*

LIAM: *"Nope, but I like stories."*

THERAPIST: *"In the place where the Vikings come from, and even here, people plant a very special guardian tree. It, of course, starts as a small tree, but they care for it, and it cares for them by providing shade, and a place for animals to hang out. As the tree grows, so does the family and they know this is their place by their tree. Your family has this very old saguaro. It started as a tiny seed, - fought off mice and other creatures who might have eaten it. It was cared for and now is home to animals, and you know you are home when you see it."*

The cactus continued to be part of Liam's therapy—how it could be prickly but have friends like owls and rabbits; how it was so strong and produced flowers and fruit, even though water was scarce. His parents reported fewer outbursts, and he found a saguaro keychain, which he kept in his pocket at school.

Summary

StoryPlay® utilizes objects of the natural worlds much like miniatures are used in Sandplay. Plants, animals, shells, and even rocks are "metaphorical miniatures containing valuable life lessons for achieving transformational healing" (Courtney & Mills, 2016). In her work with trauma, Mills developed EarthCrafts: taking broken debris and reclaiming it as personal art. Nature and story allow the therapy to adapt to time, place, and culture. Nature is also the client—the breath, the heart, even the hair can help create a path for a healing story. In his book, *The Brain's Way of Healing*, Norman Doidge (2015) speaks about "the active involvement of the whole patient in his or her own care" (p. xxi). He reminds the health professionals to look beyond deficits and take note of capacities that can aid in healing.

Utilizing nature's multisensory resources permits the story to unfold as the child sees it, without preconceived assign of value to any object, scent, sound, or texture. Nature provides stories of timing, resilience, recovery, and growth. For example, Mills refers to "butterfly wisdom" in Foundations of StoryPlay® (Mills, 2011). The story of caterpillar to butterfly offers not only the metaphors of change and healing but also of safety, timing, and felt sense. Like the tiny particles of pollen carried on the wings of butterflies from one flower to the next with the sole purpose of perpetuating regeneration and life, it is my (Mills) belief that our prayers, messages, and images are transformed into tiny particles of "spiritual pollen," carried on the wings of angels with the *soul purpose* of perpetuating healing and peace.

The heart of StoryPlay® is based on resiliency and Erickson's principle of utilization. The inner resources and strengths within each client are seen as "seeds" to be nourished during their healing process. StoryPlay® is easily adaptable to physical space, natural environment, and culture. The EarthCrafts and StoryCrafts of StoryPlay® increase the therapist's ability to reach beyond the "problem" to the "strengths" of each person. Some examples include the following: *Creating Your Playful Spirit StoryStones* (see Appendix A and Figure 16.2), *Creating a Peace Garden* (see Appendix B and Figure 16.3), *Creating your Identity Shield* (see Appendix C and Figure 16.4), *Creating Your Butterfly Mandala* (see Appendix D and Figure 16.5). The metaphors and stories from nature provide an indirect way to the neural pathways of healing. Employing the available resources within the client's world and the place of therapy, interventions are appropriate for individual, group, and family sessions.

Creating Your Playful Spirit StoryStones

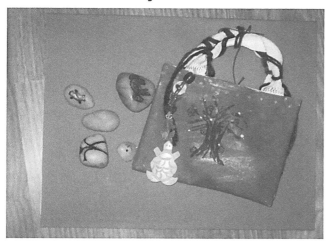

Figure 16.2 Creating your playful spirit storystones.
Source: Joyce Mills.

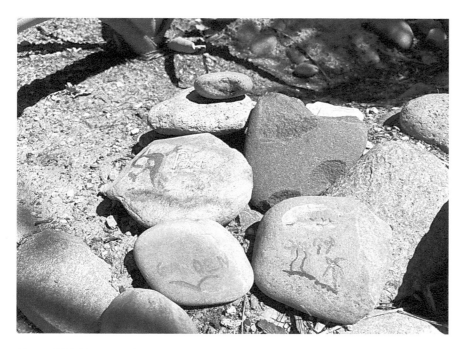

Figure 16.3 Peace garden.
Source: Joyce Mills.

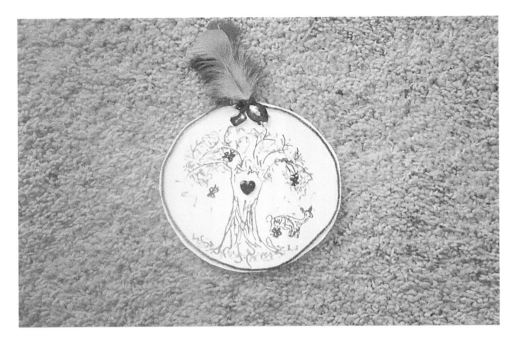

Figure 16.4 Identity shield.
Source: Joyce Mills.

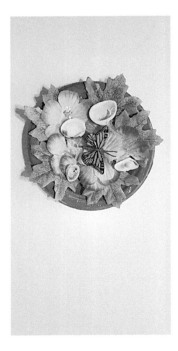

Figure 16.5 Butterfly wisdom mandala.
Source: Joyce Mills.

Reflective questions and activities:

1   Choose a natural object that attracts your attention. One that you can hold in your hand—a leaf, a rock, a small piece of wood. Hold it for a time that seems right for you, examining it. Write down what comes to mind as to what this object might teach you. (Mills, 2011)

2   Pair up with a classmate or friend. Choose an object within your view and make up a short (three minutes) story—with a beginning, middle, and end—about this object. Have your partner make note of any thoughts or metaphors that come to mind as you tell your story. Briefly talk about these ideas. Then switch roles.

3   Choose three names of natural objects, for example: tree, ant, bird. Write each object down as headings across a blank sheet of paper. In a column, under each heading, write as many attributes as possible you can think of about that object in about three minutes. Do this for each object. Next, on a separate sheet of paper, write down any stories or metaphors you find in the attributes of these objects.

Appendix A

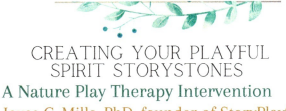

CREATING YOUR PLAYFUL SPIRIT STORYSTONES
A Nature Play Therapy Intervention
Joyce C. Mills, PhD, founder of StoryPlay®

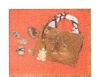

DESCRIPTION:

StoryStones are individual forms of petroglyphs "rock carvings" – petro meaning "rock" and glyph meaning "symbol." A symbolic form of communication and guidance. This sacred Indigenous art form has long been used to carve or paint images that tell stories of creation, rituals, ceremonies, etc.

SUPPLIES:

Mini-tote canvas bags; Small wooden box, or heart shaped box; Paints, brushes or paint pens; Gem stones; Heavy craft glue; Yarn; Glitter; Small river rocks.

GOAL:

Create a positive anchor. The symbols on the stones can be a link to an inner world of strength, imagination, and playfulness.

INSTRUCTIONS:

Ask child to choose the following: Choose a Mini-tote, small wooden box, or heart-shaped box; Four to seven stones. Next ask child to paint their chosen container. Then decorate each stone with a symbol that brings comfort to their hearts. It can be an animal, a religious symbol, a symbol from nature, etc.

How to use: Child chooses a stone from the container and tells a story related to the symbol painted on the stone. Stones can also be used to express an emotion and to provide comfort. It could be known as a "Way Finder" ---a marker to help children find courage within

EXTRA FUN:

As an alternative, clients can find stones outside with interesting shapes. They could be painted or plain, as part of the story

Appendix B

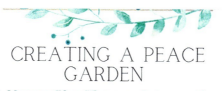

CREATING A PEACE GARDEN

A Nature Play Therapy Intervention

Joyce C. Mills, PhD, founder of StoryPlay®

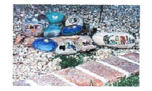

DESCRIPTION:

Gardens provide powerful metaphors for our lives. Just walking through a garden often brings us a sense of comfort, peace, and wonderment. Whether they are flower gardens, vegetable gardens, or rock gardens, we decide what we want to plant and nurture, as well as what we want to trim back or remove altogether.

SUPPLIES:

Rocks of various sizes, acrylic paints, brushes. Optional are plants, flowers, or a tree.

GOAL:

Peace gardens help to support a physical space where children can go to calm and find peace.

INSTRUCTIONS:

- Gather rocks of various sizes and put them in a pile near the area just cleared.
- Next, you and children choose a rock, hold it in your hands and meditate for a few quiet moments on the word, message, prayer, or picture you want to paint on it.
- When you and your child are finished painting the rock, place it anywhere in the Peace Garden area.
- You may wish to plant a tree, shrub or flowers in the garden also, but it is not necessary.
- Invite whomever wishes to participate in the creation and perpetuation of the Peace Garden. They can bring a rock of their own or use one from your pile.

EXTRA FUN:

If space is an issue, or they need a portable space, make it a "container" garden in a small, sturdy box

Appendix C

CREATING YOUR IDENTITY SHIELD

A Nature Play Therapy Intervention

Joyce C. Mills, PhD, founder of StoryPlay®

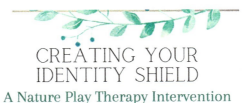

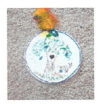

DESCRIPTION:

Native peoples created shields decorated with many symbols for various reasons; i.e., protection, healing, In today's busyness of life, we sometimes lose who we are. Our identities can become shadowed with self-doubt; we have difficulty making decisions and finding the right next step. The creation of an "Identity Shield" can help us reconnect to who "lives within."

SUPPLIES:

Large paper plate, square or round, and drawing materials.

GOAL:

Illuminate and connect with client's strengths and unique qualities

INSTRUCTIONS:

- Begin by asking your client (child, adolescent, adult, or family) to close their eyes, take a deep breath, inhaling through the nose, and exhaling through the mouth. After a moment, ask them to imagine seeing the symbols that best represent them: aspects of life and personality in terms of nature, hobbies, and interests.
- The following questions may be helpful:
- What animal or bird reminds me of myself? Example: a turtle who seeks shelter within, an eagle who views the whole picture.
- If I were a part of nature, what would I be? Example: a mighty tree, a bending willow, a a powerful ocean
- What are your hobbies or interests?

EXTRA FUN:

Use materials from nature, binding flexible branches into a circle, twine, and heavy material, along with acrylic paints, beads, and feathers

Appendix D

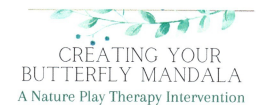

CREATING YOUR BUTTERFLY MANDALA
A Nature Play Therapy Intervention
Joyce C. Mills, PhD, founder of StoryPlay®

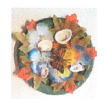

DESCRIPTION:

The word "mandala" is from the classical Indian language of Sanskrit and loosely means "circle." A mandala is a powerful symbol of unity, diversity, and peace and represents: Wholeness, a model for life itself, a design that reminds us of our relation to the world that extends both beyond and within our bodies and minds

SUPPLIES:

· Large heavy round paper plate
· Markers, acrylic paint pens, acrylic paint
· Heavy craft glue
· Silk or dried flowers, leaves, grass,
· Glitter, gem or small stones, shells, feathers
· Silk, fabric, leaves, shells to make butterflies, small or large

GOAL:
To help the client understand their unique place and purpose in the world

INSTRUCTIONS:

- Lay out all materials
- Take a few minutes to clear your mind and meditate on the four passages and seasons of your life. New beginnings, Preparing for Change, Dark Spaces, and Beautiful Butterfly.
- Next, take a paper plate and choose the supplies that best represent your passages.
- Create your Butterfly Wisdom Mandala.

EXTRA FUN:
Ask the client to relate a story, real or imaginary about Butterfly Wisdom in their world

References

Berger, R. (2017). Nature therapy: Incorporating nature into arts therapy. *Journal of Humanistic Psychology as cited in Children & Nature Network.* https://research.childrenandnature.org/research/nature-therapy-broadens-the-classical-therapeutic-relationship-between-therapist-and-client-by-introducing-nature-as-a-third-factor/

Berrera-Hernández, L., et al. (2020, February 26). Connectedness to nature: Its impact on sustainable behaviors and happiness in children. *Frontiers in Psychology, 11.* https://www.frontiersin.org/articles/10.3389/fpsyg.2020.00276/full

Brooks, R., & Goldstein, S. (2001). *Raising resilient children: Fostering strength, hope, and optimism in your child.* New York: McGraw Hill.

Courtney, J. A. & Mills, J. C. (2016, March). Utilizing the metaphor of nature as co-therapist in StoryPlay®. *Play Therapy, 11*(1), 18–21

Dankiw, K., et al. (2020, February 13). The impacts of unstructured nature play on health in early childhood development: A systematic review. *PLoS ONE, 15*(2). https://journals.plos.org/plosone/article?id=10.1371/journal.pone.0229006

Doidge, N. (2015). *The brain's way of healing.* New York: The Penguin Group.

Duran, E. (2006). *Healing the soul wound: Counseling with American Indians and other native peoples.* New York: Teachers College Press.

Goldstein, S., & Brooks, R. B. (March, 2021). *Tenacity in children.* New York: Springer.

Hulmes, D. F. (2009). Sacred Trees of Norway and Sweden: A Friluftsliv Voyage. The Birth of "Friluftsliv" - A 150 Year International Dialogue Conference Jubilee Celebration North Troendelag University College, Levanger, Norway. September 14–19, 2009.

Killert, S. (2009). Reflection on children's experience of nature. Leadership Writing Series: vol. 1:2. Children and Nature Network. *Research and Studies, Volumes I–IV.* www.childrenandnature.org.

Lai, V., et al. (2019). Concrete processing of action metaphors: Evidence from ERP as cited in Neuroscience News (2019 April). https://neurosciencenews.com/metaphor-meaning-eeg-10979

Lankton, S. (2004). *Assembling Ericksonian therapy: The collected papers of Stephen Lankton.* Phoenix, AZ: Zeig: Tucker, & Theisen.

Louv, R. (2008). *Last child in the woods: Saving our children from nature-deficit disorder.* Chapel Hill, NC: Algonquin Books.

Mills, J. C. (1999). *Reconnecting to the magic of life.* Phoenix, AZ: Imaginal Press.

Mills, J. C. (2003). *Little tree, a story for children with serious medical problems* (2nd ed.). Washington, DC: Magination Press.

Mills, J. C. (2004). *Gentle willow, a story for children about dying* (2nd ed.). Washington, D.C.: Magination Press.

Mills, J. C., (2011). *StoryPlay® foundations training manual.* Phoenix, AZ: Imaginal Press.

Mills, J. C., (2020, March). Culture, metaphors and playtherapy, rainbows of resilience in life's storms. *Play Therapy, 15*(1), 4–7.

Mills, J. C., & Crowley, R. J. (2014). *Therapeutic metaphors for children and the child within* (2nd ed.). Philadelphia, PA: Brunner-Routledge.

Oswald T.K., et al. (2018, November 29). Psychological impacts of 'screen time' and 'green time' for children and adolescents: A systematic scoping review. https://journals.plos.org/plosone/article?id=10.1371/journal.pone.0207057

Russell, E., & Fosha, D. (2008). Transformational affects and core state in AEDP: The emergence and consolidation of joy, hope, gratitude, and confidence in (the solid goodness of) the self. *Journal of Psychotherapy Integration, 18*(2), 167–190. https://doi.org/10.1037/1053-0479.18.2.167

Siegel, D. J. (2012). *The developing mind: How relationships and the brain interact to shape who we are* (2nd ed.). New York: Guildford Press.

Sobko, T., et al. (2018, November 29). Measuring connectedness to nature in preschool children in an urban setting and its relation to psychological functioning. https://journals.plos.org/plosone/article?id=10.1371/journal.pone.0207057

White Bison. (2009). *The Red road to wellbriety in the Native American way.* Colorado Springs: White Bison, Inc.

White, E. J. (2015). Seeing is believing? Insights from young children in nature. *International Journal of Early Childhood, 47,* 171–188. https://doi.org/10.1007/s13158-014-0118-5

17 Story Stone Play: Embodied Imagination in Virtual Therapy and Beyond

Cyndera Quackenbush and Janet A. Courtney

Introduction

In times of uncertainty, either personal or in a pandemic, the ancient and solid nature of stones can be comforting and dependable. Stones can also spark stories. This chapter details therapeutic breakthroughs with the use of billion-year-old stone images as a therapeutic tool. With the rise of therapy online, play therapists are exploring ways in which they can more meaningfully connect with their clients in a virtual world (Stone, 2019). The pandemic of 2020 forced practitioners across the world to welcome their child and family clients into virtual spaces instead of in-person places. As we emerge into a post-pandemic world, virtual therapies will still be necessary or desirable in certain situations. Story Stone Play utilizes the Story Through Stone Reflection Cards that have been developed for online and in-person sessions. This chapter demonstrates the use of this model within an individual child Telemental Health therapy process.

The Stones That Inspired Story Stone Play

In the Mojave Desert in 1975, a rare billion-year-old shale rock (known as Death Valley Paint Rock) was uncovered by an aspiring artist, James Quackenbush, the father of author Cyndera Quackenbush. Delicately working to carefully slice thousands of thin layers of rock with diamond saw blades, he found within the stones a variety of images occurring naturally in the mineral oxidation—ancient people, animals, landscapes, figures of mythology, and historical scenes (see Figure 17.1 as an example). In what he felt was a collaboration with the earth itself, James wanted to tell the story of the earth's history with nature's inherent imagery. His work culminated in a collection of 175 framed and named art stone masterpieces with titles alluding to art, natural, and cultural history and symbols. Inspired by the stone images crafted by her father, the author Quackenbush created the Story Through Stone Reflection Cards—54 photographs of the original art stone masterpieces. With the creation of these cards, combined with Quackenbush's professional work with children, Story Stone Play was born. This approach is a combination of nature-based rock imagery, imaginative storytelling, and embodied play, which will be listed in detailed steps later in this chapter.

Story Stone Play has foundations in Jungian theory and Narrative Therapy. The stone imagery reveals symbols and universal archetypes such as human figures, animals, and landscapes. Intended for ages five and up, children are first encouraged to use their imagination to discover their own pictures in each stone. They are then guided to tell a story using those images. This process taps into their memories, imagination, embodied selves, and feelings. Children can then act out their stories through full-body improvisational storytelling. Through this process, the inner life of the child is validated and drawn out in a creative form in which the child feels pride and ownership. The dynamic between therapist and child becomes embodied and lively, a treasured experience—even through Telemental Therapy on Zoom.

We now turn to a foundational inspiration for Story Stone Play in the experience of Carl Jung who, before he ever became the founder of analytical psychology, was shaped by the presence of stone as a child.

Stone Play in Jung's Childhood

In the early 20th century, in his autobiography *Memories, Dreams, Reflections* (1961/1989), Carl Jung details at length meaningful encounters with stone in his childhood. We turn to his early memories in this

DOI: 10.4324/9781003152767-23

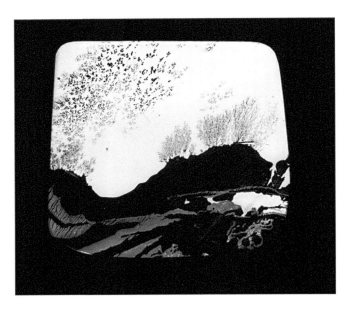

Figure 17.1 "Song of Creation," an example of death valley paint stone.

Source: Cyndera Quackenbush.

section in order to highlight the significance stone played for Jung. Jung's memories of his childhood experiences with stones are a powerful example of how stones can create meaning throughout a person's life once it has been sparked in childhood.

According to his autobiography, the extended time Jung spent playing with stones in his formative years shaped his later mid-life realizations. Having spent a significant amount of time in nature as a child, he even had a favorite stone he would return to often and sit upon for hours. In this way, stone had a comforting and stabilizing effect on him. Sitting on the stone opened his mind to the "otherness" existing in nature and who he really was. This meditation became a refuge from the doubts and uncertainties he felt amidst his family and the human world. He affirmed that there was a deep, undisturbable part of himself: "I was but the sum of my emotions, and the Other in me was the timeless, imperishable stone" (Jung, 1961/1989, p. 42). Though the stone was "other," it forged a presence within him that he felt a part of.

The stone itself sparked an interest in the great mystery of the world and the deeper, imperishable personality within Jung: "I always hoped I might be able to find something—perhaps in nature—that would give me the clue and show me where or what the secret was. At that time my interest in plants, animals, and stones grew" (p. 22). He also kept a pencil case hidden in the attic that contained a little doll and a rock that was painted both dark as night on one side and light as day on the other.

The vital play of his childhood spiraled back to help Jung profoundly during mid-life. After his split from Sigmund Freud, Jung entered a period he called his "confrontation with the unconscious" (1961/1989, p. 170). During this difficult time, he did not know what to do next with his career. He felt completely lost, as if he knew nothing at all. Surrendering to the "impulses of the unconscious," he was at first pulled toward the play he had in nature as a boy. Though feeling humiliated to return to such childish play, he found himself once again constructing castles and villages with rocks and sand:

> I began accumulating suitable stones, gathering them partly from the lake shore and partly from the water. And I started building…I caught sight of a red stone, a four-sided pyramid about an inch and a half high…I knew at once this was the altar! (1961/1989, p. 174)

In the process of this play, Jung recalled an important childhood dream and the connection gave him a deep feeling of satisfaction. Stone continued to make appearances in Jung's later works, including

The Red Book (2009), his large leather-bound journal kept private for so many years. A stone that was misdelivered during the building of one of his personal structures at his home in Bollingen became a prized stone in which he carved a mysterious figure. This was not unlike the figure he'd kept in his secret box as a child. Stones also emerged in visions that comforted him after his wife's death, as well as during a near death experience he had as an adult.

In a 21st-century world that has only grown in uncertainty, speeded up and become even more transitional in nature, there is no doubt that the presence and concept of stone can hold this same comforting influence for the children of today. The idea of stone having its own kind of inherent intelligence in the world can affirm for children that nature's archetypal patterns are numinous and accessible resources throughout one's life.

Narrative Therapy and the Use of Story

Narrative therapy was first developed by family therapists David Epston and Michael White in the 1980s. This non-pathologizing approach sees individuals as having numerous intersecting stories that make up their identity. The problems the client faces are therefore separate and distanced from defining that person completely. Individual narratives can be understood, shaped, and reauthored in order to place the client in greater control of their destinies (White, 2011).

Researcher Camilla Asplund Ingemark writes about the key therapeutic components of client narration. Narrative therapy has shown how storytelling can be therapeutic in detangling the "problem from the person" (Ingemark, 2013, p. 10). Verbalizing one's stories is itself a "ground zero" of healing. According to Ingemark (2013), placing events within a story makes them smaller and more manageable, giving the client a chance to reauthor their lives and relationships. Perhaps most importantly, metaphorical storytelling gives the client and therapist a safe buffer with which to approach difficult issues. In a process of externalization, Ingemark highlights that the client is liberated from "being defined by his or her problem...and aids in the development of a new relationship to the problem" (2013, p. 13). Through a story, a client can take a bird's eye view to their situation, and sometimes can even do so unconsciously.

There is an amusing story from Jungian analyst Robert Johnson (1986) in which a client sets out to trick him by "making up" a story of nonsense. The client intended to make a fool of Johnson's approach of active imagination. It was only after delivering the story that the client realized in amazement that it spoke directly to his situation and attitudes toward his own problems. Johnson (1986) concluded from this experience that it is nearly impossible to "produce anything in the imagination that is not an authentic representation of something in the unconscious. The whole function of the imagination is to draw up the material...clothe it in images, and transmit it to the conscious mind" (p. 150).

For children, stories are particularly important both to listen to and create. In his work *The Uses of Enchantment: The Meaning and Importance of Fairy Tales*, Bruno Bettelheim (1991) highlighted the role of story for children in gaining understanding of their conscious experiences that are impacted by unconscious forces. As children face life's disappointments, rivalries, and powerlessness in their relationship dependencies, Bettelheim (1991) advocates that daydreaming can be a powerful conduit to work out these noted issues. What is necessary is the "ruminating, rearranging, and fantasizing about suitable story elements in response to unconscious pressures. By doing this, the child fits unconscious content into conscious fantasies, which then enable him to deal with that content" (Bettelheim, 1991, pp. 6–7). He further postulated that this process allows for a sense of their own selfhood and self-worth, and a development of their own moral compass.

As you will see in the Story Stone Play case study provided in this chapter, a child feeling a sense of powerlessness and frustration can attain a more empowered perspective after a session of embodied imaginative storytelling. Further, returning to stories over time allows for the child to harness this capability of storytelling to soothe and transform their feelings.

The Steps of Story Stone Play

This section introduces the process of Story Stone Play, followed by more detailed instructions in the ten steps listed below. There are many opportunities for play in a Story Stone Play session. First, there are the Story Through Stone Reflection Cards themselves. If the sessions are virtual, the cards are mailed to the child in advance. Children are invited to shuffle the cards in any way they please, which sets the tone for a playful activity. Next, there is the engagement with the cards' imagery once the child is asked to pick a card. The practitioner then encourages the child to describe what he or she sees in the stone cards—any person, place, or thing is possible! Using his or her imagination as a guide, the child can choose what excites them. Lastly, the practitioner supports the child in incorporating aspects of their environment such as props, costumes, dolls, and home-made artwork—even pets!—in the storytelling. If this is an in-person office session, then the items of the playroom can be utilized. As seen in the numbered steps below, the child can pick multiple cards, placing them in any order of their choosing to create a story. Which stone card is first in the story? Which has the resolution or end scene?

The following ten steps are a suggested outline to be used in Story Stone Play while utilizing the Story Through Stone Reflection Cards:

Ten Steps of Story Stone Play

STEP 1   The practitioner introduces the Story Through Stone Reflection Cards to the child, mentioning that the imagery in the cards was created by the earth itself. Practitioners can describe how the imagery in the rock formed over a billion years ago—long before there were people, before there were animals, even before the dinosaurs! This was a time when the earth looked completely different, and the continents had not yet split apart. The imagery the child will observe in the stone cards has stories to tell and they, like the ancient people of every continent, can hear this story and tell their own version.

STEP 2   The child, with their deck of stone cards on the other side of a computer screen, can shuffle in any way desired. Of course, a child in-person would be invited to do the same.

STEP 3   The child picks a card and describes what they see. The practitioner writes down what the child says. In Telemental Play sessions, the child might like for the screen to be shared so that they can see the words they are speaking.

STEP 4   Repeat Step 3 for two more cards (a total of three).

STEP 5   With all three cards laid out, the child is invited to tell a story using the imagery in the cards. Common story openers can help trigger the storytelling mindset: "Once upon a time," "Long ago," even "Once Upon a Stone."

STEP 6   If the child finds this difficult and gets stuck, the practitioner can enter into the storytelling process to help. Any help should serve as a bridge to their next card or phase in the story, and not as a detour or superimposed ending created by the practitioner. It can be helpful to ask the child questions about the characters in order to guide them along.

STEP 7   The story's ending doesn't need to be neat and clean. The story can even have a dream-like, disjointed quality. If it feels necessary, more cards can be drawn, though for a young child it is recommended to stick to a one typed page per session. "The End" or "To be Continued" at the end of the story seals its closure.

STEP 8   Now it's time to bring the story to life! After the screen is un-shared, the story is read back to the child while they act it out. This is fun and playful and the child can act out every role. This process may include all kinds of movement, sound effects, different voices, nearby props or toy supporting actors. The child may even wish for the practitioner to play one of the character parts, which can build a deeper rapport between child and therapist. An entire spectrum of experience can be revealed in the process—laughter, as well as serious moments, may ensue.

STEP 9   When the story is done, the practitioner ends with a big round of applause! Now it's time for the "Writer, Director and Actor Q & A." The practitioner pretends that they are the host of a show. Being on a computer screen can prompt the child's fun feeling of being interviewed on TV. From the stance of the "Interviewer," the practitioner has the chance to ask the child questions about the story. Importantly, the questions should grow the life of the story as opposed to interpreting or dissecting the meaning of the story. The goal is for the child to feel the triumph of having created their story, not to directly or literally connect it to their life in a way that makes them feel "figured out."

STEP 10   The practitioner notices any differences in the child from when the session began.

Now that the child is warmed up through story and play, he or she may want to talk about all sorts of other details in their life. This is a great opener to a fun and meaningful session. The practitioner may expand the practice by having the child draw what they have seen in the stone picture cards.

As mentioned in Step 9, it is essential to keep within the metaphor of the story, as opposed to interpreting the material and any application to the child's literal life. Bruno Bettelheim (1991) explained how intrusive it can be to interpret a person's pre-conscious and unconscious thoughts, particularly for children:

> Adult interpretations, as correct as they may be, rob the child of the opportunity to feel that he, on his own…has coped successfully with a difficult situation. We grow, we find meaning in life, and security in ourselves by having understood and solved personal problems on our own, not by having them explained to us by others (pp. 18–19).

This point is also echoed in Ainsley Arment's book, *Wild + Free*: "What our children learn will seep out into everyday life as they process it in their own time. When you immerse yourself in a lifestyle of living learning, life becomes a never-ending narration" (p. 261).

We'll now turn to highlights of a case study with a client of author Quackenbush that transpired during the early days of the pandemic in 2020. The aforementioned steps of the Story Stone Play are at work with seven-year-old "Ella." This case, which presents selected sessions and pivotal turning points, is shared with full permission and the names are changed to protect confidentiality.

The Case of Ella

What Brought Ella to Story Stone Play?

Ella's parents arranged independent Zoom sessions with the author Quackenbush at the recommendation of the elementary school's counselor. Due to the school's closure during the COVID-19 pandemic, Ella's parents had mentioned she was particularly missing extended play time with friends at school. As an only child, at the age of 7, she was struggling to learn and adapt when the school was forced into distance learning for many months.

Ella is an incredibly bright girl—even as a Kindergartener in the school's aftercare program, she could look over the shoulders of older students playing more complicated games and figure out their strategies. She began violin early on in her school career and the music instructor marveled at her quick capacity to learn. In-person play with other children, however, was what brought her the greatest joy. Despite having a lot of inherent stoicism and resilience, Ella struggled with the pivot to distance learning brought on by the 2020 pandemic. Her father said that she missed, "the camaraderie of her classmates, the energy of the classroom environment, the little signs, gestures and words that happen naturally and spontaneously in person, and without having to 'raise one's hand' on Zoom or type in a chat" (Private Communication, August 31, 2020). On a positive note, Ella's father advised that books and stories were a great refuge for Ella during this time, in which she would be "happy to sit by herself and read, and once she is reading is really focused and doesn't like to be interrupted" (August 31, 2020). This love of story gave her parents confidence that the Story Stone Play sessions would be a good fit. The arrangement would provide her with another friendly face, in an uncertain time, which also provided an outlet for her thoughts and imagination.

The First Session

The Story Through Stone Reflection Cards were sent in the mail prior to the first virtual online session. Following Step 1 of the process mentioned earlier, the history of where the stone card images came from was explained to Ella. Quackenbush shared that her father had found these stones in the desert and that

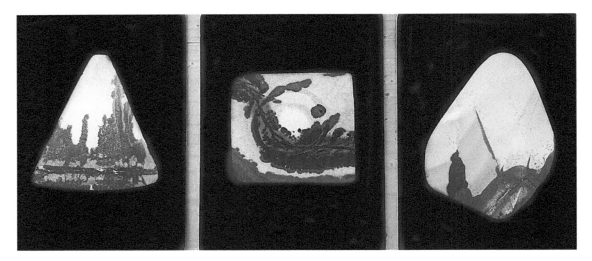

Figure 17.2 Cards from Ella's Story "The Vampire and His Werewolf Friends."
Source: Cyndera Quackenbush.

they were over a billion years old. Quackenbush then guided Ella to shuffle and pick three stone cards (see Steps 2–4). She shared what she saw in the following three stone cards (see Figure 17.2):

Card #1: "A Small Lake. Mountains and Trees and Sand. Moss."
Card #2: "A Long and Dark Tunnel. Red Rocks. A bumpy Arch."
Card #3: "A Vampire. Two long skinny rocks. Sunset."

Playing with the order of the three stone cards chosen, Ella was guided by Quackenbush to tell a story (refer to Steps 5–7). Ella liked for the screen to be shared on Zoom, so that she could see her words as Quackenbush typed them. This process reenforces to a child that they are being heard and is a powerful act of mirroring back the child's awakening imagination. The following story emerged during Ella's first session with the three cards described earlier:

ONCE A SCARY TIME…there was a forest. And in that forest lived a Vampire. And what that Vampire loved to do most on dark nights [was that] he went to his favorite place and it was an arch. And the Vampire went home at sunset for breakfast. And after he had breakfast, he went to see his friends who lived in a bat cave. One day, he didn't see them there. And he said to himself, "Where could they be?" And then, he went searching in the forest. But he couldn't find them anywhere. Then, he went to the grave. And there they were but they weren't Vampires, they were Werewolves. He could recognize their voices. But the Vampire did not know that his friends were turned into Werewolves by a Witch. Then he went to see the Witch and the Witch was his friend. But when he touched her she turned into a Skeleton. And the Skeleton turned his friends back into Vampires. And then, they went to live in the grave forever. And the people who go to that grave never return. The End.

After she told the story, Quackenbush read it back to her (refer to Step 8) followed by the "Writer, Director, Actor Q & A" to grow the story and draw out additional insights (refer to Step 9). Some finger puppets were found online that were printed and used to "perform" the story play. This is one way to bring the story to life as described in Step 8. Ella collaborated with Quackenbush on the finger puppet performance, asking her to play the part of a werewolf. As the werewolves in the story were friends, this symbolic inclusion reflected a deepening in the practitioner/client bond sparked by the first session's story.

Reflections from the First Session

The following reflections, though not shared with Ella, opened a window of understanding for Quackenbush that was valuable to the Story Stone Play process. Ella's story was impressive in how accurately, within metaphor, it captured her precise internal experience during the early jolt of change caused by the pandemic. "Once upon a scary time," as Ella chose, was appropriate to an unexpected year where all that had seemed "normal" was now untouchable because of the virus. School could not be attended in person, one could not leave the house or see one's friends because it was "unsafe" and therefore, to any child, may translate as "scary." The main character in the story, the Vampire Ella saw in the stone, had his favorite place to go and see his friends. The presence of friends in the story became a pivotal motif as she pondered their whereabouts and her own loss of contact with others. For example, in her story, the Vampire shows up and the friends are no longer there ("Where could they be?"). This speaks so directly to what Ella must have felt in her lived experience. Since the beginning of school, she had been able to play with friends. All of a sudden, they were no longer to be seen. The friends are turned into Werewolves by a Witch and the Vampire "could recognize their voices," but not their appearances. This was just what it was like to go from in-person school to the Zoom classroom, when life-like children became small familiar faces on a screen—their voices were recognizable but their relatability was completely altered. Were they even the same people she had known? She certainly could not engage with them the same way she had loved to do before. Additionally, working through the difficult acknowledgment of endings, including death, finds expression within the story: "The people who go to that grave never return." This story opened an outlet for Ella to explore and process her experience through a safe indirect channel of imagination. The story process was kept mostly in the flow of fun; however, it also naturally introduced many talking points to discuss Ella's life in more detail.

Story Stone Play During Transition: Finding Resolution Through Metaphor

Quackenbush and Ella continued to enjoy this weekly practice as the pandemic and 2020 continued, in which time Ella encountered another major transition. She moved from San Francisco back East to her parents' original home. It meant leaving behind the school and friends she had loved and beginning a new school, which was also still in distance learning. Ella's usual resilience and stoicism prevailed, though she would often wear the uniform cape of her old school. Her new school could not keep her attention very well and she often found the school work unchallenging. Her mother noticed a clinginess in her daughter—Ella never wanted to be in a separate room from her parents. Her sleep was impacted and she often could not get through the night alone. One prevailing consistency, thanks to the internet, was a continuation of the Story Stone Play process.

Ella's disappointment with school was addressed in another Story Stone Play session. In many of the sessions, Ella liked to incorporate the gods and goddesses of ancient Greece, influenced by her love of reading. Aries, God of War, was a main character of her fascination. Aries, though brave, does not show up in Ella's stories as very war-like. In fact, he is more often depicted as a son in need of his mother Hera's help. In the three stone cards, Ella shuffled and picked, she saw a "surprised elephant," a "lake with a log with mountains," and "flowers growing in a grassy field" (See Figure 17.3). Here is a highlight of the story she told:

> *Elfie, the elephant found her way to a lake with a log in it. And then she ordered the mushroom, who was surprisingly alive and said, "You find Aries and grow on his nose."*

> *So, the mushroom has grown on Aries' nose. Everyone knows it will stay there forever. Aries had a lot to think about and so, Hera was very worried and so was the mushroom, truth be told!*

In the "Writer/Director/Actor Q&A" part of the session, Quackenbush and Ella talked about the growth of the mushroom on Aries' nose. From previous experience, Quackenbush knew that directly connecting the mushroom to Ella's attitude toward school would kill the life of the story's medicine. So Quackenbush, known as Ms. Q with the children she works with, had the following exchange:

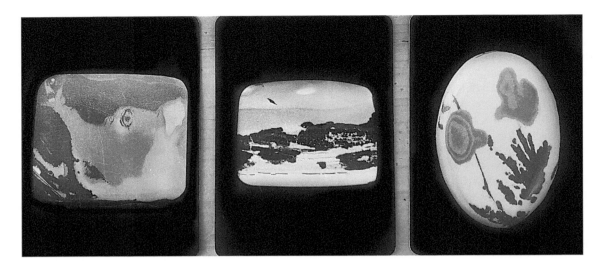

Figure 17.3 Cards from Ella's Story "The Surprised Elephant."
Source: Cyndera Quackenbush.

Ms. Q: What an awful thing to have happened to Aries! It seems neither he OR the mushroom really want to be in this situation together. What could make it better?

Ella: You'll just have to wait until later in the story! Roses will cure the mushroom!

Often if one asks the child what the resolution can be to a nightmare or problem within a story, they almost always have a straightforward answer or can create a metaphorical solution. Quackenbush related that roses also reminded her of the practice of "roses and thorns" that had been used at Ella's old school to acknowledge and speak about both the beautiful and difficult aspects that happen each day. "And the buds we are excited about!" Ella replied enthusiastically. Though Quackenbush knew this couldn't wholly resolve the dissatisfaction Ella felt toward the new school, it was a start in welcoming "more to the story" and finding resolutions within herself. In the next session, she crafted the solution for Aries, whose plight gets much worse before it gets better:

> *Then, the mushroom grew all the way out to the Log, surrounded by mountains. And then, it came across a very beautiful woman with very pretty earrings on. She told them she was going to a wedding. But when she saw Aries (Remember he's a God) and so she stopped in her tracks and just froze with fright.*

> *And it was so small, there was a baby in the woman's arms. Her name was Aurora, and she was one of the most important babies around, because she was a princess. On her dress was the most beautiful pink, with lace. With cute little arms she held them out towards Aries. Aries was stunned.*

> *Since she was a princess, she held out a rose to him. And the woman said it was from a faraway forest, which she had seen from the top of the tallest elm tree. Aries used the thorn to cut the mushroom off and he was now a normal god again.*

The archetype of the baby plays an important role in resolving Aries' issue. It is important to note that the baby was inspired by one of Ella's own dolls, which she also used in the embodied enactment of the story. The baby returns again in the next highlighted story with Ella, continuing to temper and soften the powerful forces at play within her imagination.

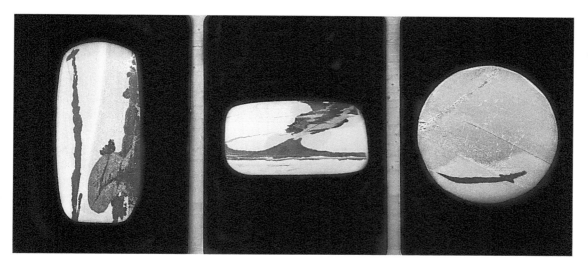

Figure 17.4 Cards from Ella's Story "The Trickster."
Source: Cyndera Quackenbush.

Encountering the Trickster During a Difficult Session

In a correspondence with Ella's mother, she indicated that Ella was continuing to struggle with certain parts of her new school's online program. The mother described that Ella would not participate in breakout sessions and would stay on mute, refusing to "chime in when kids ask her questions" (Private Communication, November 25, 2020). When Ella's mother would ask her what was wrong, Ella would reply that she "doesn't know what to say." Ella would mostly begin Story Stone Play sessions cheerfully, at other times, she was observed as frustrated and resistant to participating. In the session discussed next, she was at first nonverbal, keeping herself muted and not answering the usual welcoming check-in questions.

Once the storytelling began, Ella was like a different person. In the stone cards that she shuffled and drew, she described the following: "Frog is climbing a very steep mountain," "a monkey head with a lot of fiery hair, and a mountain," and a "sword lying on top of a table" (see Figure 17.4). Utilizing the images from the cards, here is the story she told that session:

> Once there was a Trickster and the Trickster liked to trick people. He had a very sharp sword. The people who saw him would always say, "Hi!" and quickly run. When the people ran, the Trickster would bring out his sword and chase them. The sword had special powers. It wasn't just any sword, it was a sword that could create the biggest overflows. So whenever the trickster was mad he could go to the museum and overflow the museum so that everyone would have to focus on rebuilding the museum.

> And then, the trickster would create the biggest storm. And trickster knows that storms are tricksters and storms can create storm clouds. One day a princess went up to the trickster and said, "You are going to need a regular sword, so that you can distract yourself." And off she went. The trickster didn't know where to find a regular sword so he did not go to find it.

> And then the princess came the next day and said, "You are going to have to go down in a whirlpool, down into the ocean." And so he did. About the trickster, everybody says now that the trickster is dead.

> One day, a young maiden from Jupiter came to Mars and then came to Earth. Then she visited the ocean and brought the Trickster up to be her husband. Everybody made fun of the maiden when they saw her walking hand and hand with the trickster. And so, as she did, everybody in the whole wide universe (remember she came from Jupiter) was bellowing in laughter.

And then, one day, there was a frog, climbing a very steep mountain and he said, "Don't worry, everyone is laughing but the Trickster is good." And then, one day there was a monkey face on top of the mountain with firey fur. And then, the maiden transformed into a baby and then the baby said, "Trickster."

Just then, a maiden scooped her up, and said, "Don't be around Trickster, he will teach you all kinds of funny things." And so that's the last the trickster ever saw of the baby.

Reflections from the Trickster Session

In his archetypal explorations, Jung discussed the qualities of the Trickster. In the form of the Mercurius of alchemy, the figure displays "fondness for sly jokes and malicious pranks, his powers as a shape-shifter, his dual nature, half animal, half divine, his exposure to all kinds of tortures, and—last but not least—his approximation to the figure of a saviour" (Jung, 1992, p. 135). From a Jungian perspective, the characters in the story can be viewed as different aspects of Ella's personality. She may have found a lot of power in the Trickster part of her nature—the Trickster can hold sway over others with the sword (this is like talking back). He has the capacity to "overflow," which could relate with Ella's moods and emotions. He can sabotage what is neat and orderly (places like the museum), as Ella may have been tempted to do in a well-intentioned break-out room.

During the Writer/Director/Q&A part of this session, Ella explained that the Trickster does "bad" things but is essentially good. She further elaborated that the Trickster does these things because he is "jealous of other people because they have homes and he is always having to travel around." The young Maiden sees the goodness in the Trickster, as does the Wise Frog. But the protective motherly force (in Ella's own being) helps to prevent him from taking over completely. This is a healthy response in Ella—the Trickster is a dominating force but she won't let it take over forever. Maybe even within the story itself she is facing his influence. She temporarily buries him into the whirlpool and also takes the baby away from the Trickster. Interestingly, she said in the Q&A that the Mother Maiden was her favorite character. Even though she recognizes the Trickster is not all bad, she sees that important boundaries are necessary to keep him in check. He must be controlled because it is just too hard for him to find a "regular sword" instead of the destructive one.

Feedback from Parents

In asking her mother how she was after the session mentioned earlier, she reported:

> You saw the mood when she went into the session. She was dragging her feet and talking back. After [the session] I asked her to practice violin and she just did it – no complaints. So I'd say the class [Story Stone Play Session] made a big difference!

In general, the parents reported that the Story Stone Play sessions helped:

> Our daughter work with [story stone] cards and her imagination to develop stories, write them down, illustrate them, and act them out with finger puppets. This was truly a highlight of each week and something she looked forward to…the stories [were shared] with us, helping us to better understand our child's thoughts and feelings. (Private Communication, June 16, 2020)

Conclusion

Ella's experience mirrors the challenges many children face in our modern times, and will continue to face in the future of our increasingly technologized world. The increased amount of time indoors and away from wild nature will continue to be realities in the way society is constructed. The richness of Ella's stories gives hope that embodied imagination and play is still possible with images of the natural world. The Story Stone Play process unveils a form of connection that practitioners can discover in their own way, with their own clients. Even through difficult times of distance and separation, new landscapes and ancient archetypes can be encountered in a meaningful way with the use of the Story Through Stone Reflection Cards. Like the wise old Frog in Ella's story that climbs the wall and sees the good qualities even in the Trickster, children can access their inherent sources of guidance within. The practitioner plays a key role in making space for this imaginative inquiry, and drawing out the stories as they unfold. Reading the stories back to the client and engaging in lively Q&As sets the stage for embodied expression and an ultimate understanding of the inner dramas at work. This shapes the child's sense of ownership in their developing decisions as they learn and grow.

This chapter has provided a way of working with a particular kind of stone imagery, but is in no way restrictive. It lays a path so that the reader-practitioner may find their own ways to work with natural imagery. A doctor at a children's hospital in Great Britain keeps the Story Through Stone Reflection Cards in his pocket to have on hand whenever he might need a quick, engaging go-to storytelling game with a lonely child. Another therapist uses them in her art therapy groups and noticed that the cards could calm down patients going through difficult transitions within an in-patient program, simply by looking at the imagery and naming what they see. A teacher in San Francisco uses them for her students to imagine the earth at a more ancient time, when all the continents were joined together. The stone cards can also be used by the therapist for their own personal practice and reflection—what do adults see in each billion year stone? How does this open up a world of playfulness for the practitioner? What stories do the stones wish to tell?

Reflection Questions

1   After reading about the influence stone had on Jung from childhood into his elder years, how have stones or other natural objects played a similar role within your own life? How can an early connection to stones be cultivated with your clients in their lives?
2   Narrative Therapy allows one to encapsulate an issue and find a bird's eye distance from their life through story. In what ways has story allowed you, or your clients, to find perspective or meaning?
3   In reviewing this chapter's case study, reflect on how a variety of characters can take shape within the realm of story, inspired by nature. What different aspects have you seen come alive within your clients at different times, and how might they be drawn out into realized awareness?

Appendix A

CREATING YOUR OWN STORY THROUGH STONE® CARDS
A Nature Play Therapy Intervention

Cyndera M. Quackenbush, MA, founder of Story Through Stone®

DESCRIPTION:

A deck of cards is a fun and playful way to capture the ongoing experiences a child has in nature. The art the child creates on each card will help to process their encounter and solidify its meaning in an accessible way. Children will be able to see how memories of nature evolve over time and help to propel new stories from their imagination.

SUPPLIES:

A set of blank cards or pieces of construction paper cut into equal squares. Coloring utensils. Access to entities of nature (stones, bark, leaves, etc).

GOAL:

Create storytelling cards of personal nature experiences and entities. Create new stories by drawing multiple cards from the individualized deck.

INSTRUCTIONS:

As the child engages with a new natural object each session, have them draw the object on one of the cards. They can start with things like leaves, sticks and stones, but then challenge them to look more closely at these natural objects. Can they see shapes and figures within stones, bark and the sand on their adventures? Imagination can mix with science as you discover each new entity. Over time, the child will end up with a deck that has captured their relationship with nature, and the memories of things they have encountered within their therapy sessions. Once the deck has several cards, the child can follow the Story Through Stone® method and create a story with the combined images. This story can be read back and acted out as a grand finale!

EXTRA FUN:

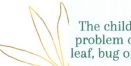

The child can also draw cards when they have a problem or question. What wisdom can the rock, leaf, bug or stick share concerning this question?

References

Arment, A. (2019). *The call of the wild + free: Reclaiming wonder in your child's education.* New York: HarperOne.

Bettelheim, B. (1991). *The uses of enchantment: The meaning and importance of fairy tales.* London: Penguin Books.

Ingemark, C. A. (Ed.). (2013). *Therapeutic uses of storytelling.* Lund: Nordic Academic Press.

Johnson, R. A. (1986). *Inner work: Using dreams & active imagination for personal growth.* New York: Harper.

Jung, C. G. (1989). *Memories, dreams, reflections* (A. Jaffe, Ed.) (R. Winston & C. Winston, Trans.). New York: Vintage Books. (Original work published 1961).

Jung, C.G. (1992). *Four archetypes: Mother/rebirth/spirit/trickster* (R.F.C. Hull, Trans.). Princeton: Princeton University Press.

Jung, C. G. (2009). *The red book* (S. Shamdasani, Ed.) (M. Kyburz, J. Peck, & S. Shamdasani, Trans.). New York: Norton.

Stone, J. (Ed.). (2019). *Integrating technology into modern therapies: A clinician's guide to developments and interventions* (1st ed.). New York: Routledge.

White, M. (2011). *Narrative practice: Continuing the conversations.* New York: WW Norton & Company.

PART VII
Closing Activities

Closing Considerations: Nature Appreciation and Gratitude

Jamie Lynn Langley and Janet A. Courtney

This book would be remiss if we did not profess our sincere gratitude for the gifts of nature we have utilized and incorporated in the activities explored within these chapters, as well as providing our readers some information regarding closing rituals. Indigenous people have long held ceremonies involving appreciation of the earth and recognition of the gifts received from nature. By maintaining this practice of gratitude, we can also help cultivate a mindset for those clients we work with to take better care of this earth we inhabit and utilize.

As play and expressive therapists who incorporate nature and materials of nature in various therapeutic ways and activities, we want to advocate for careful consideration of what materials are used, how they are used, and then returning items back to nature once no longer being used, all within a mindset of appreciation for nature. The children's book *The Giving Tree* by Shel Silverstein and first published in 1964 can be used when exploring environmental considerations. One metaphor of the book utilized is that the boy used almost of all the resources of the tree. In the story, the tree continued to give throughout the boy's life until nothing was left at the end but a stump upon which the boy, now an old man, could sit. When using this story with clients, the therapist can explore other options for getting needs met without using all of nature's resources. Using the tree as an example, we can help clients to consider ways to plant seeds for other trees to grow. This therapist (Jamie) has personally liked the idea that when apple cores were dropped by the boy in story, those seeds went into the ground to grow into other apple trees, unknowingly growing an apple orchard along his various paths (Figure Closing 1).

Play and expressive therapists can also incorporate gratitude activities such as a *Gratitude Hawaiian Lei Necklace* (see Appendix A) where clients can see something that they appreciate about themselves or others while placing a flower on a string that can be tied off for the child to wear. Another gratitude activity can utilize stones or leaves that the client can paint or decorate with words such as "Gratitude" or "Thank You." These items could also be used as the bindu (center) of a nature mandala or even a nature altar to further express the acknowledgment and appreciation for nature. Children and adolescents can be included in gratitude practices to thank nature when returning items back to the earth—such as placing the Gratitude Hawaiian Lei on a tree branch after the flowers fade. Giving back may also include planting wildflower seeds or bringing pine nettles to pour around plants and trees to help nurture them. Even picking up litter that may be found when exploring outdoors is another way to give back to nature. The gifts from nature can also be used following an activity in a gratitude ritual. For example, after completing a nature mandala, the items can be placed back in a similar area where they were originally found. Another option is to make a gratitude alter in which to place the nature items. A poem can be located or written and then recited, or a statement of gratitude can be made while returning the items back to nature (Figure Closing 2).

Another idea is to end nature-based activities with a *Wild Tea Party* (see Appendix B) to express this gratitude. There are several ingredients that can be used to make a "wild tea" such as dandelions, lavender, mint, and leaves of wild berries. This tea can be served for a quiet ending of a nature-based play and expressive therapy session, reflecting on the activity completed and appreciation for nature utilized. A further utilization of this activity is having the teacup as a transitional object at the closing of therapy. The teacup could have a succulent or other small plants placed inside with dirt. The client and therapist

DOI: 10.4324/9781003152767-25

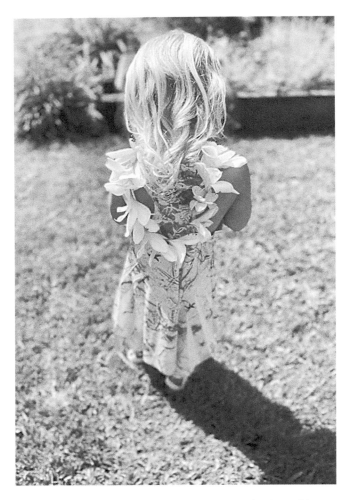

Figure Closing 1 Young girl wearing her gratitude necklace.
Source: Amber Davis.

could do this together exploring metaphors of both growth and gifts from nature. Fairy figures or other objects can also be added as a type of small fairy garden. The client can then take this teacup garden with them as a living and growing reminder of their nature-based therapy sessions and experiences. Family members could also be included as desired for this wild tea party, especially when used as a celebration for ending therapy. Our coeditor, Rose LaPiere, created a closing activity titled, *Sweet Nature Celebration* (see Appendix C), where practitioners can help to guide clients to create a nature "cake" out of mud, wet sand, or clay. This activity can help a client to identify strengths, overall gratitude to nature, and to celebrate moments shared in the play therapy process.

Together with the other editors of this book, we want to express our mutual gratitude for all the therapists who contributed to this book project to help promote nature-based play and expressive therapies. We are grateful to the earth for providing tools for healing, whether it is the wind rusting through the trees, rocks that are painted, or leaves and twigs artfully arranged to tell a story, or the many other ways we utilize the many gifts of nature. As a final perspective, the editors created a closing activity for practitioners and clients called *Gratitude for Nature* that supports an ongoing practice of thankfulness and appreciation for the environment (see Appendix D).

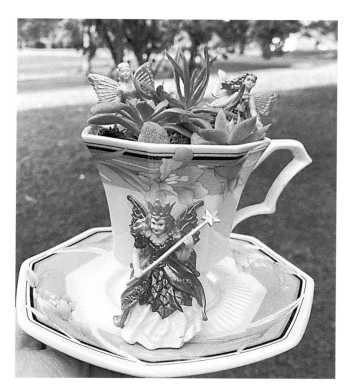

Figure Closing 2 Teacup fairy gratitude garden.
Source: Jamie Lynn Langley.

There is a saying that is attributed as an Apache Blessing that is often utilized for engraved gifts, art décor and in closing ceremonies, and we will end our book with these sentiments:

> May the sun bring you new energy by day, may the moon softly restore you by night, may the rain wash away your worries, may the breeze blow new strength into your being. May you walk gently through the world and know its beauty all the days of your life.

Appendix A

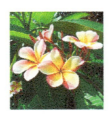

Hawaiian Lei Gratitude Necklace
A Nature Play Therapy Intervention

Janet A. Courtney, PhD, RPT-S

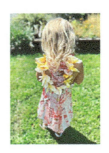

DESCRIPTION:

Working with children from a strength-based perspective to grow their sense of gratitude and elicit their hopes and dreams for themselves and others. This can be used as a closure of therapy activity.

SUPPLIES NEEDED:

- Thin sewing thread/string
- Large blunt tipped embroidery needle
- Flowers (carnations, roses, plumeria—any flower with a firm face)

GOAL:

To elicit a client's sense of gratitude for self and others.

INSTRUCTIONS:

- **Step One:** Plan ahead prior to a session. Flowers can be collected from a home garden, supermarkets, farmers' markets, plant nurseries, or donated from weddings or funeral agencies.
- **Step Two:** The stems are removed, and a blunted needle is used to pull through the middle of a flower that is placed on the string.
- **Step Three:** For each flower added, have the client express something they are thankful for.
- **Step Four:** Tie off and the client can decide to wear the gratitude flower lei. (This can also be a flower crown for the head or a bracelet).
- **Step Five:** The child is prepared that the gratitude flower necklace will fade and it can then be discussed with the child what to do with the flower lei. Children can learn that many Hawaiian people decide to return their flowers back to nature by removing the string and scattering the flowers or hanging the flowers on a tree.

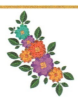

EXTRA FUN:

This can also be done in a group or family session. Clients can also list their wishes, dreams and hopes for self and others.

Appendix B

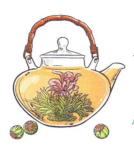

A WILD TEA PARTY

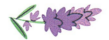

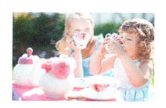

A Nature Play Therapy Intervention
Jamie Lynn Langley, LCSW, RPT-S

DESCRIPTION:

This activity is utilized as a more formal - yet fun- experience to close a nature-based therapy session and express gratitude to nature for her gifts provided.

SUPPLIES NEEDED:

A teapot (filled with hot water) and teacups for participants. Various tea recipes can be used that have ingredients from nature such as daffodils, lavender, mint or the leaves of berries. Decaffeinated or herbal tea bags may also be used.

GOAL:

Provides a closing ritual in which therapist and client(s) can express gratitude for the gifts of nature.

INSTRUCTIONS:

This "wild tea party" can be done indoors or outside for all ages. It may be a formal affair with a tablecloth, china teacups, and teapot or less formal with disposable cups (though the latter is not as environmentally friendly). Family members of the client can also be included if desired.

The therapist can prepare the "wild tea" ahead of time or can make with the client. Various recipes can be used that include different natural ingredients such as lavender, daffodils, mint and berry leaves, etc. There are also natural teas already made that can be used. There are cookies which use similar nature ingredients that can be included.

While sipping the tea, appreciation for nature is expressed by participants. Memories of nature-based experiences can be shared.

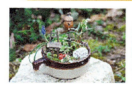

Extra Fun:

This wild tea party can be extended as a closing ceremony when completing therapy. After the tea party, the teacup can be used as a transitional object. Dirt and small plants such as succulents can be planted in the teacup. A fairy or other small figure can be added to this teacup garden.

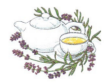

Appendix C

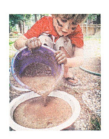

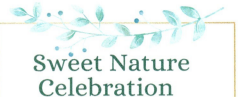

Sweet Nature Celebration

A Nature Play Therapy Intervention

ROSE LAPIERE, LPC, RPT-S

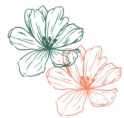

DESCRIPTION:

Cakes, cookies, and cupcakes are often used as a way to celebrate a transition. For a final therapy session, or as a transition this activity can help the client integrate their strengths and explore the gratitude they found in nature.

SUPPLIES NEEDED:

- Mud, wet sand or clay.
- Buckets, containers, and cookie cut-outs to make shapes.
- Optional tools such as whisk, large wooden spoon, markers and popsicle sticks.
- Nature items such as stones, sticks, shells, leaves, flowers, grass, pinecones, etc.

GOAL:

Closing activity for therapist and client to express gratitude for gifts of nature and strengths.

INSTRUCTIONS:

Step 1: Fill a large container of water and put sand (dirt, or clay) in a separate container.

Step 2: Invite the child by saying "today we are going to create a special cake to celebrate all the things about you, nature and the memories we shared together".

Step 3: Mix together the water and sand and begin to make a "cake" of any shape. Next, add the nature decorations such as stones, grass, leaves, flowers, acorn, etc.

Step 4: While creating and decorating the nature cake, the therapist can begin a discussion in the following areas: Strengths of the child, moments shared in the play, such as things that were fun and hard, and what in nature are they grateful for. For example, as the child is making the nature cake and adding the flowers, rocks, acorns begin asking what they appreciate about flowers, etc. Also, wonder what the animals or bugs value about those nature items to expand on different perspectives. The therapist can share what strengths they see in the child and what they notice in themselves. As the strengths and values are named, the therapist can write them on popsicle sticks and add them to the cake as pretend candles. Option: Once completed take a picture of the nature cake for the child.

EXTRA FUN:

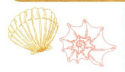

This can be a family session with everyone making one cake together in a shared experience reflecting on nature, individual, and family strengths.

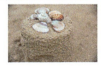

Appendix D

GRATITUDE FOR NATURE

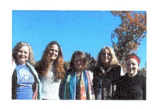

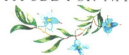

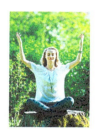

A Nature Play Therapy Practice

Jamie, Rose, Lynn, Janet and Roz

DESCRIPTION:
To assist clients with developing a practice to appreciate nature and the gifts provided from nature.

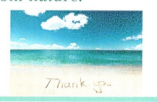

SETTING / SUPPLIES:
This can be done outside in nature or indoors using items from nature such as shells, sticks, stones, pinecones, acorns, leaves and more.

GOAL:
To promote gratitude for nature for both the benefit of the client and for nature itself.

INSTRUCTIONS:
Developing a practice of gratitude for nature is one way we can promote appreciation of nature when working with clients of all ages. This could include simply returning unused materials from nature back to the environment at the end of a session or activity. A reflection of gratitude can be stated such as, "Thank you nature for ..." Going on a walk looking for heart shapes can be fun and used as a way to tell nature what is loved and appreciated. Nature hearts can be gathered such as rocks or leaves, or even made as reminders of ways we care for and appreciate nature. Others may choose to give back to nature by picking up litter found outside, planting wildflower seeds or by watering plants.

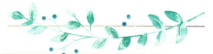

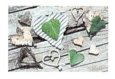

EXTRA PROCESSING:
As a gratitude ritual or closing ceremony, a sandtray depicting gratitude for nature could be made. This could include lighting a candle, reciting a poem, etc.

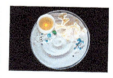

Index

Note: Page numbers in *Italic* refer to figures; and in **Bold** refer to tables.